Dietary Trace Minerals

Dietary Trace Minerals

Special Issue Editor

Elad Tako

MDPI • Basel • Beijing • Wuhan • Barcelona • Belgrade • Manchester • Tokyo • Cluj • Tianjin

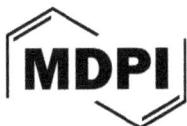

Special Issue Editor
Elad Tako
Cornell University
USA

Editorial Office
MDPI
St. Alban-Anlage 66
4052 Basel, Switzerland

This is a reprint of articles from the Special Issue published online in the open access journal *Nutrients* (ISSN 2072-6643) (available at: https://www.mdpi.com/journal/nutrients/special_issues/dietary_trace_minerals).

For citation purposes, cite each article independently as indicated on the article page online and as indicated below:

LastName, A.A.; LastName, B.B.; LastName, C.C. Article Title. *Journal Name* **Year**, *Article Number*, Page Range.

ISBN 978-3-03928-324-8 (Pbk)
ISBN 978-3-03928-325-5 (PDF)

Cover image courtesy of Elad Tako.

© 2020 by the authors. Articles in this book are Open Access and distributed under the Creative Commons Attribution (CC BY) license, which allows users to download, copy and build upon published articles, as long as the author and publisher are properly credited, which ensures maximum dissemination and a wider impact of our publications.

The book as a whole is distributed by MDPI under the terms and conditions of the Creative Commons license CC BY-NC-ND.

Contents

About the Special Issue Editor vii

Elad Tako
Dietary Trace Minerals
Reprinted from: *Nutrients* **2019**, *11*, 2823, doi:10.3390/nu11112823 1

Keren Demishtein, Ram Reifen and Moshe Shemesh
Antimicrobial Properties of Magnesium Open Opportunities to Develop Healthier Food
Reprinted from: *Nutrients* **2019**, *11*, 2363, doi:10.3390/nu11102363 5

Maria Schwarz, Kristina Lossow, Johannes F. Kopp, Tanja Schwerdtle and Anna P. Kipp
Crosstalk of Nrf2 with the Trace Elements Selenium, Iron, Zinc, and Copper
Reprinted from: *Nutrients* **2019**, *11*, 2112, doi:10.3390/nu11092112 13

Jason A. Wiesinger, Raymond P. Glahn, Karen A. Cichy, Nikolai Kolba, Jonathan J. Hart and Elad Tako
An In Vivo (*Gallus gallus*) Feeding Trial Demonstrating the Enhanced Iron Bioavailability Properties of the Fast Cooking Manteca Yellow Bean (*Phaseolus vulgaris* L.)
Reprinted from: *Nutrients* **2019**, *11*, 1768, doi:10.3390/nu11081768 31

Jesse T. Beasley, Jonathan J. Hart, Elad Tako, Raymond P. Glahn and Alexander A. T. Johnson
Investigation of Nicotianamine and 2′ Deoxymugineic Acid as Enhancers of Iron Bioavailability in Caco-2 Cells
Reprinted from: *Nutrients* **2019**, *11*, 1502, doi:10.3390/nu11071502 53

Karina M. Vermeulen, Márcia Marília G. D. Lopes, Camila X. Alves, Naira J. N. Brito, Maria das Graças Almeida, Lucia Leite-Lais, Sancha Helena L. Vale and José Brandão-Neto
Bioelectrical Impedance Vector Analysis and Phase Angle on Different Oral Zinc Supplementation in Eutrophic Children: Randomized Triple-Blind Study
Reprinted from: *Nutrients* **2019**, *11*, 1215, doi:10.3390/nu11061215 65

Anna Prescha, Katarzyna Zabłocka-Słowińska and Halina Grajeta
Dietary Silicon and Its Impact on Plasma Silicon Levels in the Polish Population
Reprinted from: *Nutrients* **2019**, *11*, 980, doi:10.3390/nu11050980 75

Youichi Ogawa, Manao Kinoshita, Takuya Sato, Shinji Shimada and Tatsuyoshi Kawamura
Biotin Is Required for the Zinc Homeostasis in the Skin
Reprinted from: *Nutrients* **2019**, *11*, 919, doi:10.3390/nu11040919 87

Raymond Glahn, Elad Tako and Michael A. Gore
The Germ Fraction Inhibits Iron Bioavailability of Maize: Identification of an Approach to Enhance Maize Nutritional Quality via Processing and Breeding
Reprinted from: *Nutrients* **2019**, *11*, 833, doi:10.3390/nu11040833 97

Julia L. Finkelstein, Saurabh Mehta, Salvador Villalpando, Veronica Mundo-Rosas, Sarah V. Luna, Maike Rahn, Teresa Shamah-Levy, Stephen E. Beebe and Jere D. Haas
A Randomized Feeding Trial of Iron-Biofortified Beans in School Children in Mexico
Reprinted from: *Nutrients* **2019**, *11*, 381, doi:10.3390/nu11020381 111

Desirrê Morais Dias, Nikolai Kolba, Dana Binyamin, Oren Ziv, Marilia Regini Nutti, Hércia Stampini Duarte Martino, Raymond P. Glahn, Omry Koren and Elad Tako
Iron Biofortified Carioca Bean (*Phaseolus vulgaris* L.)—Based Brazilian Diet Delivers More Absorbable Iron and Affects the Gut Microbiota In Vivo (*Gallus gallus*)
Reprinted from: *Nutrients* **2018**, *10*, 1970, doi:10.3390/nu10121970 . . . . **125**

Mohammad S. Masoud, Majed S. Alokail, Sobhy M. Yakout, Malak Nawaz K. Khattak, Marwan M. AlRehaili, Kaiser Wani and Nasser M. Al-Daghri
Vitamin D Supplementation Modestly Reduces Serum Iron Indices of Healthy
Arab Adolescents
Reprinted from: *Nutrients* **2018**, *10*, 1870, doi:10.3390/nu10121870 . . . . **145**

Ludmila V. Puchkova, Massimo Broggini, Elena V. Polishchuk, Ekaterina Y. Ilyechova and Roman S. Polishchuk
Silver Ions as a Tool for Understanding Different Aspects of Copper Metabolism
Reprinted from: *Nutrients* **2019**, *11*, 1364, doi:10.3390/nu11061364 . . . . **157**

Chang-Kyu Oh and Yuseok Moon
Dietary and Sentinel Factors Leading to Hemochromatosis
Reprinted from: *Nutrients* **2019**, *11*, 1047, doi:10.3390/nu11051047 . . . . **183**

About the Special Issue Editor

Elad Tako holds degrees in animal science (B.S.), endocrinology (M.S.), and physiology/nutrigenomics (Ph.D.), with previous appointments at the Hebrew University of Jerusalem, North Carolina State University, and Cornell University. As a Research Physiologist with USDA/ARS, Dr. Tako's research focuses on various aspects of trace mineral deficiencies, emphasizing molecular, physiological, and nutritional factors and practices that influence intestinal micronutrient absorption. With over 100 peer-reviewed publications and presentations, he leads a research team focused on understanding the interactions between dietary factors, physiological and molecular biomarkers, the microbiome, and intestinal functionality. His research accomplishments include the development of the Gallus gallus intra-amniotic administration procedure, and establishing recognized approaches for using animal models within mineral bioavailability and intestinal absorption screening processes. He has also developed a zinc status physiological blood biomarker (red blood cell Linoleic Acid: Dihomo–Linolenic Acid Ratio), and molecular tissue biomarkers to assess the effect of dietary mineral deficiencies on intestinal functionality, and how micronutrients dietary deficiencies alter gut microbiota composition and function.

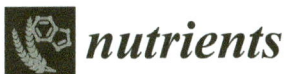

Editorial

Dietary Trace Minerals

Elad Tako

USDA-ARS, Robert W. Holley Center for Agriculture and Health, Cornell University, Ithaca, NY 14853, USA; elad.tako@ars.usda.gov or et79@cornell.edu

Received: 8 November 2019; Accepted: 14 November 2019; Published: 19 November 2019

Abstract: Dietary trace minerals are pivotal and hold a key role in numerous metabolic processes. Trace mineral deficiencies (except for iodine, iron, and zinc) do not often develop spontaneously in adults on ordinary diets; infants are more vulnerable because their growth is rapid and intake varies. Trace mineral imbalances can result from hereditary disorders (e.g., hemochromatosis, Wilson disease), kidney dialysis, parenteral nutrition, restrictive diets prescribed for people with inborn errors of metabolism, or various popular diet plans. The Special Issue "Dietary Trace Minerals" comprised 13 peer-reviewed papers on the most recent evidence regarding the dietary intake of trace minerals, as well as their effect toward the prevention and treatment of non-communicable diseases. Original contributions and literature reviews further demonstrated the crucial and central part that dietary trace minerals play in human health and development. This editorial provides a brief and concise overview that addresses and summarizes the content of the *Dietary Trace Minerals* Special Issue.

Keywords: dietary trace minerals; deficiency; iron; zinc; selenium; copper; vitamin D

This monograph, based on a Special Issue of *Nutrients*, contains 13 manuscripts—two reviews and 11 original publications—that reflect the wide spectrum of currently conducted research in the field of dietary trace minerals. The manuscripts in this Special Issue collection include populations from many countries, including the USA, Germany, Australia, Brazil, Poland, Japan, Colombia, Mexico, Saudi Arabia, Russia, Italy, South Korea, and Israel. The presented manuscripts cover a wide variety of topics in the field of dietary trace minerals, with emphasis on the antimicrobial properties of magnesium and the potential to develop healthier food [1], the link between Nrf2 and dietary selenium, iron, zinc, and copper [2], in vivo assessment of fast cooking yellow bean consumption on dietary iron bioavailability [3], the association between nicotianamine and 2′ deoxymugineic acid as enhancers of iron bioavailability in vitro [4], analysis of bioelectrical impedance vector and phase angle on various forms of oral zinc supplementation in children [5], investigation of dietary silicon and its impact on plasma silicon concentrations in human subjects [6], the role of biotin in skin zinc homeostasis [7], the maize germ fraction and its inhibitory effect on iron bioavailability in vitro [8], assessment of the iron bioavailability of iron-biofortified beans in school children [9], investigation of the dietary iron bioavailability of iron biofortified carioca beans in vivo [10], vitamin D supplementation and its effect on serum iron concentrations in adolescents [11], the demonstration of silver ions as a tool for understanding copper metabolism [12], and the dietary and sentinel potential factors that lead to hemochromatosis [13]. This wide spectrum of topics further demonstrates the importance and relevance of dietary trace minerals, as these factors are critical and have a pivotal role in organism (including human) health and physiological functions.

Minerals form only five percent of the typical human diet but are essential for normal health and function. Macrominerals are defined as minerals that are required by adults in amounts greater than 100 mg/day or make up less than one percent of total body weight. Trace elements (or trace minerals) are usually defined as minerals that are required in amounts of 1–100 mg/day by adults or make up less than 0.01 percent of total body weight. Ultra-trace minerals are generally defined as minerals that are required in amounts less than 1 microgram/day [14].

Recommended intakes for trace elements are expressed as Recommended Dietary Allowance (RDA) or Adequate Intake. The Upper Limit is the quantity of the nutrient considered to cause no adverse effects in healthy individuals. These parameters have been estimated for each trace mineral. Previous research demonstrated that: (1) Copper deficiency can be caused by an x-linked mutation of the transport protein mediating copper uptake from the intestine (Menkes disease). It can also be caused by malabsorption after gastrointestinal surgery (including gastric bypass for weight loss and gastric resection for malignancy or peptic ulcer disease), or by ingestion of high doses of zinc. Clinical manifestations include anemia, ataxia, and myeloneuropathy [15]. (2) Iodine deficiency is characterized by goiter and hypothyroidism, which in turn has effects on growth, development, and cognitive function [16]. (3) Selenium deficiency is unusual, but has been reported in parts of China where the local diet is devoid of selenium; this deficiency also occurs in individuals maintained on total parenteral nutrition without trace minerals. Clinical features of selenium deficiency are cardiomyopathy and skeletal muscle dysfunction [17]. (4) Zinc deficiency causes growth retardation in children, hypogonadism, oligospermia, alopecia, dysgeusia (impaired taste), immune dysfunction, night blindness, impaired wound healing, and skin lesions. Infants with an inherited defect in zinc absorption develop a severe deficiency state known as acrodermatitis enteropathica [18–20].

The purpose of the current Special Issue is to further expand and add research knowledge on the vital role that dietary trace minerals play in various physiological and metabolic pathways. In addition, it aims to further contribute to knowledge in regards to the relationship between dietary trace minerals' bioavailability, the microbiome, bioactive compounds, and other metabolic and physiological pathways.

I believe that this Special Issue and collection of manuscripts is a useful summary of progress in various areas related to dietary trace minerals. It also points to additional research needs, including recommendations for future research in the field, in order to better understand the dietary role that trace mineral play and also in regards to specific populations and their dietary requirements, growth and healthy development.

Conflicts of Interest: The author declares no conflict of interest.

References

1. Demishtein, K.; Reifen, R.; Shemesh, M. Antimicrobial Properties of Magnesium Open Opportunities to Develop Healthier Food. *Nutrients* **2019**, *11*, 2363. [CrossRef] [PubMed]
2. Schwarz, M.; Lossow, K.; Kopp, J.F.; Schwerdtle, T.; Kipp, A.P. Crosstalk of Nrf2 with the Trace Elements Selenium, Iron, Zinc, and Copper. *Nutrients* **2019**, *11*, 2112. [CrossRef] [PubMed]
3. Wiesinger, J.A.; Glahn, R.; Cichy, K.A.; Kolba, N.; Hart, J.J.; Tako, E. An In Vivo (*Gallus gallus*) Feeding Trial Demonstrating the Enhanced Iron Bioavailability Properties of the Fast Cooking Manteca Yellow Bean (*Phaseolus vulgaris* L.). *Nutrients* **2019**, *11*, 1768. [CrossRef] [PubMed]
4. Beasley, J.T.; Hart, J.J.; Tako, E.; Johnson, A.A.T. Investigation of Nicotianamine and 2′ Deoxymugineic Acid as Enhancers of Iron Bioavailability in Caco-2 Cells. *Nutrients* **2019**, *11*, 1502. [CrossRef] [PubMed]
5. Vermeulen, K.M.; Lopes, M.M.; Alves, C.X.; Brito, N.J.; das Graças Almeida, M.; Leite-Lais, V.S.H.; Brandão-Neto, J. Bioelectrical Impedance Vector Analysis and Phase Angle on Different Oral Zinc Supplementation in Eutrophic Children: Randomized Triple-Blind Study. *Nutrients* **2019**, *11*, 1215. [CrossRef] [PubMed]
6. Prescha, A.; Zabłocka-Słowińska, K.; Grajeta, H. Dietary Silicon and Its Impact on Plasma Silicon Levels in the Polish Population. *Nutrients* **2019**, *11*, 980. [CrossRef] [PubMed]
7. Ogawa, Y.; Kinoshita, M.; Sato, T.; Shimada, S.; Kawamura, T. Biotin Is Required for the Zinc Homeostasis in the Skin. *Nutrients* **2019**, *11*, 919. [CrossRef] [PubMed]
8. Glahn, R.; Tako, E.; Gore, M. The Germ Fraction Inhibits Iron Bioavailability of Maize: Identification of an Approach to Enhance Maize Nutritional Quality via Processing and Breeding. *Nutrients* **2019**, *11*, 833. [CrossRef] [PubMed]

9. Finkelstein, J.L.; Mehta, S.; Villalpando, S.; Mundo-Rosas, V.; Luna, S.V.; Rahn, M.; Shamah-Levy, T.; Beebe, S.E.; Haas, J.D. A Randomized Feeding Trial of Iron-Biofortified Beans in School Children in Mexico. *Nutrients* **2019**, *11*, 381. [CrossRef] [PubMed]
10. Morais Dias, D.; Kolba, N.; Binyamin, D.; Ziv, O.; Regini Nutti, M.; Stampini Duarte Martino, H.; Koren, O.; Tako, E. Iron Biofortified Carioca Bean (Phaseolus vulgaris L.)—Based Brazilian Diet Delivers More Absorbable Iron and Affects the Gut Microbiota In Vivo (Gallus gallus). *Nutrients* **2018**, *10*, 1970. [CrossRef] [PubMed]
11. Masoud, M.S.; Alokail, M.S.; Yakout, S.M.; Khattak, M.N.; AlRehaili, M.M.; Wani, K.; Al-Daghri, N.M. Vitamin D Supplementation Modestly Reduces Serum Iron Indices of Healthy Arab Adolescents. *Nutrients* **2018**, *10*, 1870. [CrossRef] [PubMed]
12. Puchkova, L.V.; Broggini, M.; Polishchuk, E.V.; Ilyechova, E.Y.; Polishchuk, R.S. Silver Ions as a Tool for Understanding Different Aspects of Copper Metabolism. *Nutrients* **2019**, *11*, 1364. [CrossRef] [PubMed]
13. Oh, C.K.; Moon, Y. Dietary and Sentinel Factors Leading to Hemochromatosis. *Nutrients* **2019**, *11*, 1047. [CrossRef] [PubMed]
14. Pazirandeh, S.; Burns, D.L.; Griffin, I.J. *Overview of Dietary Trace Minerals*; Wolters Kluwer Health: Alphen aan den Rijn, The Netherlands, 2012.
15. Kumar, N.; Gross, J.B. Mutation in the ATP7A gene may not be responsible for hypocupraemia in copper deficiency myelopathy. *Postgrad. Med. J.* **2006**, *82*, 416. [CrossRef] [PubMed]
16. Eastman, C.J.; Zimmermann, M.B. *The Iodine Deficiency Disorders*; Feingold, K.R., Anawalt, B., Boyce, A., Eds.; MDText.com, Inc.: South Dartmouth, MA, USA, 2000.
17. Jin, J.; Mulesa, L.; Carrilero Rouillet, M. Trace Elements in Parenteral Nutrition: Considerations for the Prescribing Clinician. *Nutrients* **2017**, *9*, 440. [CrossRef] [PubMed]
18. Knez, M.; Tako, E.; Kolba, N.; de Courcy-Ireland, E.; Stangoulis, J.C.R. Linoleic Acid:Dihomo-γ-Linolenic Acid Ratio Predicts the Efficacy of Zn-Biofortified Wheat in Chicken (*Gallus gallus*). *J. Agric. Food Chem.* **2018**, *66*, 1394–1400. [CrossRef] [PubMed]
19. Knez, M.; Stangoulis, J.C.R.; Glibetic, M.; Tako, E. The Linoleic Acid: Dihomo-γ-Linolenic Acid Ratio (LA:DGLA)-An Emerging Biomarker of Zn Status. *Nutrients* **2017**, *9*, 825. [CrossRef] [PubMed]
20. Reed, S.; Qin, X.; Ran-Ressler, R.; Brenna, J.T.; Tako, E. Dietary zinc deficiency affects blood linoleic acid: dihomo-γ-linolenic acid (LA:DGLA) ratio; a sensitive physiological marker of zinc status in vivo (*Gallus gallus*). *Nutrients* **2014**, *6*, 1164–1180. [CrossRef] [PubMed]

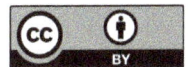

© 2019 by the author. Licensee MDPI, Basel, Switzerland. This article is an open access article distributed under the terms and conditions of the Creative Commons Attribution (CC BY) license (http://creativecommons.org/licenses/by/4.0/).

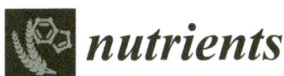

Communication

Antimicrobial Properties of Magnesium Open Opportunities to Develop Healthier Food

Keren Demishtein [1], Ram Reifen [2] and Moshe Shemesh [1,*]

1. Department of Food Sciences, Institute for Postharvest Technology and Food Sciences, Agricultural Research Organization, Volcani Center, Rishon LeZion 7528809, Israel; kerend@volcani.agri.gov.il
2. The Robert H. Smith Faculty of Agriculture, Food and Environment, Institute of Biochemistry, Food Science and Nutrition, The Hebrew University of Jerusalem, Rehovot 7610001, Israel; ram.reifen@mail.huji.ac.il
* Correspondence: moshesh@agri.gov.il; Tel.: +972-3968-3868

Received: 29 July 2019; Accepted: 21 September 2019; Published: 3 October 2019

Abstract: Magnesium is a vital mineral that takes part in hundreds of enzymatic reactions in the human body. In the past several years, new information emerged in regard to the antibacterial effect of magnesium. Here we elaborate on the recent knowledge of its antibacterial effect with emphasis on its ability to impair bacterial adherence and formation complex community of bacterial cells called biofilm. We further talk about its ability to impair biofilm formation in milk that provides opportunity for developing safer and qualitative dairy products. Finally, we describe the pronounced advantages of enrichment of food with magnesium ions, which result in healthier and more efficient food products.

Keywords: healthy food; biofilm; magnesium ions; microbial development; dairy food

1. Introduction

Magnesium represents an essential element for life and is ubiquitously found in all organisms. This important cation plays crucial roles as an enzymatic co-factor, as well as it is involved in cellular signaling, and in stabilizing cellular components [1,2]. It is not surprising that magnesium salts are typically associated with positive effects on microbial cells. However, it appears that at elevated doses, for instance at milimolar concentrations, magnesium ions become harmful for prokaryotic cell and therefore may negatively affect important cellular processes [3–7]. Although, some progress has been made in investigating the effect of magnesium ions in different microorganisms, it is still not clear how these vital ions affect the cellular processes in microbial cell. Moreover, the mode of antimicrobial action of magnesium ions remains largely unknown. In the past several years, more information emerged concerning the effect of magnesium on bacterial cells. Consequently, in this mini-review, we summarize recent advances in understanding the antimicrobial properties of magnesium ions with an emphasis on their effect on biofilm formation, which became the biggest microbiological problem in clinical as well as industrial settings. We further discuss the antimicrobial potential of magnesium ions in developing novel approaches towards improving food safety and quality. Finally, we describe new perspectives in developing healthier food for human consumption by its enrichment based on magnesium ions.

2. The Antimicrobial Properties of Magnesium

Historically, back in 1915, Professor Pierre Delbet was looking for a solution to cleanse wounds that would replace the traditional antiseptics that damage tissues. After testing several solutions, he found $MgCl_2$ solution to be most effective as it had two main advantages—it was not harmful for the tissue and it highly increased leucocyte activity and phagocytosis. Later, he found this solution to be an efficient therapy for various diseases, including diseases related to microorganisms [8]. In the past several years, new interest on this cation arose due to its antimicrobial properties. In several studies, antibiotic activity in the presence of Mg^{2+} ions was found to be more efficient [9,10]. It has been hypothesized that the divalent ions affect the membranes of bacterial cells. One study suggested that the curvature of the bacterial membrane is affected, and eventually the bacteria become more vulnerable, and the antibiotics are more efficient [11]. A different study showed that these cations permeabilize the membranes and cause them to be leakier [5]. Other studies tested the potential antimicrobial effect of coating different surfaces with magnesium or magnesium compounds. These surfaces were found as effective in prevention of bacteria adherence as well as biofilm formation. Some of these compounds were suggested to disrupt the membrane potential, again strengthening the idea that magnesium permeabilizes membranes and eventually cause the bacteria to be more sensitive [6,12–14]. Moreover, metal oxide nanoparticles of MgO were tested as antibacterial agents as well [3,6]. Indeed, these particles were found to be effective against yeast and planktonic bacteria as well as against biofilms [3]. In addition, these nanoparticles were found to be of low cytotoxicity and relatively safe. Since biofilm formation is considered as a major problem in the food industry as well as in the biomedical field, a lot of effort is put into dealing with this phenomenon [15,16]. Therefore, the effect of magnesium ions was also tested recently as a potential solution for the biofilm problem.

2.1. The Effect of Magnesium on Bacterial Survival and Biofilm Formation

Biofilms are highly structured multicellular communities [17–19]. Biofilm formation is a multistage process in which bacterial cells adhere to a surface and/or to each other through production of an extracellular matrix that is typically composed of exopolymeric substances (EPS) such as polysaccharides, proteins, and nucleic acids, which surround and may protect the enclosed bacteria [19–21]. They form highly structured multicellular communities that are capable of coordinated and collective behavior [17,18,22]. Bacterial cells in biofilms are characterized by increased resistance to unfavorable environmental conditions, antimicrobial agents, and cleaning chemicals [19,23,24]. It appears that the major source of the contamination of food products is often associated with biofilms on the surfaces of food processing equipment [15,25,26]. Therefore, biofilm formation is considered as a major problem in the food industry [15,26,27].

Several approaches were suggested to deal with biofilm formation in the food industry [15,26]. Environmental factors such as electrolyte concentrations and medium composition were shown to have important impact on biofilm formation [28]. Divalent cations can influence biofilm formation directly through their effect on electro-static interactions and indirectly via physiology-dependent attachment processes by acting as important cellular cations and enzyme cofactors [28–31]. Due to its potentially important role, the effect of Mg^{2+} ions on biofilm formation has been tested. These ions are crucial for the physiology of bacterial cells, although their excess can be harmful for them. Bacterial cells maintain the tolerable concentrations of Mg^{2+} ions by influx and efflux strategies based on their availability. Bacteria overcome limitations in those ions or respond to excess levels, and this helps to maintain the metal homeostasis within the cell. It appears that Mg^{2+} ions are vital for membrane stabilization and function as a cofactor for diverse enzymatic reactions. Bacteria achieve Mg^{2+} homeostasis by regulating the Mg^{2+} transporters and sensors that coordinate the influx and efflux of Mg^{2+} from the bacterial cell. The Gram-negative bacterium *Salmonella enterica* serovar Typhimurium is one of the best-understood models for explaining the Mg^{2+} homeostasis [32,33]. In *Staphylococcus aureus*, Mg^{2+} was shown to increase the rigidity of cell wall by binding to teichoic acids (TA). TA, bind the positively charged Mg^{2+} ions to mitigate the electrostatic repulsive interactions between the negatively charged neighboring phosphates. In addition, the Mg^{2+} ions start a signaling cascade, which results in expression of biofilm related genes [34]. Furthermore, studies have shown that Mg^{2+} ions have varying effects on bacterial adhesion and biofilm formation [4,28,35–37] (Table 1), which could be explained by differences in bacterial species and Mg^{2+} concentrations used in the various studies. Since EPS possesses an anionic nature, it was proposed previously that certain Mg^{2+} concentration might contribute to an increase in exopolysaccharide (EPS) production and biofilm stabilization [38]. It was also reported that Mg^{2+} limitation is an important environmental trigger of *Pseudomonas aeruginosa* biofilm development [39]. However, it was found that biofilm formation decreased with increasing concentration of Mg^{2+} in *Enterobacter cloacae* [40]. Moreover, another recent study demonstrated how Mg^{2+} ions affected *Bacillus subtilis* biofilm formation by down-regulating the expression of extracellular matrix genes by more than 10-fold [4]. Taken together, the literatures up to now suggest that, in low concentrations, Mg^{2+} ions seem to induce adherence of bacteria to surfaces and subsequent biofilm formation, while higher concentrations seem to reduce the biofilm formation.

Table 1. Varying effects of magnesium ions on bacterial adhesion and biofilm formation.

Bacteria	Influence of Magnesium Ions	Reference
Staphylococcus aureus	High concentrations of magnesium bind TA, which increases cell wall rigidity and results in better adherence.	[30]
Pseudomonas aeruginosa	Adherence of two of three tested *P. aeruginosa* strains was enhanced by magnesium ions	[32]
	Magnesium ions limitation represses the expression of retS which leads to increased aggregation, exopolysaccharide (EPS) production and biofilm formation	[36]
	Diverse effect of divalent ions on *Pseudomonas aeruginosa* strains of various origins	[38]
Staphylococcus epidermidis	Adherence of all tested strains was enhanced in low concentrations of magnesium	[31]
Group b streptococci	Magnesium had no effect on adherence at physiologic concentrations	[33]
Pseudomonas fluorescens	Magnesium ions increased initial attachment and altered subsequent biofilm formation and structure	[24]
Bacillus species	Magnesium ions are significantly inhibited biofilm formation of Bacillus species at 50 mM concentration and higher. The expression of the two matrix operons was reduced drastically in response to magnesium ions	[34]
	Fortification of milk with magnesium mitigated biofilm formation by *Bacillus* species	[39]
Enterobacter cloacae	Biofilm formation decreased with increasing concentration of magnesium ions	[37]
Arthrobacter sp.	Mg^{2+} induced biofilm development through the removal of toxic hexavalent chromium	[40,41]

Thus, magnesium ions have a reasonable potential in affecting the food associated biofilm formation and by this preventing food spoilage and losses in the food industry. The exact mechanism as to how exactly the magnesium ions operate and delay biofilm formation remains unclear, yet several suggestions arise [5,11,41,42] (Figure 1). They could directly interact with the membrane and in some way prevent biofilm formation. Alternatively, they could also directly or indirectly influence the regulation of biofilm formation and delay biofilm formation. Due to the promising results obtained with magnesium ions in prevention of biofilm formation, the effect of Mg^{2+} ions on biofilm formation in the context of food matrices has also been recently studied.

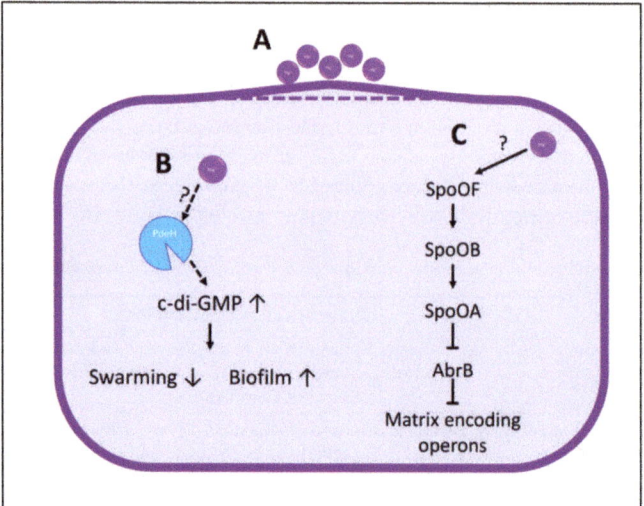

Figure 1. Possible mechanisms for the influence of Mg^{2+} ions on biofilm formation. **A**: Mg^{2+} can affect the membranes curvature, which results in a more sensitive bacterial population. **B**: Elevation of c-di-GMP levels leads to inhibition of the swarming motility and increased biofilm formation. The activity of PdeH, the enzyme that degrades c-di-GMP, is Mg^{2+} dependent. Therefore, Mg^{2+} ions could possibly enhance c-di-GMP degradation and hence decrease biofilm formation that results in heat sensitive bacteria. **C**: A third possible explanation is that the Mg^{2+} ions directly regulate the pathway leading to biofilm formation, which would again result in heat sensitive bacteria.

2.2. The Effect of Magnesium on Microbiological and Technological Properties of Milk

Milk is highly nutritious as it contains abundant water and nutrients, such as lactose, proteins, and lipids, and has a nearly neutral pH. This makes it an ideal medium for the growth of different microorganisms. Since microorganisms in milk may hold spoilage and health risks, milk manufacturing is subject to extremely stringent regulations. These regulations include pasteurization at high temperatures, which kills most bacteria, and milk storage at low temperatures, which limits the growth of many bacteria. It has been shown that in several *Bacillus* strains, milk triggers the formation of biofilm [43], and this might make the bacteria more resistant to pasteurization. A recent study has shown that supplementation of milk by 5mM $MgCl_2$ and above is capable of impairment of biofilm formation [44]. The impairment of the biofilm eventually results in about a two-log reduction in survival rate of bacterial cells once exposed to heat-pasteurization [44]. Accordingly, enrichment of milk and its products with magnesium would eventually result in safer dairy products as well as this would enable a longer shelf life of the products. In addition, enrichment of food with Mg^{2+} ions may also influence its technological properties as well [44,45]. It was also suggested that in the presence of Mg^{2+} ions the milk clotting starts significantly earlier, and the obtained curd is notably firmer [44]. This finding indicates that the curdling process appears to be improved in the presence of Mg^{2+} ions; i.e., in order to obtain cheeses in a desired hardness, the curdling process in the presence of Mg^{2+} ions is shorter. In another study in which magnesium lactate was added to fat free milk to produce yogurts, the hardness of the yogurts was increased [45]. Moreover, it was also demonstrated that fortified cheeses with Mg^{2+} ions had higher protein quantity [44]. Therefore, enrichment of milk with magnesium not only makes the dairy products healthier, but also improves their technological properties and increases potential availability of this essential mineral for absorption from the magnesium-enriched products. Taking into account also the antimicrobial effect of magnesium, which results in longer shelf life, enrichment of food with magnesium would result in healthier and inexpensive food (Figure 2).

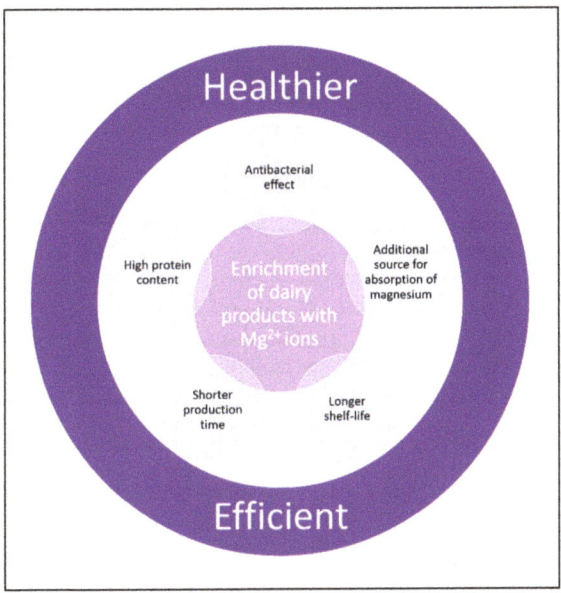

Figure 2. Enrichment of food products, for instance, dairy products, with magnesium would provide pronounced advantages and eventually result in healthier and efficient food products.

3. The Existing Need for the Enrichment of Food with Magnesium

Magnesium is a vital mineral that takes part in hundreds of enzymatic activities, and consumption of a sufficient amount magnesium is highly important for human health. This vital cation also plays important roles in the physiological functioning of the brain, heart, and skeletal muscles and has anti-inflammatory properties. Low levels of magnesium are associated with a wide range of diseases such as migraine, Alzheimer's disease, hypertension, insulin resistance, pre-eclampsia and cardiovascular diseases [1,46]. The recommended daily allowance of Mg^{2+} according to the US Food and Nutrition Board is 420 mg for men and 320 mg for women. However, it is estimated that most people do not consume the recommended daily allowance of magnesium [2,47,48], and about 10% to 30% of a given population are in a condition of Mg^{2+} deficiency (MGD) [49]. MGD as a result of low intake of magnesium could potentially increase risks for various diseases. Hence, finding new means to supply magnesium to humans is essential. According to [44] an evaluation of the bioavailability potential of magnesium in milk enriched with 5–10 mM $MgCl_2$, is ~75–90 mg/L. Hence, one needs to consume over 3.5 L of fortified milk to reach the lower limit of the recommended daily allowance. Nevertheless, consumption of milk fortified with Mg^{2+} will enable to increase the daily consumption of magnesium. Enrichment of food products with magnesium may provide a novel mean to deliver this important mineral to humans and other mammals [50].

4. Discussion

As mentioned above, magnesium plays a vital role as a cofactor in numerous enzymatic reactions in the cell [1,2,51]. These include phosphorylation and catalytic reactions, carbohydrate metabolism, lipid metabolism, as well as protein and nucleic acid synthesis. It also plays a role in the active transport of calcium and potassium ions across cell membranes. This vital cation is highly important for the human health [2,52,53]. Here, we elaborated on magnesium in the aspect of its antimicrobial effects. At high concentrations, magnesium ions decrease adherence of bacteria to surfaces and impair biofilm assembly. This makes the bacterial cells more sensitive to heat treatments. In dairy products, lower concentrations (~5mM) are required, maybe due to additional antimicrobial molecules found in the milk. Therefore, addition of magnesium ions to food and especially to dairy products would result in safer food with a longer shelf-life. Moreover, the magnesium ions also improve the technological properties of the products, which eventually results in cheaper production costs. Most importantly, enrichment of food products with magnesium ions would enable a new efficient source of consumption of this important mineral.

5. Conclusions

Magnesium is a vital mineral, which is not consumed to a sufficient quantity. Addition of magnesium to food matrices, for instance, to dairy products has several added benefits. First, the antibacterial effect of Mg^{2+} ions enables development of the safer and healthier food. Second, improvements in the technological properties of the magnesium supplemented food enables shorter production time and high protein content of the food products. Finally, enrichment of the food with Mg^{2+} ions provides a new source for the delivery of this vital mineral to humans.

Author Contributions: K.D. and M.S. originated the draft. K.D. prepared the illustrations for the manuscript. M.S. and K.D. developed the section on the antimicrobial and technological properties of magnesium ions. K.D. and R.R. discussed and elaborated on the role of magnesium in human health. All authors approved the final version of the manuscript.

Funding: This work was partially funded by the Nitzan Grant No. 4210342 of the Chief Scientist of the Ministry of Agriculture and Rural Development (Israel). This work was also supported by the Copia Agro & Food Technologies Fund, grant number 4210360.

Conflicts of Interest: The authors declare no conflict of interest.

References

1. Glasdam, S.M.; Glasdam, S.; Peters, G.H. The Importance of Magnesium in the Human Body: A Systematic Literature Review. *Adv. Clin. Chem.* **2016**, *73*, 169–193. [CrossRef] [PubMed]
2. De Baaij, J.H.; Hoenderop, J.G.; Bindels, R.J. Magnesium in man: Implications for health and disease. *Physiol. Rev.* **2015**, *95*, 1–46. [CrossRef] [PubMed]
3. Nguyen, N.T.; Grelling, N.; Wetteland, C.L.; Rosario, R.; Liu, H. Antimicrobial Activities and Mechanisms of Magnesium Oxide Nanoparticles (nMgO) against Pathogenic Bacteria, Yeasts, and Biofilms. *Sci. Rep.* **2018**, *8*, 16260. [CrossRef]
4. Oknin, H.; Steinberg, D.; Shemesh, M. Magnesium ions mitigate biofilm formation of *Bacillus* species via downregulation of matrix genes expression. *Front. Microbiol.* **2015**, *6*, 907. [CrossRef] [PubMed]
5. Xie, Y.; Yang, L. Calcium and Magnesium Ions Are Membrane-Active against Stationary-Phase *Staphylococcus aureus* with High Specificity. *Sci. Rep.* **2016**, *6*, 20628. [CrossRef]
6. Hayat, S.; Muzammil, S.; Rasool, M.H.; Nisar, Z.; Hussain, S.Z.; Sabri, A.N.; Jamil, S. *In vitro* antibiofilm and anti-Adhesion effects of magnesium oxide nanoparticles against antibiotic resistant bacteria. *Microbiol. Immunol.* **2018**, *62*, 211–220. [CrossRef] [PubMed]
7. Oyarzua Alarcon, P.; Sossa, K.; Contreras, D.; Urrutia, H.; Nocker, A. Antimicrobial properties of magnesium chloride at low pH in the presence of anionic bases. *Magnes. Res.* **2014**, *27*, 57–68. [CrossRef] [PubMed]
8. Delbet, P. *Politique Préventive du Cancer: Cytophylaxie*; Denoël: Paris, France, 1944.
9. Houlihan, A.J.; Russell, J.B. The effect of calcium and magnesium on the activity of bovicin HC5 and nisin. *Curr. Microbiol.* **2006**, *53*, 365–369. [CrossRef]
10. Khan, F.; Patoare, Y.; Karim, P.; Rayhan, I.; Quadir, M.A.; Hasnat, A. Effect of magnesium and zinc on antimicrobial activities of some antibiotics. *Pak. J. Pharm. Sci.* **2005**, *18*, 57–61.
11. Som, A.; Yang, L.; Wong, G.C.; Tew, G.N. Divalent metal ion triggered activity of a synthetic antimicrobial in cardiolipin membranes. *J. Am. Chem. Soc.* **2009**, *131*, 15102–15103. [CrossRef]
12. Zaatreh, S.; Haffner, D.; Strauss, M.; Dauben, T.; Zamponi, C.; Mittelmeier, W.; Quandt, E.; Kreikemeyer, B.; Bader, R. Thin magnesium layer confirmed as an antibacterial and biocompatible implant coating in a coculture model. *Mol. Med. Rep.* **2017**, *15*, 1624–1630. [CrossRef] [PubMed]

13. Zaatreh, S.; Haffner, D.; Strauss, M.; Wegner, K.; Warkentin, M.; Lurtz, C.; Zamponi, C.; Mittelmeier, W.; Kreikemeyer, B.; Willumeit-Romer, R.; et al. Fast corroding, thin magnesium coating displays antibacterial effects and low cytotoxicity. *Biofouling* **2017**, *33*, 294–305. [CrossRef] [PubMed]
14. Lellouche, J.; Kahana, E.; Elias, S.; Gedanken, A.; Banin, E. Antibiofilm activity of nanosized magnesium fluoride. *Biomaterials* **2009**, *30*, 5969–5978. [CrossRef] [PubMed]
15. Alvarez-Ordonez, A.; Coughlan, L.M.; Briandet, R.; Cotter, P.D. Biofilms in Food Processing Environments: Challenges and Opportunities. *Ann. Rev. Food Sci. Technol.* **2019**, *10*, 173–195. [CrossRef] [PubMed]
16. Bridier, A.; Sanchez-Vizuete, P.; Guilbaud, M.; Piard, J.C.; Naitali, M.; Briandet, R. Biofilm-Associated persistence of food-Borne pathogens. *Food Microbiol.* **2015**, *45*, 167–178. [CrossRef]
17. Hall-Stoodley, L.; Costerton, J.W.; Stoodley, P. Bacterial biofilms: From the natural environment to infectious diseases. *Nat. Rev. Microbiol.* **2004**, *2*, 95–108. [CrossRef] [PubMed]
18. Kolter, R.; Greenberg, E.P. Microbial sciences: The superficial life of microbes. *Nature* **2006**, *441*, 300–302. [CrossRef]
19. Saxena, P.; Joshi, Y.; Rawat, K.; Bisht, R. Biofilms: Architecture, Resistance, Quorum Sensing and Control Mechanisms. *Indian J. Microbiol.* **2019**, *59*, 3–12. [CrossRef]
20. Allison, D.G. The biofilm matrix. *Biofouling* **2003**, *19*, 139–150. [CrossRef]
21. Shemesh, M.; Kolter, R.; Losick, R. The biocide chlorine dioxide stimulates biofilm formation in *Bacillus subtilis* by activation of the histidine kinase KinC. *J. Bacteriol.* **2010**, *192*, 6352–6356. [CrossRef]
22. Kalamara, M.; Spacapan, M.; Mandic-Mulec, I.; Stanley-Wall, N.R. Social behaviours by *Bacillus subtilis*: Quorum sensing, kin discrimination and beyond. *Mol. Microbiol.* **2018**, *110*, 863–878. [CrossRef] [PubMed]
23. Checinska, A.; Paszczynski, A.; Burbank, M. Bacillus and other spore-Forming genera: Variations in responses and mechanisms for survival. *Ann. Rev. Food Sci. Technol.* **2015**, *6*, 351–369. [CrossRef] [PubMed]
24. Shaheen, R.; Svensson, B.; Andersson, M.A.; Christiansson, A.; Salkinoja-Salonen, M. Persistence strategies of *Bacillus cereus* spores isolated from dairy silo tanks. *Food Microbiol.* **2010**, *27*, 347–355. [CrossRef] [PubMed]
25. Flint, S.H.; Bremer, P.J.; Brooks, J.D. Biofilms in dairy manufacturing plant—description, current concerns and methods of control. *Biofouling* **1997**, *11*, 81–97. [CrossRef]
26. Yuan, L.; Hansen, M.F.; Roder, H.L.; Wang, N.; Burmolle, M.; He, G. Mixed-Species biofilms in the food industry: Current knowledge and novel control strategies. *Crit. Rev. Food Sci. Nutr.* **2019**, 1–17. [CrossRef] [PubMed]
27. Maukonen, J.; Matto, J.; Wirtanen, G.; Raaska, L.; Mattila-Sandholm, T.; Saarela, M. Methodologies for the characterization of microbes in industrial environments: A review. *J. Ind. Microbiol. Biotechnol.* **2003**, *30*, 327–356. [CrossRef] [PubMed]
28. Song, B.; Leff, L.G. Influence of magnesium ions on biofilm formation by *Pseudomonas fluorescens*. *Microbiol. Res.* **2006**, *161*, 355–361. [CrossRef]
29. Fletcher, M. Attachment of Pseudomonas fluorescens to glass and influence of electrolytes on bacterium-Substratum separation distance. *J. Bacteriol.* **1988**, *170*, 2027–2030. [CrossRef]
30. Mhatre, E.; Sundaram, A.; Holscher, T.; Muhlstadt, M.; Bossert, J.; Kovacs, A.T. Presence of Calcium Lowers the Expansion of *Bacillus subtilis* Colony Biofilms. *Microorganisms* **2017**, *5*. [CrossRef] [PubMed]
31. Polyudova, T.V.; Eroshenko, D.V.; Korobov, V.P. Plasma, serum, albumin, and divalent metal ions inhibit the adhesion and the biofilm formation of *Cutibacterium (Propionibacterium) acnes*. *AIMS Microbiol.* **2018**, *4*, 165–172. [CrossRef]
32. Cromie, M.J.; Shi, Y.; Latifi, T.; Groisman, E.A. An RNA sensor for intracellular Mg^{2+}. *Cell* **2006**, *125*, 71–84. [CrossRef] [PubMed]
33. Groisman, E.A.; Hollands, K.; Kriner, M.A.; Lee, E.J.; Park, S.Y.; Pontes, M.H. Bacterial Mg^{2+} homeostasis, transport, and virulence. *Ann. Rev. Genet.* **2013**, *47*, 625–646. [CrossRef] [PubMed]
34. Garcia-Betancur, J.C.; Goni-Moreno, A.; Horger, T.; Schott, M.; Sharan, M.; Eikmeier, J.; Wohlmuth, B.; Zernecke, A.; Ohlsen, K.; Kuttler, C.; et al. Cell differentiation defines acute and chronic infection cell types in *Staphylococcus aureus*. *eLife* **2017**, *6*. [CrossRef] [PubMed]
35. Dunne, W.M., Jr.; Burd, E.M. The effects of magnesium, calcium, EDTA, and pH on the *in vitro* adhesion of *Staphylococcus epidermidis* to plastic. *Microbiol. Immunol.* **1992**, *36*, 1019–1027. [CrossRef] [PubMed]
36. Marcus, H.; Austria, A.; Baker, N.R. Adherence of *Pseudomonas aeruginosa* to tracheal epithelium. *Infect. Immun.* **1989**, *57*, 1050–1053.

37. Tamura, G.S.; Kuypers, J.M.; Smith, S.; Raff, H.; Rubens, C.E. Adherence of group B streptococci to cultured epithelial cells: Roles of environmental factors and bacterial surface components. *Infect. Immun.* **1994**, *62*, 2450–2458.
38. Costerton, J.W.; Lewandowski, Z.; Caldwell, D.E.; Korber, D.R.; Lappin-Scott, H.M. Microbial biofilms. *Ann. Rev. Microbiol.* **1995**, *49*, 711–745. [CrossRef]
39. Mulcahy, H.; Lewenza, S. Magnesium limitation is an environmental trigger of the *Pseudomonas aeruginosa* biofilm lifestyle. *PLoS ONE* **2011**, *6*, e23307. [CrossRef]
40. Zhou, G.; Li, L.J.; Shi, Q.S.; Ouyang, Y.S.; Chen, Y.B.; Hu, W.F. Efficacy of metal ions and isothiazolones in inhibiting *Enterobacter cloacae* BF-17 biofilm formation. *Can. J. Microbiol.* **2014**, *60*, 5–14. [CrossRef]
41. Gao, X.; Mukherjee, S.; Matthews, P.M.; Hammad, L.A.; Kearns, D.B.; Dann, C.E. Functional characterization of core components of the *Bacillus subtilis* cyclic-di-GMP signaling pathway. *J. Bacteriol.* **2013**, *195*, 4782–4792. [CrossRef]
42. Chen, Y.; Chai, Y.; Guo, J.H.; Losick, R. Evidence for cyclic Di-GMP-Mediated signaling in *Bacillus subtilis*. *J. Bacteriol.* **2012**, *194*, 5080–5090. [CrossRef] [PubMed]
43. Pasvolsky, R.; Zakin, V.; Ostrova, I.; Shemesh, M. Butyric acid released during milk lipolysis triggers biofilm formation of *Bacillus* species. *Int. J. Food Microbiol.* **2014**, *181*, 19–27. [CrossRef]
44. Ben-Ishay, N.; Oknin, H.; Steinberg, D.; Berkovich, Z.; Reifen, R.; Shemesh, M. Enrichment of milk with magnesium provides healthier and safer dairy products. *NPJ Biofilms Microb.* **2017**, *3*, 24. [CrossRef] [PubMed]
45. Szajnar, K.; Znamirowska, A.; Kalicka, D.; Kuzniar, P.; Najgebauer-Lejko, D. Quality of yogurt fortified with magnesium lactate. *Acta Sci. Pol. Technol. Aliment.* **2018**, *17*, 247–255. [CrossRef] [PubMed]
46. Grober, U.; Schmidt, J.; Kisters, K. Magnesium in Prevention and Therapy. *Nutrients* **2015**, *7*, 8199–8226. [CrossRef]
47. King, D.E.; Mainous, A.G., III; Geesey, M.E.; Woolson, R.F. Dietary magnesium and C-Reactive protein levels. *J. Am. Coll. Nutr.* **2005**, *24*, 166–171. [CrossRef]
48. Razzaque, M.S. Magnesium: Are We Consuming Enough? *Nutrients* **2018**, *10*, 1863. [CrossRef]
49. Costello, R.B.; Elin, R.J.; Rosanoff, A.; Wallace, T.C.; Guerrero-Romero, F.; Hruby, A.; Lutsey, P.L.; Nielsen, F.H.; Rodriguez-Moran, M.; Song, Y. Perspective: The Case for an Evidence-Based Reference Interval for Serum Magnesium: The Time Has Come. *Adv. Nutr.* **2016**, *15*, 977–993. [CrossRef]
50. Sacco, J.E.; Tarasuk, V. Discretionary addition of vitamins and minerals to foods: Implications for healthy eating. *Eur. J. Clin. Nutr.* **2011**, *65*, 313–320. [CrossRef]
51. Uwitonze, A.M.; Razzaque, M.S. Role of Magnesium in Vitamin D Activation and Function. *J. Am. Osteopath. Assoc.* **2018**, *118*, 181–189. [CrossRef]
52. Gant, C.M.; Soedamah-Muthu, S.S.; Binnenmars, S.H.; Bakker, S.J.L.; Navis, G.; Laverman, G.D. Higher Dietary Magnesium Intake and Higher Magnesium Status Are Associated with Lower Prevalence of Coronary Heart Disease in Patients with Type 2 Diabetes. *Nutrients* **2018**, *10*, 307. [CrossRef] [PubMed]
53. DiNicolantonio, J.J.; Liu, J.; O'Keefe, J.H. Magnesium for the prevention and treatment of cardiovascular disease. *Open Heart* **2018**, *5*, e000775. [CrossRef] [PubMed]

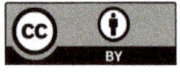

© 2019 by the authors. Licensee MDPI, Basel, Switzerland. This article is an open access article distributed under the terms and conditions of the Creative Commons Attribution (CC BY) license (http://creativecommons.org/licenses/by/4.0/).

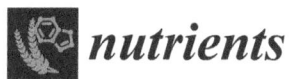

Article

Crosstalk of Nrf2 with the Trace Elements Selenium, Iron, Zinc, and Copper

Maria Schwarz [1,2,†], **Kristina Lossow** [1,2,3,4,†], **Johannes F. Kopp** [2,4], **Tanja Schwerdtle** [2,4] **and Anna P. Kipp** [1,2,*]

1. Department of Molecular Nutritional Physiology, Institute of Nutritional Sciences, Friedrich Schiller University Jena, Dornburger Str. 24, 07743 Jena, Germany
2. TraceAge-DFG Research Unit on Interactions of Essential Trace Elements in Healthy and Diseased Elderly, D-13353 Potsdam-Berlin-Jena, Germany
3. German Institute of Human Nutrition, Arthur-Scheunert-Allee 114-116, 14558 Nuthetal, Germany
4. Department of Food Chemistry, Institute of Nutritional Science, University of Potsdam, Arthur-Scheunert-Allee 114-116, 14558 Nuthetal, Germany
* Correspondence: anna.kipp@uni-jena.de; Tel.: +49-3641-949609
† These authors equally contributed to the manuscript.

Received: 10 July 2019; Accepted: 23 August 2019; Published: 5 September 2019

Abstract: Trace elements, like Cu, Zn, Fe, or Se, are important for the proper functioning of antioxidant enzymes. However, in excessive amounts, they can also act as pro-oxidants. Accordingly, trace elements influence redox-modulated signaling pathways, such as the Nrf2 pathway. Vice versa, Nrf2 target genes belong to the group of transport and metal binding proteins. In order to investigate whether Nrf2 directly regulates the systemic trace element status, we used mice to study the effect of a constitutive, whole-body Nrf2 knockout on the systemic status of Cu, Zn, Fe, and Se. As the loss of selenoproteins under Se-deprived conditions has been described to further enhance Nrf2 activity, we additionally analyzed the combination of Nrf2 knockout with feeding diets that provide either suboptimal, adequate, or supplemented amounts of Se. Experiments revealed that the Nrf2 knockout partially affected the trace element concentrations of Cu, Zn, Fe, or Se in the intestine, liver, and/or plasma. However, aside from Fe, the other three trace elements were only marginally modulated in an Nrf2-dependent manner. Selenium deficiency mainly resulted in increased plasma Zn levels. One putative mediator could be the metal regulatory transcription factor 1, which was up-regulated with an increasing Se supply and downregulated in Se-supplemented Nrf2 knockout mice.

Keywords: Nrf2; selenium; iron; copper; zinc; homeostasis

1. Introduction

Essential trace elements (TEs) are micronutrients with indispensable roles in enzymatic reactions, which consequently modify signaling pathways. The effects of TEs are mostly attributed to their redox-modulatory properties. TEs, such as Cu, Zn, and Fe but also Se, can act as pro-oxidants if present in excess or if available as free unbound ions. Otherwise, antioxidant and protective enzymes, such as the selenoproteins, glutathione peroxidases (GPX) and thioredoxin reductases (TXNRD) and also Cu/Zn superoxide dismutase (SOD1), catalase, and metallothioneins (MT), depend on the supply with specific TEs. Via both ways, TEs have the potential to influence redox-modulated signaling pathways. Until now, many transcription factors have been shown to be sensitive towards the cellular redox status. Among them, nuclear factor erythroid 2 p45-related factor 2 (Nrf2) is a better characterized one [1].

Under basal conditions the transcription factor Nrf2 is kept in the cytosol by its binding partner, Kelch-like ECH-associated protein 1 (Keap1), which is anchored to the actin cytoskeleton and acts as a scaffold for the cullin3-dependent E3 ubiquitin ligase complex. After poly-ubiquitination,

Nrf2 is degraded via the proteasome. There are several ways to induce the nuclear translocation and DNA binding of Nrf2. Of those, the best understood mechanism is the redox-dependent modification of thiol groups in the Keap1 protein, which results in a conformational change locking Nrf2 at Keap1. Newly synthesized Nrf2 can no longer be degraded and translocates to the nucleus. Besides Keap1, caveolin 1, the ubiquitin ligase Skp, cullin, F-box containing complex (SCF), and the retinoid X receptor α (RXRα) also interact with and repress Nrf2. Nrf2 target genes contain so-called antioxidant-responsive elements (ARE) within their promoter regions (reviewed in [2]). The list of Nrf2-regulated genes is further increasing continuously and comprises genes involved in antioxidant defense, NADPH regeneration, glutathione synthesis, and drug detoxification, as well as in metabolic control, including carbohydrate and lipid metabolism [3]. Nrf2 has previously been shown to be modulated by changes in the cellular status of single TEs, e.g., Zn. Zn binding triggers a conformational switch in the cullin3 substrate adaptor function of Keap1, thus Nrf2 becomes stabilized and can activate the transcription of target genes [4]. Furthermore, Zn modulates the activity of several kinases and phosphatases, which accordingly enhances Nrf2 activity (Table 1).

Vice versa, Nrf2 target genes belong to the group of selenoproteins or are involved in regulating the systemic TE status (Table 1). This has already been studied for Fe [3]. In mice, Nrf2 is activated in response to increased hepatic Fe levels [5]. Accordingly, Nrf2 protects the murine liver against the toxicity of dietary Fe overload by preventing cell death of hepatocytes and enhancing Fe release [6]. During inflammation, Nrf2 induces ferroportin (Fpn1), the sole Fe exporter, to enhance Fe efflux from macrophages or enterocytes [7]. Several Fe transport and binding proteins, like Fpn1, hepcidin (Hamp), and ferritin, are Nrf2 target genes [8]. In addition, key enzymes of heme biosynthesis are induced via Nrf2 (Table 1). Altogether, this battery of proteins reduces the pool of free intracellular Fe. A comparable approach is the upregulation of MTs, a family of cysteine-rich proteins that bind Zn and Cu via their thiol groups [9]. Another important mediator of Cu homeostasis is the Cu-transporting ATPase 2 (Atp7b), the Wilson's ATPase. Being primarily expressed in hepatocytes, Atp7b supports the incorporation of Cu into ceruloplasmin (Cp) and enhances the excretion of Cu from the liver into the bile [10,11].

Table 1. Effects of single trace elements on Nrf2 signaling (overview in [12]).

TE	Nrf2 Pathway Activity	TE-Related Nrf2 Target Genes
Cu	$CuCl_2$ activates Nrf2; Nrf2 is crucial for MRE/ARE-mediated transcription in response to Cu [13]	MT1/2, SOD1
Fe	cytotoxic concentrations of Fe activate Nrf2 in murine primary astrocytes [14] and hepatocytes [6]	Fpn1, heme oxygenase (Hmox1) [15], Hamp, ferritin (FTH-1, FTL) [16], heme transporter (Slc48a1/HRG1), ferrochelatase (Fech), biliverdin reductases (BlvrA/B)
Se	a suboptimal Se status activates Nrf2 in mice [17]; high selenite concentrations enhance Nrf2 target gene expression [18]	GPX2 [19], TXNRD1 [20]
Zn	Zn upregulates Nrf2 function, e.g., via phosphorylation signals [21]	MT1/2, SOD1

There is substantial cross-talk between Nrf2 and other transcription factors, including the aryl hydrocarbon receptor (AhR), nuclear factor κ-light-chain-enhancer of activated B cells (NF-κB), tumor suppressor protein p53, and Notch making Nrf2, an important factor in regulating immune defense, differentiation, and tissue regeneration, as well as cell death [22]. Another interesting interaction could take place with the metal regulatory transcription factor 1 (MTF1), which senses Cu and Zn and binds to metal-responsive elements (MREs) in the promoter of target genes. These include the zinc transporter solute carrier family 30 member 1 Slc30A1, encoding for ZnT1, as well as MT1 and 2, but also selenoproteins, like Selenoh, Selenow, and TXNRD2, modulators of the Fe status, like Fpn1 and Hamp [23], and Atp7b [24]. In particular, MT genes often contain AREs next to MREs and are activated via Nrf family members. For MT1, this activation has been shown by Nrf1 as well as by Nrf2, especially in response to the cellular Zn status, albeit to a smaller extent [25]. Thus, MTF1 could be a potential link between Nrf2 signaling and regulation of TE homeostasis.

In most previous studies, the authors focused on high concentrations and pro-oxidant effects of overloading single TEs, e.g., Se. However, we have previously shown that Nrf2 becomes activated under conditions of a suboptimal Se status in the duodenum [17] and liver [26] of mice. NAD(P)H quinone dehydrogenase 1 (NQO1) activity was analyzed as one of the most strongly regulated target genes of Nrf2. Most probably, the Nrf2 activation is an attempt to compensate for the reduced expression of antioxidant selenoproteins. This condition has a much higher physiological relevance than Se supplementation because of the suboptimal nutritional Se supply prevailing in Europe [27]. The U-shaped effect on Nrf2 activity observed for Se could also be true for other TEs; however, this has not been studied systematically so far.

Based on the results obtained for single TEs, we aimed to study the effect of a whole-body Nrf2 knockout (KO) in mice on the systemic TE status of Fe, Se, Cu, and Zn. A suboptimal Se status results in limited expression of Se-sensitive selenoproteins. As reduced expression of selenoproteins, such as TXNRD1, under Se-deprived conditions further enhances Nrf2 activity [28], we also studied the combination of Nrf2 KO mice with feeding diets that provide either a suboptimal, adequate, or supplemented amount of Se. Focusing only on wild type (WT) mice with different Se statuses allowed the question of whether changes in a single TE (in this case Se) affect the homeostasis of three other TEs to be addressed. In addition to markers for the TE status, TE-related Nrf2 target genes were analyzed in the liver of those mice.

2. Materials and Methods

2.1. Animal Experiment

Animal experiments were approved by the ethics committee of the Ministry of Agriculture and Environment (State Brandenburg, Germany) and all methods were carried out in accordance to permission number V3-2437-29-2012. Nrf2 KO mice on a C57BL/6J background were kindly provided by Masayuki Yamamoto (Tohoku University Graduate School of Medicine) and genotyped as previously described [29]. Adult male and female mice were used for the animal experiments that were group-housed and random-caged with ad libitum access to a standard chow diet (Ssniff, Soest, Germany, Table 2), with an Se content of 0.3 mg/kg diet, deionized water, 23 °C, and a 12:12 h dark:light cycle. Those mice were sacrificed at an age of 6 months.

Table 2. Estimated trace element requirements of mice [30] and trace elements in the diets used.

TE	Requirement (mg/kg)	Chow (Ssniff) (mg/kg)	Altromin C1045 (mg/kg)
Cu	6	8.8	2.7
Fe	35	215	151
Se	0.15	0.3	0.03
Zn	10	97	57

In the second experiment, male WT and Nrf2 KO mice were weaned onto a diet based on torula yeast (Altromin C1045; Lage, Germany, Table 2) with a low basal selenium content of 0.03 mg/kg. For the selenium adequate (+Se) and the supplemented (++Se) diets, the basal chow was enriched with L (+)-selenomethionine (Fisher Scientific, Schwerte, Germany) to a final selenium content of 0.15 or 0.6 mg/kg, respectively. The Se, Fe, Cu, and Zn concentration of the diets was measured by ICP-MS/MS. Diets were fed for 6 weeks until an age of 10 weeks before mice were anesthetized by isoflurane (Abbot, Wiesbaden, Germany), and blood was withdrawn by heart puncture. Plasma was obtained after centrifugation of the blood for 15 min (1200× g and 4 °C).

2.2. ICP-MS/MS Analysis of TE

Frozen tissue (liver or duodenum) was pulverized using a TissueLyser (Qiagen, Hilden, Germany) for 2 × 30 s at maximum speed. Feed samples were pulverized by mortar and pestle. About 50 mg of each sample were weighed precisely into polytetrafluoroethylene (PTFE) microwave vessels. For mouse tissue, the variance was found to be far below 5% between replicates of the same mouse (data not shown); therefore, only one replicate was analyzed to preserve tissue for other experiments. However, in the case of obvious outliers, the sample was digested and analyzed again. Due to high in-batch variance in the chow diets from some manufacturers, at least three independent replicates were prepared in the case of feed samples. For tissue samples, 1000 µL of concentrated HNO_3 (65%, suprapure, Merck, Darmstadt, Germany), 50 µL of a solution containing 100 µg Rh/L (made from 10 mg/L single-element stock solution, Carl Roth, Karlsruhe, Germany) as the internal standard, and 950 µL ultrapure water were added. For feed samples, 900 µL of concentrated HNO_3, 250 µL of H_2O_2 (30%, Merck/Sigma-Aldrich, Darmstadt, Germany), and 810 µL of ultrapure water were added. In addition, 20 µL of a solution containing 1000 µg Rh/L and 20 µL of 10,000 µg ^{77}Se/L (made from a 10,000 mg/L stock solution, prepared from isotopically enriched ^{77}Se (97.20 ± 0.20% ^{77}Se; 0.10% ^{74}Se; 0.40 ± 0.10% ^{76}Se; 2.40 ± 0.10% ^{78}Se; 0.10% ^{80}Se; 0.10% ^{82}Se as certified by Trace Sciences International, ON, Canada), purchased from Eurisotop SAS (Saarbrücken, Germany), were added as internal standard or isotope dilution standard, respectively. The samples were then digested in a Mars 6 microwave digestion system (CEM, Kamp-Lintfort, Germany) by heating to 200 °C over a period of 10 min and holding this temperature for 20 min. In each digestion, two blank samples and 50 mg of certified reference material ERM-BB 422 (fish muscle) or ERM BB 186 (pig kidney, Merck/Sigma-Aldrich) were carried along to ensure accuracy of results. Samples were repeated if the recovery for any analyzed element deviated by more than 10% from the reference value and/or was outside the error range of the material. After digestion, samples were quantitatively transferred to 15-mL polypropylene tubes combined with two times 475 µL (tissue) or 1 mL (feed) of ultrapure water from vessel rinsing. The samples were kept at 4 °C until one day prior to measurement, when they were further diluted 1 + 4 in 15-mL polypropylene tubes to give a final concentration of 2.93% HNO_3, as well as either 2.5 µg Rh/L (tissue) or 1 µg Rh/L and 10 µg ^{77}Se/L (feed). Mixed-element calibration standards were made to match the concentration of HNO_3 and the internal standard in the diluted digests from 1000 mg/L single-element stock solutions (Carl Roth). Calibration ranges were Fe: 5–1000 µg/L, Cu: 0.5–100 µg/L, Zn: 2.5–500 µg/L, Se: 0.05–10 µg/L. For Se isotope dilution analysis (IDA), a solution containing 10 µg ^{77}Se/L, as well as a 1 + 1 mixture of 10 µg ^{77}Se/L and 10 µg naturally distributed Se/L was prepared. Solutions were then analyzed via ICP-MS/MS (8800 ICP-QQQ-MS, Agilent Technologies, Waldbronn, Germany at 1550 W plasma Rf power, equipped with Ni-cones, MicroMist nebulizer at 1.2 L Ar/min and Scott-type spraychamber) monitoring the following mass to charge ratios (Q1→Q2): He-mode: Fe (56→56), Cu (63→63), Zn (66→66), Rh (103→103); O2-mode: Se (77→93), Se (80→96), Rh (103→103). Elements in He-mode were determined via external calibration after internal standard correction using Rh and Se was also determined either via external calibration (tissue) or via isotope dilution analysis (IDA) (feed) as described previously [31]. The instrument was optimized on a daily basis for maximum sensitivity across the relevant mass range (He: Co (59→59), Y (89→89), Tl (205→205); O2: Co (59→59), Y (89→95), Tl (205→205)), an oxide ratio of <1.5% ($^{156}(CeO)^+/^{140}Ce^+$), and a doubly charged ratio of <2% ($^{140}Ce^{2+}/^{140}Ce^+$), as well as a background of <0.1 CPS prior to measurement.

The applied method for the analysis of TEs in murine plasma has been described previously [32]. In brief, 50 µL of murine plasma were diluted 1 + 9 with a dilution mix (5 vol.-% butanol (99%, Alfa Aesar, Karlsruhe, Germany), 0.05 m.-% Na-EDTA (Titriplex® III, pro analysis, Merck), 0.05 vol.-% Triton™ X-100 (Merck Sigma-Aldrich), and 0.25 vol.-% ammonium hydroxide (puriss. p.a. plus, 25% in water, Fluka, Buchs, Germany)), as well as internal standards (final concentrations: 1 µg Rh/L and 30 µg ^{77}Se/L). The diluted sample was then subjected to analysis for Fe, Cu, Zn, and Se (IDA) via ICP MS/MS.

2.3. RNA Isolation, Reverse Transcription, and Quantitative Real-Time PCR

The mRNA was isolated from frozen and pulverized (TissueLyser; Qiagen) tissues with the Dynabeads mRNA DIRECT Kit (Life Technologies, Fisher Scientific) according to the manufacturer's protocol. Reverse transcription (RT) was performed with 150 ng mRNA, 0.15 pmol oligo(dT)15 primers, 1× RT buffer, 700 µM dNTPs, 0.1 mg/mL BSA, 30 U RNasin® (Promega, Mannheim, Germany), and 180 U Moloney murine leukemia virus reverse transcriptase (M-MLV RT, Promega) in a total volume of 45 µL. Real-time PCR was performed in a total volume of 25 µL with 1 µL of 1 + 9 diluted cDNA measured in triplicates using a Mx3005P QPCR System (Agilent). SYBR Green I (Molecular Probes, Eugene, OR, USA) served as the fluorescent reporter. The annealing temperature was 60 °C for all PCR reactions and specificity was confirmed by a melting curve analysis. All PCR products were quantified with a standard curve to correct for differences in PCR efficiencies. Primer sequences (Sigma-Aldrich, Steinheim, Germany) are listed in Table 3. A normalization factor was calculated from the two reference genes, *Epcam* and *Rpl13a*, and used for normalization.

Table 3. Primer sequences (5'→3').

Gene	RefSeq-ID	Sequence
Atp7b, ATPase copper transporting beta	NM_007511.2	CAGATGTCAAAGGCTCCCATTCAG CCAATGACGATCCACACCACC
Cp, ceruloplasmin	NM_001276248.1	GTACTACTCTGGCGTTGACCC TTGTCTACATCTTTCTGTCTCCCA
DMT1, divalent metal transporter 1	NM_001146161.1	CTCAGCCATCGCCATCAATCTC TTCCGCAAGCCATATTTGTCCA
Epcam, epithelial cell adhesion molecule	NM_008532.2	TCATCGCTGTCATTGTGGTGGT TCACCCATCTCCTTTATCTCAGCC
Fpn1, ferroportin	NM_016917.2	CTGGTGGTTCAGAATGTGTCCGT AGCAGACAGTAAGGACCCATCCA
Fth1, ferritin heavy polypeptide 1	NM_010239.2	CGCCAGAACTACCACCAGGA TTCTTCAGAGCCACATCATCTCGG
Hamp, hepcidin	NM_032541.1	AAGCAGGGCAGACATTGCGA TGCAACAGATACCACACTGGGA
MT2, metallothionein 2	NM_008630.2	CTGTGCCTCCGATGGATCCT CTTGTCGGAAGCCTCTTTGCAG
NQO1, NAD(P)H quinone dehydrogenase 1	NM_008706.4	ATGTACGACAACGGTCCTTTCCAG GATGCCACTCTGAATCGGCCA
Rpl13a, ribosomal protein L13a	NM_009438.5	GTTCGGCTGAAGCCTACCAG TTCCGTAACCTCAAGATCTGCT
Selenow, selenoprotein W	NM_009156.2	ATGCCTGGACATTTGTGGCGA GCAGCTTTGATGGCGGTCAC
Tfrc, transferrin receptor	NM_011638.4	GGCTGAAACGGAGGAGACAGA CTGGCTCAGCTGCTTGATGGT
Zip14, solute carrier family 39 member 14	NM_001135151.1	GCCTCACCATCCTGGTATCCGT AGCAGACGAGGCATGAGTCTGG

2.4. ELISA

Ferritin and transferrin were measured in plasma samples using Mouse Ferritin and Transferrin ELISA (ALPCO, Salem, MA, USA) following the manufacturer's instruction. Therefore, plasma samples were either diluted 1:20 or 1:200,000, respectively.

2.5. Western Blot

To obtain protein lysates, frozen liver samples were homogenized in Tris buffer (100 mM Tris, 300 mM KCl, pH 7.6 with 0.1% Triton X-100 (Serva, Heidelberg, Germany)) using a TissueLyser (Qiagen) for 2 × 30 s at maximum speed. Cellular debris was removed by centrifugation (14,000× g, 15 min, 4 °C) and protein concentrations were determined by Bradford analysis (Biorad, München, Germany). After SDS polyacrylamide gel electrophoresis, gels were immunoblotted to nitrocellulose and blots were blocked in 5% non-fat dry milk in Tris-buffered saline containing 0.1% Tween 20 at room temperature for 1 h. The following antibodies were used: Rabbit anti-Ferritin-H (151023, Abcam, Cambridge, UK; 1:500), rabbit anti-MT (192385, Abcam; 1:1000), rabbit anti-Ctr1 (129067, Abcam; 1:2000), rabbit anti-MTF-1 antibody (86380, Novus Biologicals, Centennials, US; 1:250), and rabbit anti-β-Actin (8227, Abcam; 1:10,000). Horseradish peroxidase-conjugated goat anti-rabbit IgG (Chemicon, Hofheim, Germany; 1:50,000) served as secondary antibody. Intensities of identified bands were quantified densitometrically with the Luminescent Image Analyzer LAS-3000 system (Fujifilm, Tokyo, Japan). Protein expression was normalized to β-actin expression or Ponceau staining.

2.6. Enzyme Activities

Protein lysates were prepared as described in the section 'Western Blot'. Measurements of NQO1 [17], TXNRD [33], GPX [34], and glutathione S transferase (GST) [35] activities have been described previously. Briefly, NQO1 activity was examined by a menadione-mediated reduction of 3-(4,5-dimethylthiazol-2-yl)-2,5-diphenyltetrazolium bromide (MTT). TXNRD activity was measured by the NADPH-dependent reduction of 5,5′-dithiobis (2-nitrobenzoic acid) (DTNB). GPX activity was determined in an NADPH-consuming glutathione reductase coupled assay. GST activity was conducted using 1-chloro-2,4-dinitrobenzene (CDNB) as substrate in the presence of reduced glutathione. All measurements were performed in triplicates using 96-well plates and a microplate reader (Synergy2, BioTek, Bad Friedrichshall, Germany).

2.7. Statistics

Data are shown as mean + SD. Statistical significance was calculated by GraphPad Prism version 5 (San Diego, CA, USA) using two-way analysis of variance (ANOVA) with Bonferroni's post-test as indicated in the figure legends. A p-value below 0.05 was considered statistically significant.

3. Results

To address the question of whether Nrf2 not only modulates the status of single TEs, such as Fe, but also of several TEs in parallel, we analyzed Se, Fe, Cu, and Zn in male and female Nrf2 KO mice fed a standard chow diet. TE concentrations were assessed in the intestine, liver, and plasma. Fe was retained more in the liver and small intestine of Nrf2 KO than in WT mice (Figure 1A,B). Consequently, plasma Fe levels were reduced but only in female mice (Figure 1C).

No changes were observed concerning the Fe markers, ferritin and transferrin (Figure S1A,B). In parallel, intestinal Se (Figure 1D) and Zn (Figure 1G) concentrations were reduced in Nrf2 KO compared to WT mice. This was also partially reflected in the Se and Zn plasma and liver values but less consistently. Nrf2-mediated changes of the Cu status appear to be sex specific as only female mice showed lower plasma Cu levels upon loss of Nrf2 (Figure 1L). Overall, Nrf2 reduced the systemic Fe status but increased Se and Zn. Female WT mice had higher plasma levels of Fe, Zn, and Cu. In the liver, amounts of Fe and Se were increased in female mice. In general, chow diets contain high amounts of all TEs, usually at least twice the recommended amounts. Thus, Nrf2-modulated effects might be more pronounced under conditions of limited TE access.

To analyze the role of the Se status on other TEs in combination with loss of Nrf2, both WT and Nrf2 KO mice were weaned onto one of three diets containing suboptimal (0.03 ppm), adequate (0.15 ppm), or supplemented (0.6 ppm) amounts of Se. The experimental set-up was chosen according to previous feeding experiments to efficiently reduce the Se status in the –Se group. For better comparability with previous experiments, only male mice were studied [17]. In addition, the remaining three TEs were reduced in the torula yeast-based diet as compared to the chow diet (Table 2).

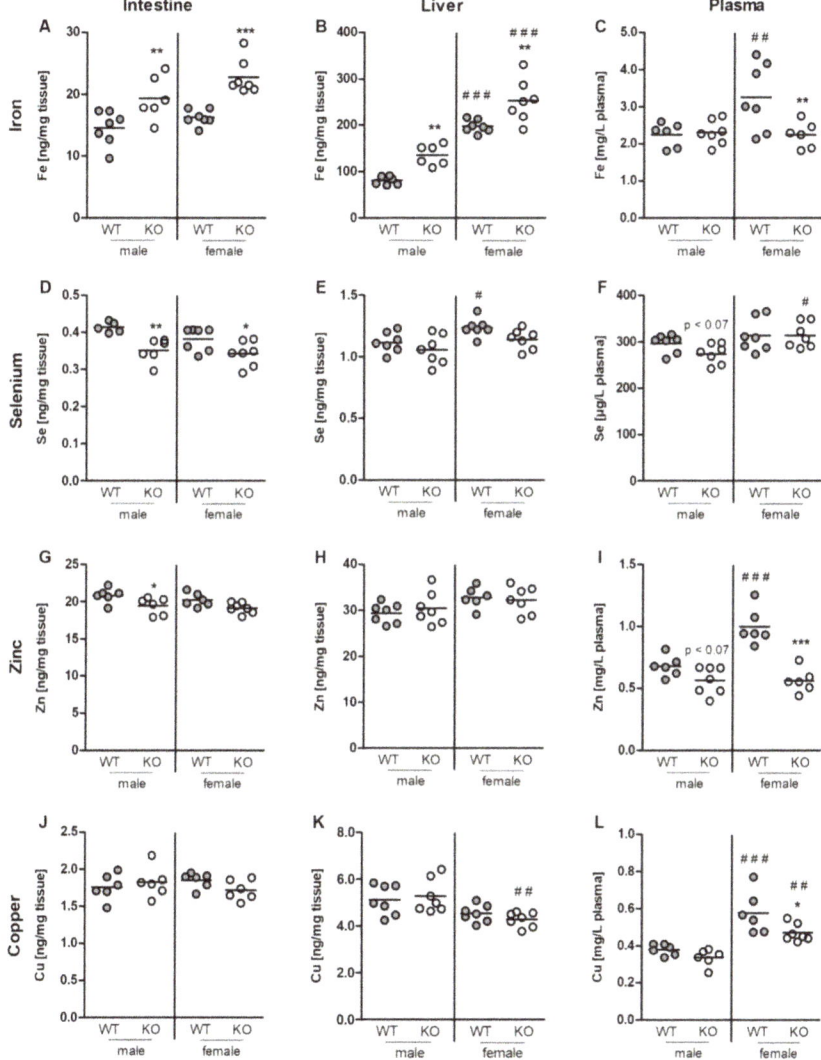

Figure 1. Fe (**A–C**), Se (**D–F**), Zn (**G-I**), and Cu (**J–L**) concentrations in the jejunum (**A,D,G,J**), liver (**B,E,H,K**), and plasma (**C,F,I,L**) of six-month-old male and female Nrf2 KO and WT mice fed a standard chow diet with 0.3 ppm Se. The TE profile was analyzed using ICP-MS/MS. Scatter dot plots with mean (n = 6–7). * $p < 0.05$; ** $p < 0.01$; *** $p < 0.001$ vs. WT and # $p < 0.05$; ## $p < 0.01$; ### $p < 0.001$ vs. male (two-way ANOVA with Bonferroni's post-test).

As expected, the dietary approach successfully modulated the Se status of the different feeding groups (Figure 2A,B). The Se content of the chow diet fed in experiment one was 0.3 ppm and thus between the amount of the +Se (0.15 ppm) and the ++Se (0.6 ppm) diets. Comparing the plasma Se content in both experiments (Figures 1F and 2A) revealed that the +Se diet with 0.15 ppm was already able to set the plasma Se concentration to almost 300 µg/L, which was nearly the same amount as measured in the 0.3 (Figure 1F) or 0.6 ppm Se groups (++Se, Figure 2A).

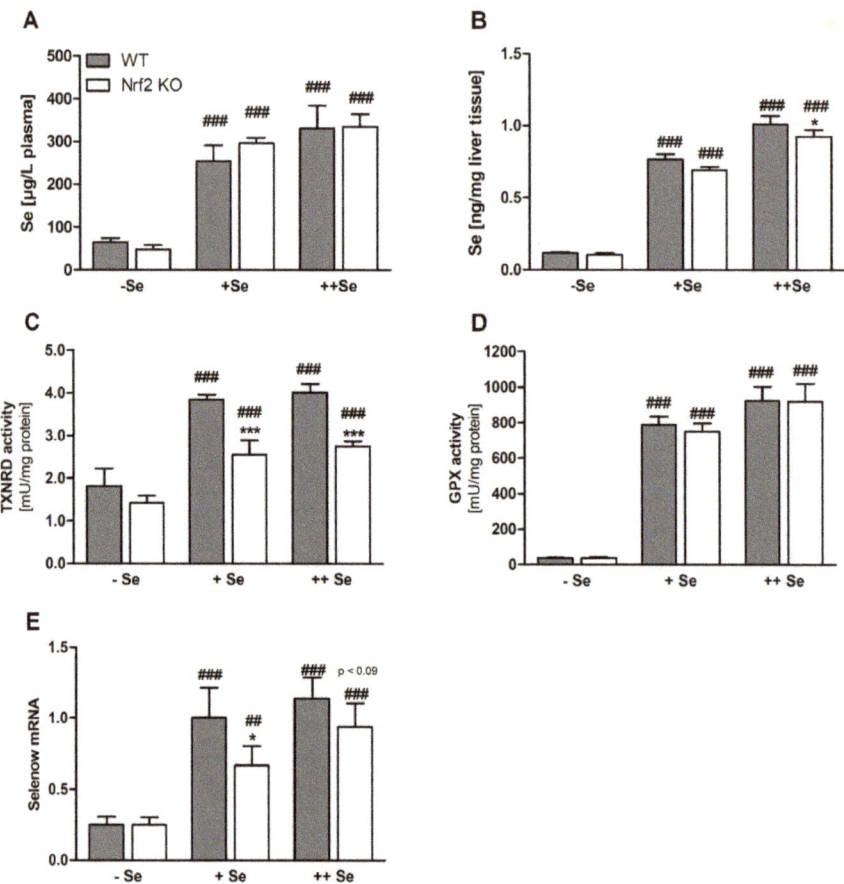

Figure 2. Biomarkers of the Se status. Se concentrations in the plasma (**A**) and liver (**B**) of Nrf2 KO and WT male mice fed diets with defined Se contents (−Se: 0.03 ppm; +Se: 0.15 ppm; ++Se: 0.6 ppm). The TE profile was analyzed using ICP-MS/MS. Enzyme activity of TXNRD (**C**) and GPX (**D**) was analyzed together with mRNA expression of Selenow (**E**) from liver samples of male Nrf2 KO and WT mice. Bars represent means + SD (n = 4-5). * $p < 0.05$; *** $p < 0.001$ vs. WT and ## $p < 0.01$; ### $p < 0.001$ vs. −Se (two-way ANOVA with Bonferroni's post-test).

In order to confirm that loss of Nrf2 resulted in diminished expression of classical Nrf2 target genes, NQO1 activity (Figure 3A) was analyzed. Enzyme activity was substantially decreased in Nrf2 KO mice. Basal NQO1 mRNA levels were much higher in female than in male mice (Figure S1C). To our surprise, NQO1 activity was not increased under −Se conditions but was significantly decreased in comparison to the +Se or ++Se groups. In Nrf2 KO mice, no Se-dependent effect was detectable. Comparable results were obtained for total GST activity (Figure 3B).

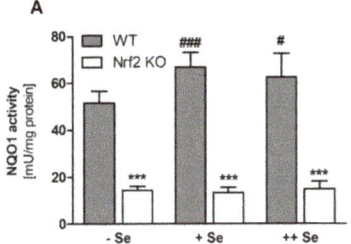 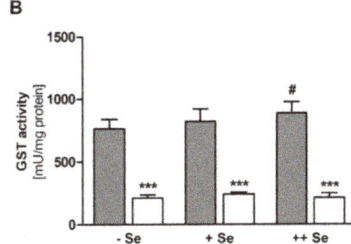

Figure 3. Hepatic enzyme activities as markers for Nrf2 activity. The Nrf2 target gene *NQO1* was measured by an activity assay (**A**). Total enzyme activity of all GST isoforms was measured by an activity assay (**B**). Samples were the liver of Nrf2 KO and WT male mice fed diets with defined Se contents (–Se: 0.03 ppm; +Se: 0.15 ppm; ++Se: 0.6 ppm). Bars represent means + SD ($n = 4$–5). *** $p < 0.001$ vs. WT and # $p < 0.05$; ### $p < 0.001$ vs. –Se (two-way ANOVA with Bonferroni's post-test).

Besides Nrf2 target genes, selenoprotein expression was also studied. Classical biomarkers of the murine Se status, such as TXNRD and GPX activity, already reached a plateau in the +Se groups and could not be further increased by the ++Se supply (Figure 2C,D). Total TXNRD activity was reduced in Nrf2 KO mice, because TXNRD1 expression is regulated via Nrf2 (Figure 2C). Total hepatic GPX activity, mainly reflecting GPX1 activity, was not affected by the loss of Nrf2 (Figure 2D). Under certain conditions, selenoprotein mRNAs could also serve as biomarkers of the Se status, which is the case for Selenow, showing a four-fold increase in the Se-treated groups in comparison to the –Se group (Figure 2E). Under +Se conditions, Selenow expression was significantly lower in Nrf2 KO than in WT mice and in the ++Se groups there was a trend ($p < 0.09$; Figure 2E). Together with a small reduction of the hepatic Se content, this might indicate that the Se status is lower in Nrf2 KO than in WT mice.

As shown before (Figure 1C and Figure S1A,B), Fe, ferritin, and transferrin plasma levels were unaffected by Nrf2 in male mice (Figure 4A–C). In addition, all three parameters were independent of the Se status. The increased Fe tissue retention described under chow diet conditions (Figure 1) was only significant under –Se conditions in the liver in this case (Figure 4D). To study putative mechanisms for the observed Fe accumulation in the liver, the expression of different Fe-related genes/proteins were tested.

First, we tested Hamp expression in the liver, because Hamp is the major regulator of Fe homeostasis, which is upregulated in response to an increase in Fe levels. Recently, it has been shown that this upregulation is partially impaired in Nrf2 KO livers [36]. Herein, we could not observe an upregulation in –Se Nrf2 KO livers (Figure 4E). Hamp is known to limit the expression of the Fe exporter Fpn1 in the intestine to reduce systemic Fe levels. Indeed, Fpn1 expression was reduced in the duodenum of both –Se and ++Se Nrf2 KO mice (Figure 4F). Under physiological conditions, Fe is transported in the plasma bound to transferrin, which is taken up by the hepatocytes by binding to the transferrin receptor (TfR). The mRNA expression of TfR was only upregulated in the –Se Nrf2 KO mice (Figure 4G) together with expression levels of the Fe transporter DMT1 (Figure 4H), which is consistent with higher Fe levels in the liver. In the plasma, ferrous Fe is immediately oxidized to ferric Fe by Cu-dependent Cp, and then bound to transferrin. Also, Cp was upregulated in the –Se Nrf2 KO group (Figure 4I). Cp is an acute phase protein, which is known to be sensitive towards inflammation. However, no increase in hepatic inflammatory cells has been detected in Nrf2 KO mice previously [37]. Intracellularly, Fe is efficiently bound to ferritin. The subunit ferritin H (FTH) is regulated by Nrf2 [16]. Herein, mRNA of FTH was only reduced under +Se and ++Se conditions (Figure 4J). However, ferritin H protein levels were almost undetectable also in –Se Nrf2 KO mice (Figure 4K,L). In addition, ferritin H protein was upregulated under –Se conditions in WT mice in comparison to +Se WT mice.

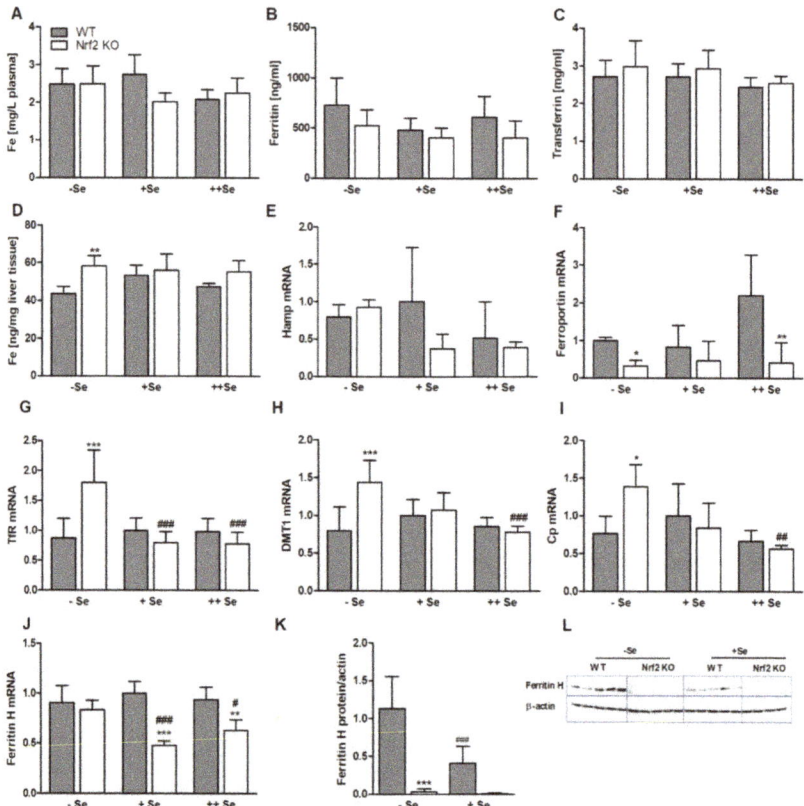

Figure 4. Biomarkers of the Fe status. Fe (**A**), ferritin (**B**), and transferrin (**C**) concentrations in the plasma of male Nrf2 KO and WT mice fed diets with defined Se contents (−Se: 0.03 ppm; +Se: 0.15 ppm; ++Se: 0.6 ppm). Additionally, Fe concentration in the liver (**D**) as well as mRNA and protein expression of Fe-related genes/proteins in the liver were determined by qPCR or western blot, respectively (**E,G–L**). Ferroportin mRNA was measured in the duodenum (**F**). The TE profile was analyzed using ICP-MS/MS (**A,D**). Further Fe plasma parameters were detected by ELISA (**B,C**). Bars represent means + SD (n = 4–5). * $p < 0.05$; ** $p < 0.01$; *** $p < 0.001$ vs. WT and # $p < 0.05$; ## $p < 0.01$; ### $p < 0.001$ vs. −Se (two-way ANOVA with Bonferroni's post-test).

As in the previous experiment (Figure 1), there was no effect of Nrf2 on hepatic or plasma Cu levels under ++Se conditions, but under −Se and +Se conditions hepatic Cu levels were reduced (Figure 5B) while plasma values were increased in the −Se Nrf2 KO group (Figure 5A). The latter obviously resulted from lower Cu levels of −Se WT mice in comparison to +Se WT mice. Higher expression levels of Atp7b (Figure 5G) might be the reason for lower Cu levels in −Se Nrf2 KO mice, while at the same time, higher Cu plasma levels could be explained by more efficient binding of Cu to Cp (Figure 4I) being excreted from hepatocytes. The Cu transporter 1 (Ctr1) is important for Cu as well as Zn absorption in the intestine; however, hepatocytes also express Ctr1 in relevant amounts to take up Cu from the circulation. Ctr1 protein expression was completely unaffected by the Nrf2 genotype or Se supply (Figure 5C).

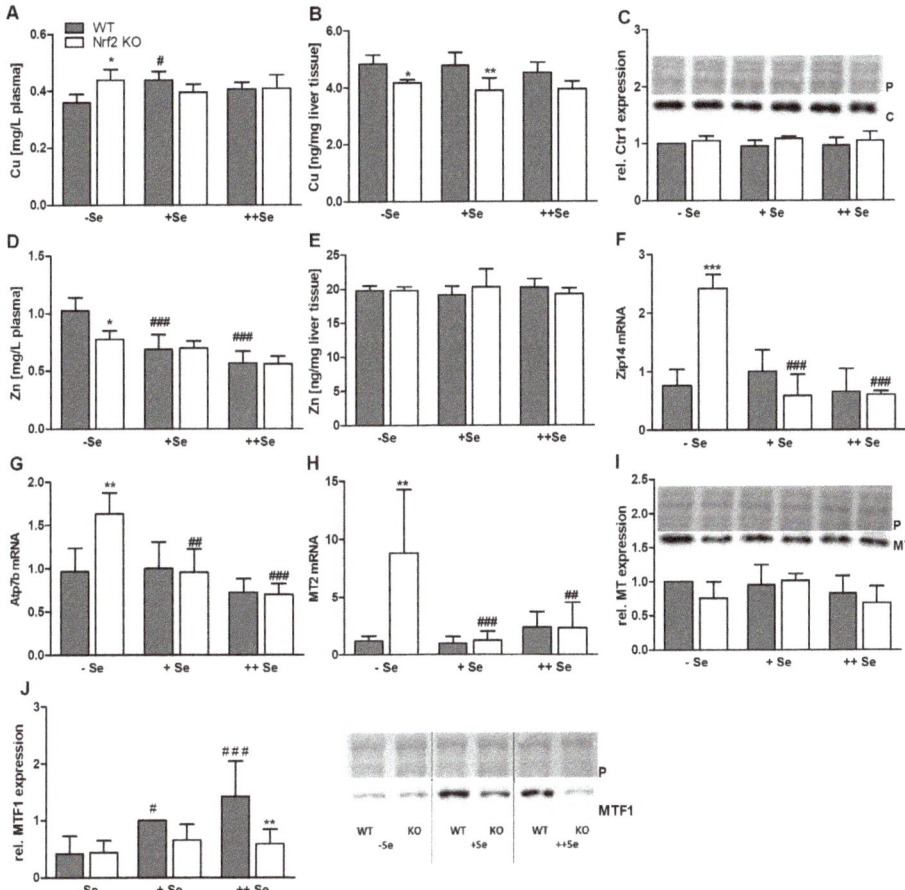

Figure 5. Biomarkers of the Cu and Zn status. Cu and Zn concentrations in the plasma (**A,C**) and liver (**B,D**) of male Nrf2 KO and WT mice fed diets with defined Se contents (–Se: 0.03 ppm; +Se: 0.15 ppm; ++Se: 0.6 ppm), analyzed by ICP-MS/MS. Additionally, mRNA (**F–H**) and protein expression (**C, I–J**) of Cu- and Zn-related genes/proteins in the liver of these animals were determined. Western blots were normalized to the Ponceau staining (P). Bars represent means + SD (n = 4–5). * $p < 0.05$; ** $p < 0.01$; *** $p < 0.001$ vs. WT and # $p < 0.05$; ## $p < 0.01$; ### $p < 0.001$ vs. –Se (two-way ANOVA with Bonferroni's post-test). C = Ctr1.

As seen before, hepatic Zn levels were neither affected by Nrf2 nor by Se status (Figure 5E). However, plasma concentrations were substantially reduced in Nrf2 KO mice under –Se conditions (Figure 5D). There was a concentration-dependent decrease of plasma Zn values with an increasing Se supply. In contrast to other members of the Zip family, Zip14 transports not only Zn but also Fe. Herein, intracellular Fe concentrations were increased in –Se Nrf2 KO mice, and at the same time, Zip14 mRNA levels were upregulated under these conditions (Figure 5F). Also, MT2 shows a very similar mRNA expression pattern (Figure 5H) to Zip14. It was highly upregulated in –Se Nrf2 KO livers. However, western blots with an antibody against all MT isoforms could not confirm the effect observed for MT2 mRNA expression (Figure 5I). As a potential mechanistic link between regulated genes and the Nrf2 and Se status, MTF1 expression was analyzed in the liver. MTF1 was significantly downregulated in ++Se Nrf2 KO mice (Figure 5J), but MTF1 levels declined with reduction of the Se status and thus the Nrf2 KO effect was lost under +Se and –Se conditions.

4. Discussion

It is well established that the transcription factor Nrf2 is an important mediator of Fe homeostasis [8]. In this study, we addressed the question of whether other trace elements, such as Se, Zn, and Cu, are modulated by Nrf2 as well. A reduction of Nrf2 levels and responsiveness is a relevant health condition that physiologically takes place during aging [38]. Thus, the question arises whether age-specific changes in TE profiles [39] might be related to Nrf2. Recently, it has been examined that Nrf2 activity levels strongly differ in the liver of male and female mice [40]. Also, herein, we were able to show that basal NQO1 mRNA expression in WT livers is much higher in female than in male mice (Figure S1C). Thus, sex differences of TEs could be attributed to higher Nrf2 activity as well. All three TEs, Fe, Cu, and Zn, were indeed higher in the plasma of female than in male mice (Table 4), but the underlying mechanisms are unclear so far. Also, MT2 mRNA levels were substantially higher in female livers but at the same time independent of the Nrf2 status (Figure S1E).

Table 4. Effects of Nrf2 genotype, sex, and a suboptimal Se status on homeostasis of Fe, Zn, and Cu.

TE	Nrf2 Genotype (KO vs. WT)	Sex in WT Mice (Female vs. Male)	Se Effect in WT Mice (−Se vs. +/++Se)
Cu	intracellular Cu → plasma Cu (↓)	plasma Cu ↑	plasma Cu →
Fe	intracellular Fe ↑ plasma Fe biomarkers →	liver and plasma Fe ↑	only hepatic ferritin H ↑
Se	intracellular Se ↓ plasma Se →	liver Se ↑	↓ as expected
Zn	intestinal and plasma Zn ↓ liver Zn →	plasma Zn ↑	plasma Zn ↓

We observed an increase in Fe tissue levels upon loss of Nrf2 (Figure 1A,B and Figure 4D). Vice versa, Nrf2 protects the murine liver against dietary Fe overload by enhancing Fe release [6]. Combining a genetic mouse model for hereditary hemochromatosis with an Nrf2 KO results in hepatic fibrosis, which could otherwise be prohibited by upregulation of Nrf2 target genes [41]. Furthermore, under conditions of nutritional steatohepatitis, Nrf2 inhibits hepatic Fe accumulation and thereby counteracts oxidative stress [42]. Recently, it has been shown that Fe-induced Nrf2 activation enhances bone morphogenetic protein 6 (Bmp6) signaling, which upregulates hepcidin expression to fine-tune Fe homeostasis [36]. One of the first observations indicating a change in Fe homeostasis in Nrf2 KO mice was the finding that Nrf2 KO mice have abnormally white teeth in comparison to WT mice due to defective Fe utilization during tooth development [43]. Higher Fe tissue levels can be attributed to the Fe exporter Fpn1, which was downregulated in male Nrf2 KO mice (Figure 4F and Figure S1D), and to the hepatic Fe importers, TfR and DMT1 [44], which were upregulated in −Se Nrf2 KO mice (Figure 4G,H). Also, Zip14 was strongly induced in −Se Nrf2 KO mice (Figure 5F). Zip14 was originally described as a Zn importer with the highest expression in the jejunum and liver, but it is now established that it transports further TEs, such as Fe [45]. Under conditions of Fe depletion, Zip14 membrane localization is impaired based on post-translational modifications [46]. Under physiological conditions, Fe is mainly transported bound to transferrin. Thus, TfR appears to be of major relevance for Fe uptake into the liver. To get an idea of the putative crosstalk between several TEs, we included DMT1 and Zip14, as those not only transport Fe but also additional TEs. Usually, the intracellular free labile Fe pool is tightly regulated. One of the most important regulating proteins is ferritin, which is able to bind up to 4,500 Fe atoms in its core [47]. The amount of intracellular ferritin H was strongly reduced in Nrf2 KO mice (Figure 4J–L), especially on the protein level, indicating that the labile free Fe pool is substantially increased under those conditions. Ferritin can be secreted from both hepatocytes and Kupffer cells to contribute to plasma ferritin levels in addition to the relevant amounts secreted by macrophages [48]. Surprisingly, plasma ferritin levels stayed unaffected by the Nrf2 genotype

(Figure 4B and Figure S1A). This might be explained by the fact that plasma ferritin mostly consists of the ferritin L subunit and not H [49], even though ferritin L has been identified as an Nrf2 target gene as well [50]. Based on the observed substantial downregulation of ferritin H, effects of Fe on the liver are supposed to be stronger than detected. Eventually, Fe availability to the systemic circulation is also reduced in Nrf2 KO mice, counteracting the loss of Nrf2-mediated limitation of the intracellular free Fe pool. Indeed, intestinal Fpn1 expression was reduced in Nrf2 KO mice (Figure 4F), indicating that absorbed Fe might be retained there and released back into the intestinal lumen when enterocytes go into apoptosis. In line with this, Fe plasma levels were reduced in Nrf2 KO mice but only in females (Figure 1F).

In parallel to Fe, intracellular levels of Se and Zn were affected by loss of Nrf2 as well. In this case, both were reduced. Also, plasma Cu levels were slightly reduced in Nrf2 KO mice (overview in Table 4). Overall, these effects were rather small. For Se, the small reduction in liver Se levels could not be confirmed by analyzing selenoproteins, which respond very sensitively towards changes in the Se status. This was the case for total GPX activity. Only Selenow mRNA expression, which might be a useful additional biomarker for the Se status [51], was slightly reduced in Nrf2 KO mice under +Se conditions (Figure 2E). Thus, Nrf2 does not appear to be a major regulator of the Se status.

Comparable to Zip14, mRNA levels of Atp7b, the essential ATPase for Cu export into the bile [10], were upregulated under −Se Nrf2 KO conditions (Figure 5F,G). Additionally, DMT1 (Figure 4F) and MT2 revealed a similar expression pattern (Figure 5H), which could not be confirmed on the protein level when using an antibody capable of detecting all MT isoforms (Figure 5I). MT isoforms are cysteine-rich proteins that efficiently bind Cu and Zn to reduce the amount of both TEs in their free form [9]. Feeding of rats with the Nrf2 activator sulforaphane resulted in a robust induction of genes encoding for MT-1/2 and MT1a [52]. The MT1 promoter contains an ARE that is activated by Nrf1 and Nrf2, but in the latter case, not to the same extent. In Nrf1 KO mice, basal levels of both MT1 and MT2 genes were reduced [25]. Herein, we did not detect any downregulation of MT2 mRNA upon loss of Nrf2. As several genes (*MT2*, *Atp7b*, *Zip14*, *Cp*, *TfR*, and *Dmt1*) showed a comparable expression pattern, being induced specifically under −Se Nrf2 KO conditions, the question arose if there is a common regulator. One possibility would be MTF1, which regulates MT expression in response to Zn or Cu [53]. Recently, it has been shown that the disruption of an MTF1 binding site by a homozygous variant in the promoter of Atp7b likely causes Wilson disease [24]. In addition, the induction of Fpn1 transcription by MTF1 has been shown [54]. However, there was no detectable MTF1 activation in −Se Nrf2 KO livers. In contrast, MTF1 was upregulated in a concentration-dependent manner as a response to Se. Only under ++Se conditions, an Nrf2 genotype effect was detectable, showing lower MTF1 levels upon loss of Nrf2. Thus, MTF1 expression does not provide an obvious explanation for the observed mRNA expression pattern of some MTF1 target genes.

Besides DMT1, Ctr1 is the main universal Cu importer in mammalian cells. A KO of Ctr1 in the intestine resulted in peripheral Cu hypoaccumulation. In parallel, hepatic Fe levels were upregulated [55]. Expression of Ctr1 was unaffected by the Nrf2 genotype and hepatic Se levels (Figure 5C). Furthermore, an Se-dependent reduction of plasma Zn concentration was observed (Figure 5D). An intestine-specific Ctr1 KO did not modulate the systemic Zn status [55], while liver-specific Ctr1 KO mice showed a transient increase in hepatic Zn levels but not in serum [56]. Taken together, homeostasis of Zn and Cu also appears to be regulated rather independently of Nrf2. However, it is possible that there are short-term effects of Nrf2 on TE homeostasis, which might be undetectable in constitutive KO mice because of putative adaptation processes in response to a loss of Nrf2 over time.

We and others have shown previously that a suboptimal selenium supply results in Nrf2 activation predominantly in the liver and intestine of mice [17,57]. This can be attributed mainly to low levels of the selenoproteins TXNRD1 and GPX4, as single KOs of one of these two selenoproteins also activate Nrf2 [28,58–60]. Patients with Kaschin–Beck disease, a disease diagnosed under conditions of Se deficiency, have been characterized by higher expression of Nrf2 and its target gene *Hmox1* in whole blood samples as compared to healthy controls, indicating potential Nrf2 activation in humans under Se deficient conditions [61]. However, in this case, we could not confirm previous results and observed no Nrf2 activation indicated by NQO1 and GST activity in the liver (Figure 3) or intestine (Figure S2) of mice fed an −Se diet, even though the levels of TXNRD and GPX activity were in a comparable range to previous experiments [17,26]. Only the Nrf2 target gene *ferritin H* was clearly upregulated in −Se WT livers and was almost lost in Nrf2 KO mice (Figure 4K,L). This phenomenon has also been described in another recent study analyzing the response to lifelong dietary Se interventions in mice. Additionally, in this study, no effect of an Se-deficient diet could be observed on hepatic Nrf2 response genes considering whole transcriptome analyses [62]. Another study found that Se deficiency affected the expression of neither Hmox1 nor NQO1 [63]. In those two studies, and similar to our study, Se deficiency decreased the expression of important selenoproteins but did not activate Nrf2. Thus, it has been suggested that a low Se status interacts with another dietary or environmental component to regulate the Nrf2 response but is not sufficient by itself [62].

Therefore, the initial aim of studying the crosstalk between Nrf2 and selenium status in modulating three other TEs is difficult to address under the present conditions. Herein, it is relatively clear that Se effects observed on Zn appear to be regulated independently of Nrf2. However, when only considering WT mice, we could still draw conclusions towards the role of the Se status on TE status of Zn, Fe, and Cu. Most strikingly, Zn plasma levels were higher in mice with low Se status and vice versa (Figure 5D). In comparison to that, Cu and Fe were rather unaffected by Se. At the same time, hepatic Zn levels were unaffected by the Se status, indicating that Zn appears to be taken up by other tissues besides the liver when Se levels are rising. As MTF1 shows the complete opposite effect than plasma Zn levels and also as most of the MTF1 target genes, it might be an attempt to compensate for the low Se status. Any underlying mechanisms, however, are unclear so far.

5. Conclusions

Overall, only Fe was substantially regulated in response to Nrf2 while the impact of Nrf2 on homeostasis of Se, Cu, and Zn appeared to be rather marginal. Nevertheless, crosstalk between Se and MTF1 is a promising idea that needs to be followed up in the future and might provide an explanation for the observed counter regulation of plasma Se and Zn levels.

The mammalian ionome has been evaluated in 26 species and across several tissues [64]. In this study, Zn levels in the liver and kidney were positively correlated with maximum lifespan while hepatic Se was negatively correlated with longevity, albeit in a relatively weak manner. The Nrf2 responsiveness is reduced during aging, which provides a putative explanation for changes in TE profiles in the elderly and for TE effects on longevity. We have recently shown in a reinvited sub-cohort of the EPIC Potsdam study that Cu and Fe serum levels increased over time, while Zn and Se levels showed an age-dependent decline [39]. This is supposed to be associated with a reduction in Nrf2 activity for which, herein, Nrf2 KO mice were used as a model. Also, in Nrf2 KO mice, Se and Zn levels were reduced; however, there was no upregulation but rather a slight downregulation of the systemic Cu status (Table 4). Systemic Fe levels increased in Nrf2 KO mice but that was shown herein for intracellular amounts and not for plasma biomarkers as done in the EPIC study. Thus, it needs to be further clarified how age-dependent changes in the TE status are modulated on the molecular level.

Supplementary Materials: The following are available online at http://www.mdpi.com/2072-6643/11/9/2112/s1, Figure S1: Ferritin and transferrin concentrations in the plasma and mRNA expression in the livers of male and female Nrf2 KO and WT mice fed a standard chow diet. Figure S2: NQO1 mRNA (A) and activity (B) in the duodenum of male Nrf2 KO and WT mice fed diets with defined Se content (−Se: 0.03 ppm; +Se: 0.15 ppm; ++Se: 0.6 ppm).

Author Contributions: A.P.K. and T.S. were responsible for the conceptualization of the study, supervision, and funding acquisition; M.S., K.L. and J.F.K. established the methodology, performed the analyses and prepared the original draft.

Funding: This research was funded by German Research Foundation (DFG), FOR 2558.

Acknowledgments: The authors highly acknowledge the support of Franziska Hiller in organizing the animal experiment and excellent technical support by Stefanie Deubel, Gabriele Pohl, and Sören Meyer. In addition, we thank Masayuki Yamamoto for providing the Nrf2 KO mice.

Conflicts of Interest: The authors declare no conflict of interest.

References

1. Brigelius-Flohé, R.; Flohé, L. Basic principles and emerging concepts in the redox control of transcription factors. *Antioxid. Redox. Signal.* **2011**, *15*, 2335–2381. [CrossRef]
2. Tebay, L.E.; Robertson, H.; Durant, S.T.; Vitale, S.R.; Penning, T.M.; Dinkova-Kostova, A.T.; Hayes, J.D. Mechanisms of activation of the transcription factor Nrf2 by redox stressors, nutrient cues, and energy status and the pathways through which it attenuates degenerative disease. *Free. Radic. Biol. Med.* **2015**, *88*, 108–146. [CrossRef]
3. Hayes, J.D.; Dinkova-Kostova, A.T. The Nrf2 regulatory network provides an interface between redox and intermediary metabolism. *Trends. Biochem. Sci.* **2014**, *39*, 199–218. [CrossRef]
4. McMahon, M.; Swift, S.R.; Hayes, J.D. Zinc-binding triggers a conformational-switch in the cullin-3 substrate adaptor protein KEAP1 that controls transcription factor NRF2. *Toxicol. Appl. Pharmacol.* **2018**, *360*, 45–57. [CrossRef]
5. Moon, M.S.; McDevitt, E.I.; Zhu, J.; Stanley, B.; Krzeminski, J.; Amin, S.; Aliaga, C.; Miller, T.G.; Isom, H.C. Elevated hepatic iron activates NF-E2-related factor 2-regulated pathway in a dietary iron overload mouse model. *Toxicol. Sci.* **2012**, *129*, 74–85. [CrossRef]
6. Silva-Gomes, S.; Santos, A.G.; Caldas, C.; Silva, C.M.; Neves, J.V.; Lopes, J.; Carneiro, F.; Rodrigues, P.N.; Duarte, T.L. Transcription factor NRF2 protects mice against dietary iron-induced liver injury by preventing hepatocytic cell death. *J. Hepatol.* **2014**, *60*, 354–361. [CrossRef]
7. Harada, N.; Kanayama, M.; Maruyama, A.; Yoshida, A.; Tazumi, K.; Hosoya, T.; Mimura, J.; Toki, T.; Maher, J.M.; Yamamoto, M.; et al. Nrf2 regulates ferroportin 1-mediated iron efflux and counteracts lipopolysaccharide-induced ferroportin 1 mRNA suppression in macrophages. *Arch. Biochem. Biophys.* **2011**, *508*, 101–109. [CrossRef]
8. Kerins, M.J.; Ooi, A. The Roles of NRF2 in Modulating Cellular Iron Homeostasis. *Antioxid. Redox Signal.* **2018**, *29*, 1756–1773. [CrossRef]
9. Davis, S.R.; Cousins, R.J. Metallothionein expression in animals: A physiological perspective on function. *J. Nutr.* **2000**, *130*, 1085–1088. [CrossRef]
10. Polishchuk, E.V.; Concilli, M.; Iacobacci, S.; Chesi, G.; Pastore, N.; Piccolo, P.; Paladino, S.; Baldantoni, D.; van, I.S.C.; Chan, J.; et al. Wilson disease protein ATP7B utilizes lysosomal exocytosis to maintain copper homeostasis. *Dev. Cell* **2014**, *29*, 686–700. [CrossRef]
11. Lutsenko, S. Human copper homeostasis: A network of interconnected pathways. *Curr. Opin. Chem. Biol.* **2010**, *14*, 211–217. [CrossRef]
12. Mocchegiani, E.; Costarelli, L.; Giacconi, R.; Malavolta, M.; Basso, A.; Piacenza, F.; Ostan, R.; Cevenini, E.; Gonos, E.S.; Monti, D. Micronutrient-gene interactions related to inflammatory/immune response and antioxidant activity in ageing and inflammation. A systematic review. *Mech. Ageing Dev.* **2014**, *136–137*, 29–49. [CrossRef]
13. Song, M.O.; Mattie, M.D.; Lee, C.H.; Freedman, J.H. The role of Nrf1 and Nrf2 in the regulation of copper-responsive transcription. *Exp. Cell. Res.* **2014**, *322*, 39–50. [CrossRef]
14. Cui, Z.; Zhong, Z.; Yang, Y.; Wang, B.; Sun, Y.; Sun, Q.; Yang, G.Y.; Bian, L. Ferrous Iron Induces Nrf2 Expression in Mouse Brain Astrocytes to Prevent Neurotoxicity. *J. Biochem. Mol. Toxicol.* **2016**, *30*, 396–403. [CrossRef]
15. Alam, J.; Cook, J.L. Transcriptional regulation of the heme oxygenase-1 gene via the stress response element pathway. *Curr. Pharm. Des.* **2003**, *9*, 2499–2511. [CrossRef]
16. Pietsch, E.C.; Chan, J.Y.; Torti, F.M.; Torti, S.V. Nrf2 mediates the induction of ferritin H in response to xenobiotics and cancer chemopreventive dithiolethiones. *J. Biol. Chem.* **2003**, *278*, 2361–2369. [CrossRef]
17. Müller, M.; Banning, A.; Brigelius-Flohé, R.; Kipp, A. Nrf2 target genes are induced under marginal selenium-deficiency. *Genes. Nutr.* **2010**, *5*, 297–307. [CrossRef]

18. Zhang, J.; Wang, H.; Peng, D.; Taylor, E.W. Further insight into the impact of sodium selenite on selenoenzymes: High-dose selenite enhances hepatic thioredoxin reductase 1 activity as a consequence of liver injury. *Toxicol. Lett.* **2008**, *176*, 223–229. [CrossRef]
19. Banning, A.; Deubel, S.; Kluth, D.; Zhou, Z.; Brigelius-Flohé, R. The GI-GPx gene is a target for Nrf2. *Mol. Cell. Biol.* **2005**, *25*, 4914–4923. [CrossRef]
20. Sakurai, A.; Nishimoto, M.; Himeno, S.; Imura, N.; Tsujimoto, M.; Kunimoto, M.; Hara, S. Transcriptional regulation of thioredoxin reductase 1 expression by cadmium in vascular endothelial cells: Role of NF-E2-related factor-2. *J. Cell. Physiol.* **2005**, *203*, 529–537. [CrossRef]
21. Li, B.; Cui, W.; Tan, Y.; Luo, P.; Chen, Q.; Zhang, C.; Qu, W.; Miao, L.; Cai, L. Zinc is essential for the transcription function of Nrf2 in human renal tubule cells in vitro and mouse kidney in vivo under the diabetic condition. *J. Cell. Mol. Med.* **2014**, *18*, 895–906. [CrossRef]
22. Wakabayashi, N.; Slocum, S.L.; Skoko, J.J.; Shin, S.; Kensler, T.W. When NRF2 talks, who's listening? *Antioxid. Redox. Signal.* **2010**, *13*, 1649–1663. [CrossRef]
23. Gunther, V.; Lindert, U.; Schaffner, W. The taste of heavy metals: Gene regulation by MTF-1. *Biochim. Biophys. Acta* **2012**, *1823*, 1416–1425. [CrossRef]
24. Chen, H.I.; Jagadeesh, K.A.; Birgmeier, J.; Wenger, A.M.; Guturu, H.; Schelley, S.; Bernstein, J.A.; Bejerano, G. An MTF1 binding site disrupted by a homozygous variant in the promoter of ATP7B likely causes Wilson Disease. *Eur. J. Hum. Genet.* **2018**, *26*, 1810–1818. [CrossRef]
25. Ohtsuji, M.; Katsuoka, F.; Kobayashi, A.; Aburatani, H.; Hayes, J.D.; Yamamoto, M. Nrf1 and Nrf2 play distinct roles in activation of antioxidant response element-dependent genes. *J. Biol. Chem.* **2008**, *283*, 33554–33562. [CrossRef]
26. Lennicke, C.; Rahn, J.; Kipp, A.P.; Dojcinovic, B.P.; Müller, A.S.; Wessjohann, L.A.; Lichtenfels, R.; Seliger, B. Individual effects of different selenocompounds on the hepatic proteome and energy metabolism of mice. *Biochim. Biophys. Acta.* **2017**, *1861*, 3323–3334. [CrossRef]
27. Rayman, M.P. Selenium and human health. *Lancet* **2012**, *379*, 1256–1268. [CrossRef]
28. Cebula, M.; Schmidt, E.E.; Arnér, E.S. TrxR1 as a potent regulator of the Nrf2-Keap1 response system. *Antioxid. Redox Signal.* **2015**, *23*, 823–853. [CrossRef]
29. Itoh, K.; Chiba, T.; Takahashi, S.; Ishii, T.; Igarashi, K.; Katoh, Y.; Oyake, T.; Hayashi, N.; Satoh, K.; Hatayama, I.; et al. An Nrf2/small Maf heterodimer mediates the induction of phase II detoxifying enzyme genes through antioxidant response elements. *Biochem. Biophys. Res. Commun.* **1997**, *236*, 313–322. [CrossRef]
30. Ritskes-Hoitinga, M. Nutrition of the laboratory mouse. In *The Laboratory Mouse*; Academic Press, Elsevier: London, UK, 2012; pp. 567–596.
31. Marschall, T.A.; Kroepfl, N.; Jensen, K.B.; Bornhorst, J.; Meermann, B.; Kuehnelt, D.; Schwerdtle, T. Tracing cytotoxic effects of small organic Se species in human liver cells back to total cellular Se and Se metabolites. *Metallomics* **2017**, *9*, 268–277. [CrossRef]
32. Kopp, J.F.; Müller, S.M.; Pohl, G.; Lossow, K.; Kipp, A.P.; Schwerdtle, T. A quick and simple method for the determination of six trace elements in mammalian serum samples using ICP-MS/MS. *J. Trace Elem. Med. Biol.* **2019**, *54*, 221–225. [CrossRef]
33. Krehl, S.; Loewinger, M.; Florian, S.; Kipp, A.P.; Banning, A.; Wessjohann, L.A.; Brauer, M.N.; Iori, R.; Esworthy, R.S.; Chu, F.F.; et al. Glutathione peroxidase-2 and selenium decreased inflammation and tumors in a mouse model of inflammation-associated carcinogenesis whereas sulforaphane effects differed with selenium supply. *Carcinogenesis* **2012**, *33*, 620–628. [CrossRef]
34. Florian, S.; Krehl, S.; Loewinger, M.; Kipp, A.; Banning, A.; Esworthy, S.; Chu, F.F.; Brigelius-Flohé, R. Loss of GPx2 increases apoptosis, mitosis and GPx1 expression in the intestine of mice. *Free. Radic. Biol. Med.* **2010**, *49*, 1694–1702. [CrossRef]
35. Habig, W.H.; Pabst, M.J.; Jakoby, W.B. Glutathione S-transferases. The first enzymatic step in mercapturic acid formation. *J. Biol. Chem.* **1974**, *249*, 7130–7139.
36. Lim, P.J.; Duarte, T.L.; Arezes, J.; Garcia-Santos, D.; Hamdi, A.; Pasricha, S.R.; Armitage, A.E.; Mehta, H.; Wideman, S.; Santos, A.G.; et al. Nrf2 controls iron homeostasis in haemochromatosis and thalassaemia via Bmp6 and hepcidin. *Nat. Metab.* **2019**, *1*, 519–531. [CrossRef]
37. Köhler, U.A.; Böhm, F.; Rolfs, F.; Egger, M.; Hornemann, T.; Pasparakis, M.; Weber, A.; Werner, S. NF-kappaB/RelA and Nrf2 cooperate to maintain hepatocyte integrity and to prevent development of hepatocellular adenoma. *J. Hepatol.* **2016**, *64*, 94–102. [CrossRef]

38. Huang, D.D.; Fan, S.D.; Chen, X.Y.; Yan, X.L.; Zhang, X.Z.; Ma, B.W.; Yu, D.Y.; Xiao, W.Y.; Zhuang, C.L.; Yu, Z. Nrf2 deficiency exacerbates frailty and sarcopenia by impairing skeletal muscle mitochondrial biogenesis and dynamics in an age-dependent manner. *Exp. Gerontol.* **2019**, *119*, 61–73. [CrossRef]
39. Baudry, J.; Kopp, J.F.; Boeing, H.; Kipp, A.P.; Schwerdtle, T.; Schulze, M.B. Changes of trace element status during aging: Results of the EPIC-Potsdam cohort study. *Eur. J. Nutr.* **2019**. submitted.
40. Rooney, J.; Oshida, K.; Vasani, N.; Vallanat, B.; Ryan, N.; Chorley, B.N.; Wang, X.; Bell, D.A.; Wu, K.C.; Aleksunes, L.M.; et al. Activation of Nrf2 in the liver is associated with stress resistance mediated by suppression of the growth hormone-regulated STAT5b transcription factor. *PLoS ONE* **2018**, *13*, e0200004. [CrossRef]
41. Duarte, T.L.; Caldas, C.; Santos, A.G.; Silva-Gomes, S.; Santos-Goncalves, A.; Martins, M.J.; Porto, G.; Lopes, J.M. Genetic disruption of NRF2 promotes the development of necroinflammation and liver fibrosis in a mouse model of HFE-hereditary hemochromatosis. *Redox Biol.* **2017**, *11*, 157–169. [CrossRef]
42. Okada, K.; Warabi, E.; Sugimoto, H.; Horie, M.; Tokushige, K.; Ueda, T.; Harada, N.; Taguchi, K.; Hashimoto, E.; Itoh, K.; et al. Nrf2 inhibits hepatic iron accumulation and counteracts oxidative stress-induced liver injury in nutritional steatohepatitis. *J. Gastroenterol.* **2012**, *47*, 924–935. [CrossRef]
43. Yanagawa, T.; Itoh, K.; Uwayama, J.; Shibata, Y.; Yamaguchi, A.; Sano, T.; Ishii, T.; Yoshida, H.; Yamamoto, M. Nrf2 deficiency causes tooth decolourization due to iron transport disorder in enamel organ. *Genes Cells* **2004**, *9*, 641–651. [CrossRef]
44. Shindo, M.; Torimoto, Y.; Saito, H.; Motomura, W.; Ikuta, K.; Sato, K.; Fujimoto, Y.; Kohgo, Y. Functional role of DMT1 in transferrin-independent iron uptake by human hepatocyte and hepatocellular carcinoma cell, HLF. *Hepatol. Res.* **2006**, *35*, 152–162. [CrossRef]
45. Liuzzi, J.P.; Aydemir, F.; Nam, H.; Knutson, M.D.; Cousins, R.J. Zip14 (Slc39a14) mediates non-transferrin-bound iron uptake into cells. *Proc. Natl. Acad. Sci. USA* **2006**, *103*, 13612–13617. [CrossRef]
46. Aydemir, T.B.; Cousins, R.J. The Multiple Faces of the Metal Transporter ZIP14 (SLC39A14). *J. Nutr.* **2018**, *148*, 174–184. [CrossRef]
47. Macara, I.G.; Hoy, T.G.; Harrison, P.M. The formation of ferritin from apoferritin. Kinetics and mechanism of iron uptake. *Biochem. J.* **1972**, *126*, 151–162. [CrossRef]
48. Wang, W.; Knovich, M.A.; Coffman, L.G.; Torti, F.M.; Torti, S.V. Serum ferritin: Past, present and future. *Biochim. Biophys. Acta* **2010**, *1800*, 760–769. [CrossRef]
49. Santambrogio, P.; Cozzi, A.; Levi, S.; Arosio, P. Human serum ferritin G-peptide is recognized by anti-L ferritin subunit antibodies and concanavalin-A. *Br. J. Haematol.* **1987**, *65*, 235–237. [CrossRef]
50. Kuosmanen, S.M.; Viitala, S.; Laitinen, T.; Perakyla, M.; Polonen, P.; Kansanen, E.; Leinonen, H.; Raju, S.; Wienecke-Baldacchino, A.; Narvanen, A.; et al. The Effects of Sequence Variation on Genome-wide NRF2 Binding–New Target Genes and Regulatory SNPs. *Nucleic Acids Res.* **2016**, *44*, 1760–1775. [CrossRef]
51. Kipp, A.P.; Frombach, J.; Deubel, S.; Brigelius-Flohé, R. Selenoprotein W as biomarker for the efficacy of selenium compounds to act as source for selenoprotein biosynthesis. *Methods Enzymol.* **2013**, *527*, 87–112.
52. Hu, R.; Hebbar, V.; Kim, B.R.; Chen, C.; Winnik, B.; Buckley, B.; Soteropoulos, P.; Tolias, P.; Hart, R.P.; Kong, A.N. In vivo pharmacokinetics and regulation of gene expression profiles by isothiocyanate sulforaphane in the rat. *J. Pharmacol. Exp. Ther.* **2004**, *310*, 263–271. [CrossRef]
53. Hardyman, J.E.; Tyson, J.; Jackson, K.A.; Aldridge, C.; Cockell, S.J.; Wakeling, L.A.; Valentine, R.A.; Ford, D. Zinc sensing by metal-responsive transcription factor 1 (MTF1) controls metallothionein and ZnT1 expression to buffer the sensitivity of the transcriptome response to zinc. *Metallomics* **2016**, *8*, 337–343. [CrossRef]
54. Troadec, M.B.; Ward, D.M.; Lo, E.; Kaplan, J.; De Domenico, I. Induction of FPN1 transcription by MTF-1 reveals a role for ferroportin in transition metal efflux. *Blood* **2010**, *116*, 4657–4664. [CrossRef]
55. Nose, Y.; Kim, B.E.; Thiele, D.J. Ctr1 drives intestinal copper absorption and is essential for growth, iron metabolism, and neonatal cardiac function. *Cell Metab.* **2006**, *4*, 235–244. [CrossRef]
56. Kim, H.; Son, H.Y.; Bailey, S.M.; Lee, J. Deletion of hepatic Ctr1 reveals its function in copper acquisition and compensatory mechanisms for copper homeostasis. *Am. J. Physiol. Gastrointest. Liver Physiol.* **2009**, *296*, G356–G364. [CrossRef]
57. Burk, R.F.; Hill, K.E.; Nakayama, A.; Mostert, V.; Levander, X.A.; Motley, A.K.; Johnson, D.A.; Johnson, J.A.; Freeman, M.L.; Austin, L.M. Selenium deficiency activates mouse liver Nrf2-ARE but vitamin E deficiency does not. *Free Radic. Biol. Med.* **2008**, *44*, 1617–1623. [CrossRef]

58. Carlson, B.A.; Tobe, R.; Yefremova, E.; Tsuji, P.A.; Hoffmann, V.J.; Schweizer, U.; Gladyshev, V.N.; Hatfield, D.L.; Conrad, M. Glutathione peroxidase 4 and vitamin E cooperatively prevent hepatocellular degeneration. *Redox Biol.* **2016**, *9*, 22–31. [CrossRef]
59. Patterson, A.D.; Carlson, B.A.; Li, F.; Bonzo, J.A.; Yoo, M.H.; Krausz, K.W.; Conrad, M.; Chen, C.; Gonzalez, F.J.; Hatfield, D.L. Disruption of thioredoxin reductase 1 protects mice from acute acetaminophen-induced hepatotoxicity through enhanced NRF2 activity. *Chem. Res. Toxicol.* **2013**, *26*, 1088–1096. [CrossRef]
60. Suvorova, E.S.; Lucas, O.; Weisend, C.M.; Rollins, M.F.; Merrill, G.F.; Capecchi, M.R.; Schmidt, E.E. Cytoprotective Nrf2 pathway is induced in chronically txnrd 1-deficient hepatocytes. *PLoS ONE* **2009**, *4*, e6158. [CrossRef]
61. Li, Y.; Mo, X.; Xiong, Y. The Study on Polymorphism of TrxR and Nrf2/HO-1 Signaling Pathway in Kaschin-Beck Disease. *Biol. Trace Elem. Res.* **2018**, *190*, 303–308. [CrossRef]
62. Yim, S.H.; Clish, C.B.; Gladyshev, V.N. Selenium Deficiency Is Associated with Pro-longevity Mechanisms. *Cell Rep.* **2019**, *27*, 2785–2797 e3. [CrossRef]
63. Dong, R.; Wang, D.; Wang, X.; Zhang, K.; Chen, P.; Yang, C.S.; Zhang, J. Epigallocatechin-3-gallate enhances key enzymatic activities of hepatic thioredoxin and glutathione systems in selenium-optimal mice but activates hepatic Nrf2 responses in selenium-deficient mice. *Redox Biol.* **2016**, *10*, 221–232. [CrossRef]
64. Ma, S.; Lee, S.G.; Kim, E.B.; Park, T.J.; Seluanov, A.; Gorbunova, V.; Buffenstein, R.; Seravalli, J.; Gladyshev, V.N. Organization of the Mammalian Ionome According to Organ Origin, Lineage Specialization and Longevity. *Cell. Rep.* **2015**, *13*, 1319–1326. [CrossRef]

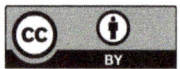

© 2019 by the authors. Licensee MDPI, Basel, Switzerland. This article is an open access article distributed under the terms and conditions of the Creative Commons Attribution (CC BY) license (http://creativecommons.org/licenses/by/4.0/).

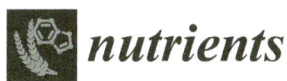

Article

An In Vivo (*Gallus gallus*) Feeding Trial Demonstrating the Enhanced Iron Bioavailability Properties of the Fast Cooking Manteca Yellow Bean (*Phaseolus vulgaris* L.)

Jason A. Wiesinger [1], Raymond P. Glahn [1], Karen A. Cichy [2], Nikolai Kolba [1], Jonathan J. Hart [1] and Elad Tako [1,*]

1 USDA-ARS, Robert W. Holley Center for Agriculture and Health, Cornell University, Ithaca, NY 14853, USA
2 USDA-ARS, Sugarbeet and Bean Research, Michigan State University, East Lansing, MI 48824, USA
* Correspondence: elad.tako@ars.usda.gov or et79@cornell.edu; Tel.: +1-607-255-5434

Received: 21 June 2019; Accepted: 27 July 2019; Published: 1 August 2019

Abstract: The common dry bean (*Phaseolus vulgaris* L.) is a globally produced pulse crop and an important source of micronutrients for millions of people across Latin America and Africa. Many of the preferred black and red seed types in these regions have seed coat polyphenols that inhibit the absorption of iron. Yellow beans are distinct from other market classes because they accumulate the antioxidant kaempferol 3-glucoside in their seed coats. Due to their fast cooking tendencies, yellow beans are often marketed at premium prices in the same geographical regions where dietary iron deficiency is a major health concern. Hence, this study compared the iron bioavailability of three faster cooking yellow beans with contrasting seed coat colors from Africa (Manteca, Amarillo, and Njano) to slower cooking white and red kidney commercial varieties. Iron status and iron bioavailability was assessed by the capacity of a bean based diet to generate and maintain total body hemoglobin iron (Hb-Fe) during a 6 week in vivo (*Gallus gallus*) feeding trial. Over the course of the experiment, animals fed yellow bean diets had significantly ($p \leq 0.05$) higher Hb-Fe than animals fed the white or red kidney bean diet. This study shows that the Manteca yellow bean possess a rare combination of biochemical traits that result in faster cooking times and improved iron bioavailability. The Manteca yellow bean is worthy of germplasm enhancement to address iron deficiency in regions where beans are consumed as a dietary staple.

Keywords: *Phaseolus vulgaris* L.; yellow bean; cooking time; iron; iron bioavailability; phytate; polyphenols; kaempferol 3-glucoside; Caco-2 cell bioassay; *Gallus gallus*

---

1. Introduction

The common dry bean (*Phaseolus vulgaris* L.) is a globally produced pulse crop that serves as an important source of protein and micronutrients for millions of people across Africa, the Caribbean, Latin America, and Southern Europe [1]. Dry beans accumulate trace minerals, such as iron and zinc, into their seed by using a complex network of ion transporters and chelating molecules that include phytate, nicotianamine, and polyphenols [2]. Traditional breeding practices can be used to generate bean seeds with very high iron concentrations [3]. This lead to the conception of using biofortified bean varieties as a vehicle to alleviate trace mineral deficiencies in resource-limited regions of Latin America and Sub-Saharan Africa, where beans are widely accepted as a dietary staple [4]. Many of the preferred seed types in these regions are black and red beans, which contain polyphenolic compounds that inhibit the absorption of iron in the upper intestine, potentially limiting their nutritional impact [5–8]. Polyphenols and other prebiotic molecules that survive enzymatic digestion in the small intestine, however, can stimulate the growth of beneficial microbiota in the lower intestine, improving the overall health of the digestive system [9–14].

Iron uptake assays in Caco-2 cells indicate that not all polyphenols are inhibitors of iron absorption [7]. Certain polyphenolic compounds, such as kaempferol and kaempferol 3-glucoside are shown to promote iron uptake in vitro [5,7]. Kaempferol is a flavonoid expressed in the seed coats of many bean seed types including black, carioca, cranberry, pinto, kidney, and small red [15,16]. While the concentrations of kaempferol compounds vary between the different bean market classes, the most dominant polyphenol measured in seed coats of yellow beans is kaempferol 3-glucoside [17,18]. Alleles in the color genes of yellow beans direct polyphenol pathways in the seed coat to create a vast array of color combinations that range from bright neon yellow to orange and green [19,20].

Originating from the Peruano coast, yellow beans were cultivated very early in human history [21] and over the centuries have diversified into many different market classes that are sold throughout Central and South America, as well as Sub-Saharan Africa [22,23]. Yellow beans owe their long heritage to smallholder farmers selecting for unique seed coat colors that would appeal to consumers at the marketplace, and are often marketed at premium prices in Africa for their fast cooking tendencies [23,24]. Iron uptake studies measuring the formation of ferritin protein in Caco-2 cells recently showed that a set of fast cooking yellow beans from Africa have more bioavailable iron than slower cooking yellow and red mottled beans from Africa and the Caribbean [25]. Exploring the yellow bean's unique market classes to develop new fast cooking varieties that could potentially deliver more absorbable iron would be a useful strategy; especially for regions where long cooking times often deter consumers purchasing beans and where micronutrient deficiencies, such as iron deficiency anemia are highly prevalent [26,27].

The purpose of this research was to further evaluate the iron nutrition and iron bioavailability of different yellow bean market classes by incorporating cooked beans into diets for a long-term in vivo feeding trial. The objective of this study was to compare the nutritional properties, polyphenolic profiles, and iron bioavailability of three yellow beans with contrasting seed coat colors from Africa (Manteca, Amarillo, Njano) to slower cooking white and red kidney commercial varieties from North America. Bean based diets were formulated with cooked beans as the major ingredient and included the complementary food crops of potato, rice, and cabbage. Iron bioavailability was evaluated for each of bean based diets with a Caco-2 bioassay and by the ability to maintain total body hemoglobin iron (Hb-Fe) during a 6 week in vivo (*Gallus gallus*) feeding trial.

2. Materials and Methods

2.1. Plant Materials—African Yellow Beans and Commercial Kidney Bean Varieties

Three yellow and two kidney *P. vulgaris* genotypes with contrasting seed coat colors were selected for this study. Ervilha is a fast cooking Manteca (pale-lemon) landrace collected from the Instituto de Investigação Agronómica located in the Huambo province of Angola [25]. Uyole 98 is an Amarillo (yellow-orange) variety release by the Tanzanian Breeding Program in 1999, renowned for its strong agronomic performance, disease resistance, and consumer quality traits, such as fast cooking times and excellent taste [28]. PI527538 is a Njano (yellow-green) landrace collected from Burundi. Selected for generations among farmers throughout Sub-Saharan Africa, the Njano and Soya Njano market classes are preferred seed types among consumers in East Africa [29]. Snowdon is a white kidney bean released by Michigan State University AgBioResearch in 2012. Snowdon is an early maturing, disease tolerant white bean with good canning qualities [30]. Red Hawk is a dark red kidney variety jointly released by Michigan State University and USDA-ARS in 1998. Red Hawk is an early maturing, disease-resistant red kidney bean with excellent canning and processing qualities [31]. Photographs depicting the different seed coat colors of each bean are shown in Figure 1. A summary of the collection sites, sources and cultivation status of each genotype is presented in Table 1.

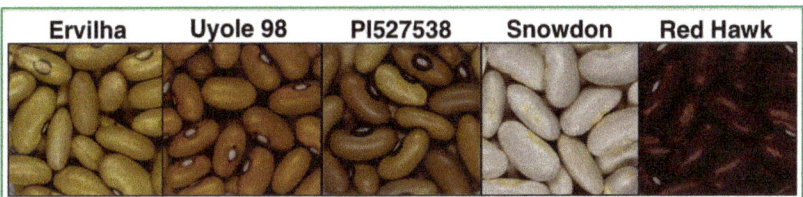

Figure 1. Photographs depicting the five genotypes used to evaluate the iron bioavailability of the African yellow bean. To compare differences in seed sizes, all photographs were taking to scale under standardized lighting conditions.

Table 1. Description, Sources, Cultivation Status, and Cooking Times of the Five Genotypes Used to Evaluate the Iron Bioavailability of Yellow Beans from Africa and Kidney Beans from North America. [1]

Name	Seed Type (*Market Class*)	Source	Cultivation	Cooking Time (Min) [2]
Ervilha	Yellow (*Manteca*)	IIA; Huambo, Angola	Landrace	15.3 ± 0.22 [e]
Uyole 98	Yellow (*Amarillo*)	Tanzania Breeding	Variety	22.3 ± 0.37 [d]
PI527538	Yellow (*Njano*)	Burundi; US GRIN	Landrace	26.0 ± 0.63 [c]
Snowdon	White Kidney	Michigan State Unv.	Variety	29.4 ± 0.37 [b]
Red Hawk	Dark Red Kidney	Michigan State Unv.	Variety	36.8 ± 0.92 [a]

[1] This panel consists of medium to large Andean beans ranging from 58 to 81 g/100 seed. IIA, Instituto de Investigação Agronómica; US GRIN, U.S. Germplasm Resources Information Network. [2] Raw seed were soaked in distilled water for 12 h prior to determining the number of minutes to reach 80% cooking time with an automated Mattson pin-drop device. Values are means ± SEM of four field replicates, each measured in duplicate (n = 8). Means sharing the same letter are not significantly different at $p \leq 0.05$.

2.2. Field Design, Growing Conditions and Post Harvest Handling

Genotypes were planted side-by-side with 0.5 m spacing between rows at the Michigan State University Montcalm Research Farm near Entrican, MI in 2017. The soil type at the Montcalm Research Farm is Eutric Glossoboralfs (coarse-loamy, mixed) and Alfic Fragiorthods (coarse-loamy, mixed, frigid). Rainfall was supplemented with overhead irrigation as needed. Weeds and pests were controlled by hand or with herbicides if needed. Upon maturity, bean plants were pulled by hand and then threshed with a Hege 140 plot harvester (Wintersteiger Inc., Salt Lake City, UT, USA). Immediately after harvest, seeds were hand sorted to eliminate any immature, wrinkled, discolored, or damaged seeds. To equilibrate moisture content, sorted seed was placed into dark storage under ambient conditions (20–22 °C, 50–60% relative humidity) at standard atmospheric pressure and monitored for eight weeks with a John Deere Grain Moisture Tester (Moisture Chek-Plus™; Deere & Company, Watseka, IL, USA) until the moisture content reached 10–12% [32].

2.3. Cooking Time Determination

Growing conditions and post-harvest handling ensured the differences in cooking times between the yellow and kidney beans were under genetic control and not influenced by the growing or processing conditions of the seed after harvest [25]. Subsets of 50 seed from four randomly selected field replicates for each genotype were evaluated for cooking time. Prior to cooking, bean seeds were pre-soaked in distilled water (1:6 *w/w*) for 12 h at room temperature. Cooking time was measured with a Mattson pin drop cooking device, which fits into a 4 L stainless steel beaker heated over an electric portable burner containing 1.8 L of boiling distilled water. Cooking time was standardized as the number of minutes required for twenty out of twenty-five piercing tip rods (70 g, 2 mm diameter) to pass completely through each seed under a steady boil at 100 °C [33].

2.4. Ingredient Preparation and Diet Composition

To prepare beans for diet formulation, 35 kg of raw seed were first rinsed and cleaned thoroughly in distilled water to remove dust, debris, and non-edible material. Beans were pre-soaked in distilled water (1:6 w/w) for 12 h at room temperature before cooking at the Food Processing and Development Laboratory (FPDL) located at Cornell University, Ithaca, New York. Beans were cooked according to their predetermined cooking times in boiling distilled water using large (20 gallon) stainless steel steam kettles at the processing facility. Drained beans were spread evenly in stainless steel trays and allowed to cool for thirty minutes at room temperature. Cooked beans were then stored in a −20 °C cold room for 24 h prior to freeze-drying (VirTis Research Equipment, Gardiner, NY, USA). Basmati rice was purchased from Wegmans™ food store located in Ithaca, NY, USA. Large quantities of rice (25 kg) were cooked with distilled water at the FPDL in stainless steel steam kettles. Cooked rice was cooled to room temperature on stainless steel trays and stored at −20 °C for 24 h before freeze-drying. Cooked/air-dried potatoes and white cabbage were purchased from North Bay Trading Co. (Brule, WI, USA). Dried ingredients were milled into a course powder using a Waring Commercial® CB15 stainless steel blender (Torrington, CT, USA). Chick Vitamin Mixture 330,002 and Salt Mix for Chick Diet 230,000 (without iron) was purchased from Dyets Inc. (Bethlehem, PA, USA). DL-Methionine and choline chloride were purchased from Sigma–Aldrich (St. Louis, MO, USA). Ingredients were mixed with corn oil (0.5 L/kg) and stored at 4 °C during the duration of the feeding trial. The final composition of each bean based diet is presented in Table 2.

Table 2. Ingredient Formulation, Iron Concentrations and Phytate Analysis of Bean Based Diets.

Ingredient [1]	Iron (µg/g) [2]	Diet Formulation (g/kg)				
		Ervilha	Uyole 98	PI527538	Snowdon	Red Hawk
Ervilha (Manteca)	83.0 ± 0.78 [a]	420	–	–	–	–
Uyole 98 (Amarillo)	79.1 ± 0.75 [b]	–	420	–	–	–
PI527538 (Njano)	84.8 ± 0.70 [a]	–	–	420	–	–
Snowdon (white kidney)	75.3 ± 0.50 [b]	–	–	–	420	–
Red Hawk (red kidney)	81.9 ± 0.76 [a]	–	–	–	–	420
Potato (white)	14.6 ± 0.27 [d]	330	330	330	330	330
Rice (white/polished)	6.55 ± 0.54 [e]	90	90	90	90	90
Cabbage (white)	19.8 ± 0.74 [c]	90	90	90	90	90
Vitamin/mineral premix [3]	0.00 ± 0.0 [f]	70	70	70	70	70
DL-Methionine	0.00 ± 0.0 [f]	2.5	2.5	2.5	2.5	2.5
Choline Chloride	0.00 ± 0.0 [f]	0.75	0.75	0.75	0.75	0.75
Total Composition (g)		1000	1000	1000	1000	1000
Dietary Analysis [4]						
Iron concentration (µg/g)		53.7 ± 1.5 [a]	46.5 ± 0.36 [b]	54.5 ± 0.91 [a]	47.4 ± 0.37 [b]	52.4 ± 1.1 [a]
Phytate concentration (mg/g)		7.55 ± 0.22 [a]	7.30 ± 0.01 [a]	6.91 ± 0.12 [b]	7.19 ± 0.11 [a,b]	7.16 ± 0.08 [a,b]
Phytate-iron molar ratio		12.1 ± 0.69 [b,c]	13.9 ± 0.16 [a]	11.3 ± 0.49 [c]	12.9 ± 0.92 [a,b]	12.6 ± 0.86 [b,c]

[1] Food ingredients were cooked, drained, and lyophilized prior to milling into a course powder for chemical analysis. [2] Values are means ± SEM of five replicates for each ingredient. Means sharing the same letter are not significantly different at ($p \leq 0.05$). [3] Vitamin and mineral premix: #330,002 Chick vitamin mixture; #230,000 Salt mix (no iron) for chick diet (Dyets Inc., Bethlehem, PA, USA). [4] Values are means ± SEM of five replicates for each of the bean-based diets. Means sharing the same letter in each row are not significantly different at $p \leq 0.05$.

2.5. Iron Analysis

For iron analysis, either a 500 mg sample of each ingredient, a 500 mg sample of each bean based diet or a 100 mg sample of liver tissue (wet weight) were pre-digested in boro–silicate glass tubes with 3 mL of a concentrated ultra-pure nitric acid and perchloric acid mixture (60:40 v/v) for 16 h at room temperature. Samples were then placed in a digestion block (Martin Machine, Ivesdale, IL, USA) and heated incrementally over 4 h to a temperature of 120 °C with refluxing. After incubating at 120 °C for 2 h, 2 mL of concentrated ultra-pure nitric acid was subsequently added to each sample before raising the digestion block temperature to 145 °C for an additional 2 h. The temperature of the digestion block was then raised to 190 °C and maintained for at least ten minutes before samples were allowed to cool at room temperature. Digested samples were re-suspended in 20 mL of ultrapure water prior to analysis using ICP-AES (inductively coupled plasma-atomic emission spectroscopy; Thermo iCAP 6500 Series, Thermo Scientific, Cambridge, UK) with quality control standards (High Purity Standards, Charleston, SC, USA) following every 10 samples. Yttrium purchased from High Purity Standards (10M67-1) was used as an internal standard. All samples were digested and measured with 0.5 µg/mL of Yttrium (final concentration) to ensure batch-to-batch accuracy and to correct for matrix inference during digestion.

2.6. Phytate Analysis

For phytate (phytic acid) determination, a 500 mg sample from each ingredient and a 500 mg sample from each of the bean based diets were first extracted in 10 mL of 0.66 M hydrochloric acid under constant motion for 16 h at room temperature. A 1 mL aliquot of total extract was collected using a wide bore pipet tip, and then centrifuged (16,000 g) for 10 min to pellet debris. A 0.5 mL sample of supernatant was then neutralized with 0.5 mL 0.75 M sodium hydroxide and stored at −20 °C until the day of analysis. A phytate/total phosphorous kit (K-PHYT; Megazyme International, Bray, Ireland) was used to measure liberated phosphorous by phytase and alkaline phosphatase. Phosphorous was quantified by colorimetric analysis as molybdenum blue with phosphorous standards read at a wavelength of 655 nm against the absorbance of a reagent blank. Total phytate concentrations were calculated with Mega-Calc™ by subtracting free phosphate concentrations in the extracts from the total amount of phosphorous that is exclusively released after enzymatic digestion.

2.7. Protein and Fiber Analysis

Total nitrogen concentrations were measured in a 500 mg sample of cooked beans by the Dumas combustion method at A&L Great Lakes Laboratories (Fort Wayne, IN, USA) in accordance with AOAC method 968.06 [34]. The percentage of crude protein was estimated by multiplying the dry weight total nitrogen concentration by a factor of 6.25 [35]. Insoluble, soluble and total fiber concentrations were determined by the enzymatic-gravimetric AOAC method 985.29 [36], using enzymatic hydrolysis with heat-resistant amylase, protease, and amyloglucosidase (Total Dietary Fiber Assay Kit, Sigma Aldrich Co., St. Louis, MO, USA).

2.8. Polyphenolic Extraction

For polyphenol extraction, 5 mL of methanol:water (50:50 *v/v*) was added to either 500 mg of cooked beans or to 500 mg of bean based diet, and vortexed for one minute before incubating in a sonication water bath for 20 min at room temperature. Samples were again vortexed and placed on a compact digital Rocker (Labnet International, Inc., Edison, NJ, USA) at room temperature for 60 min before centrifuging at 4000 g for 15 min. Supernatants were filtered with a 0.2 µm Teflon™ syringe filter and stored at −20 °C until chemical analysis.

Liquid Chromatography—Mass Spectrometry (LC–MS) Analysis of Polyphenols

Extracts and standards were analyzed by an Agilent 1220 Infinity Liquid Chromatograph (LC; Agilent Technologies, Inc., Santa Clara, CA, USA) coupled to an Advion expressionL® compact mass spectrometer (CMS; Advion Inc., Ithaca, NY, USA). Two-µL samples were injected and passed through an Acquity™ UPLC BEH Shield RP18 1.7 µm 2.1 × 100 mm column (Waters, Milford, MA, USA) at 0.35 mL/min. The column was temperature-controlled at 45 °C. The mobile phase consisted of ultra-pure water with 0.10% formic acid (solvent A) and acetonitrile with 0.10% formic acid (solvent B). Polyphenols were eluted using linear gradients of 86.7 to 77.0% A in 0.50 min, 77.0 to 46.0% A in 5.50 min, 46.0 to 0% A in 0.50 min, held at 0% A for 3.50 min, 0 to 86.7% A in 0.50 min, and held at 86.7% A for 3.50 min, for a total run time of 14 min. From the column, flow was directed into a variable wavelength UV detector set at 278 nm. Flow was then directed into the source of an Advion expressionL® CMS, and electro spray ionization (ESI) mass spectrometry was performed in negative ionization mode using selected ion monitoring with a scan time of 50 milliseconds for the 18 polyphenol masses of interest. Capillary temperature and voltages were 300 °C and 100 volts, respectively. ESI source voltage and gas temperature were 2.6 kilovolts and 240 °C respectively. Desolvation gas flow was 240 L/h. Advion Mass Express™ software was used to control the LC and CMS instrumentation and data acquisition. Individual polyphenols were identified and confirmed by comparison of m/z and LC retention times with authentic standards. Polyphenol standard curves for flavonoids were derived from integrated areas under UV absorption peaks from 8 replications. Standard curves for catechin and 3.4-dihydroxybenzoic acid were constructed from MS ion intensities using 8 replications.

2.9. In Vitro Iron Bioavailability Assessment (Caco-2 Cell Bioassay)

An established in vitro digestion/Caco-2 cell culture model was initially used to assess the iron bioavailability of cooked beans and bean based diets [37–39]. A 500 mg sample of lyophilized powder from either whole cooked beans or bean based diets were subjected to a simulated gastric and intestinal digestion as described previously [37,39]. The bioassay was performed according to the detailed methods described in Glahn et al., 1998 [37]. The bioassay works according to the following principle. In response to increases in cellular iron concentrations, Caco-2 cells produce more ferritin protein. Therefore, iron bioavailability was determined as the increase in Caco-2 cell ferritin production expressed as a ratio to total protein (ng ferritin per mg of total cell protein) after exposure to a digested sample [37–39]. Ferritin was measured by enzyme linked immunoassay (Human Ferritin ELISA kit S-22, Ramco Laboratories Inc., Stafford, TX, USA) and total cell protein concentrations were quantified using the Bio-Rad DC™ protein assay kit (Bio-Rad Laboratories Inc., Hercules, CA, USA).

To confirm the responsiveness of the bioassay, each experiment was run with several quality controls. These include a blank-digest, which is only the physiologically balanced saline and the gastrointestinal enzymes. The blank-digest was used to ensure there was no iron contamination in the bioassay. Ferritin values of Caco-2 cells were exposed to the blank-digest averaged 2.5 ± 0.08 ng ferritin/mg cell protein (mean ± Standard Deviation; SD) over the course of two cell culture experiments. The responsiveness of the bioassay was monitored by: (1) a blank-digest with $FeCl_3$ (66 µM) and (2) a blank-digest of $FeCl_3$ (66 µM) plus the addition of 1.3 mM ascorbic acid (Sigma Aldrich Co., St. Louis, MO, USA). Ferritin values for the $FeCl_3$ digest and the $FeCl_3$ digest with ascorbic acid averaged 68 ± 5.3 and 234 ± 17 ng/mg cell protein (mean ± SD), respectively. The quality controls could be utilized as a reference standard because they do not contain the same food matrix properties as the cooked beans. Therefore, a cooked/lyophilized/milled navy bean control (commercial variety Merlin) was run with each assay as a reference standard to index the ferritin/total cell protein ratios of the Caco-2 cells over the course of several cell culture experiments. Ferritin values for the Merlin navy bean control averaged 8.07 ± 0.63 ng/mg cell protein (mean ± SD).

2.10. Animals and Feeding Trial Design

Cornish-cross fertile broiler eggs were obtained from a commercial hatchery (Moyer's Chicks, Quakertown, PA, USA). The eggs were incubated under optimal conditions at the Cornell University Animal Science poultry farm incubator. On the day of hatching (hatchability = 95%) chicks were randomly allocated into five treatment groups (n = 13) shown in Table 2 and given ad libitum access to food and water (iron concentration <0.4 µg/L). Chicks were housed in a total confinement building (3–4 animals per 1 m^2 metal cage) under controlled temperatures and humidity with 16 h of light. Each cage was equipped with an automatic watering dish and a manual self-feeder. Feed intakes were measured daily starting from the day of hatching and body weights were recorded each week. All animal protocols were approved by the Cornell University Institutional Animal Care and Use Committee (protocol# 2007-0129).

2.11. Blood Collection, Hemoglobin and Index of Iron Absorption Calculations

Blood samples were collected from the wing vein of each animal with heparinized capillary tubes and stored on ice in BD Vacutainer® vials (lithium heparin; 95 USP Units). For Hemoglobin (Hb) determination, whole blood samples were diluted 100-fold in distilled water and measured colorimetrically with BioAssay Systems Quantichrom™ hemoglobin assay (DIHB-250) following the manufacturer's instructions (BioAssay Systems, Hayward, CA, USA). Total body hemoglobin iron (Hb-Fe) is an index of iron absorption, and is calculated from hemoglobin concentrations and total blood volume based on body weight (85 mL per kg of body weight) [6,40–42]:

$$\text{Hb-Fe (mg)} = \text{Body Weight (kg)} \times 0.085 \text{ L/kg} \times \text{Hb (g/L)} \times 3.35 \text{ mg Fe/g Hb}. \tag{1}$$

Hemoglobin maintenance efficiency (HME) is calculated as the cumulative difference in total body hemoglobin iron from the start of the experiment, divided by total dietary iron intake. Dietary iron intakes were determined by multiplying the cumulative amount of diet consumed over the course of the experiment with the iron concentrations measured for each diet shown in Table 2 [6,40–42]:

$$\text{HME} = \frac{\text{Hb Fe (final) mg} - \text{Hb Fe (initial) mg}}{\text{Total Fe Intake (mg)}} \times [100\%]. \tag{2}$$

At the end of the experiment (42 days), animals were euthanized by CO_2 exposure and their blood, small intestine, cecum, and liver were quickly collected. Tissue was immediately frozen in liquid nitrogen and stored at −80 °C until further analysis.

2.12. Liver Iron and Ferritin

The quantification of liver Fe (ICP-AES) and liver ferritin were conducted as previously described [40,43,44]. Polyacrylamide gels were scanned with a Bio-Rad® densitometer and the measurement of band intensity conducted with Quantity-One 1-D analysis program (Bio-Rad Laboratories Inc., Hercules, CA, USA). Local background was subtracted from each sample and horse spleen ferritin (Sigma Aldrich Co., St. Louis, MO, USA) was used as a standard for identifying and calibrating ferritin protein.

2.13. Isolation of Total RNA from Duodenum

Total RNA was extracted using Qiagen RNeasy Mini Kit (RNeasy Mini Kit, Qiagen Inc., Valencia, CA, USA) according to the manufacturer's protocol. Proximal duodenal tissue (30 mg) was disrupted and homogenized with a rotor-stator homogenizer in buffer RLT®, containing β-mercaptoethanol. The tissue lysate was centrifuged for 3 min at 8000 g in a microcentrifuge. An aliquot of the supernatant was transferred to another tube, combined with 1 volume of 70% ethanol and mixed immediately. Each sample (700 µL) was applied to an RNeasy mini column, centrifuged for 15 s at 8000 g, and the flow through material was discarded. The RNeasy columns were transferred to new 2 mL collection tubes, and 500 µL of buffer RPE® was pipetted onto the RNeasy column followed by centrifugation for 15 s at 8000 g. An additional 500 µL of buffer RPE were pipetted onto the RNeasy column and centrifuged for 2 min at 8000 g. Total RNA was eluted in 50 µL of RNase free water. All steps were carried out under RNase free conditions. RNA was quantified by absorbance at A 260/280. Integrity of the 28S and 18S ribosomal RNAs was verified by 1.5% agarose gel electrophoresis followed by ethidium bromide staining. DNA contamination was removed using TURBO DNase treatment and removal kit from AMBION (Austin, TX, USA).

2.14. Real Time Polymerase Chain Reaction (RT-PCR)

To create the cDNA, a 20 µL reverse transcriptase (RT) reaction was completed in a BioRad C1000 touch thermocycler using the Improm-II Reverse Transcriptase Kit (Catalog #A1250; Promega Corp.,

Madison, WI, USA). The first step consisted of 1 μg of total RNA template, 10 μM of random hexamer primers, and 2 mM of oligo-dT primers. The RT protocol was used to anneal primers to RNA at 94 °C for 5 min. The first strand was copied for 60 min at 42 °C (optimum temperature for the enzyme), followed by exposure to 70 °C (15 min) for enzymatic inactivation, samples were then held at 4 °C until quantification by a Nanodrop™ ND-1000 (Thermo Fisher Scientific, Wilmington, DE, USA). The concentration of cDNA obtained was determined by measuring the absorbance at 260 nm and 280 nm using an extinction coefficient of 33 (for single stranded DNA). Genomic DNA contamination was assessed by a real-time RT-PCR assay for the reference gene samples.

2.15. Primer Design for Divalent Metal Transporter 1, Duodenal Cytochrome B, and Ferroportin Gene Expression Analysis

The primers used in the real-time PCR to measure the duodenum gene expression of the iron import proteins divalent metal transporter 1 (DMT-1) and duodenal cytochrome B (DcytB), as well as the iron export protein ferroportin were designed according gene sequences obtained from the National Center for Biotechnology Information (NCBI) Genbank® database, using Real-Time Primer Design Tool software (IDT DNA, Coralvilla, IA, USA). The sequences and the description of the forward and reverse primers used for PCR reactions in this study are summarized in Table S1. The amplicon length was limited to 90 to 150 base pairs. The length of the primers was 17–25 bp, and the GC content was between 41% and 55%. The *Gallus gallus* primer 18S Ribosomal subunit 18S rRNA was designed as a reference gene (Table S1).

2.16. Real-Time qPCR Design

Isolated cDNA was used for each 10 μL reaction together with 2× BioRad® SSO Advanced Universal SYBR Green Supermix (Cat. #1725274, Hercules, CA, USA) which included buffer, Taq DNA polymerase, dNTPs and SYBR green dye. Specific primers (Table S1) and cDNA or water (for no template control) were added to each PCR reaction. For each gene, the optimal $MgCl_2$ concentration produced the amplification plot with the lowest cycle product (Cq), the highest fluorescence intensity and the steepest amplification slope. Master mix (8 μL) was pipetted into the 96-well plate and 2 μL cDNA was added as PCR template. Each run contained seven standard curve points in duplicate. A no template control of nuclease-free water was included to exclude DNA contamination in the PCR mix. The double stranded DNA was amplified in the Bio-Rad® CFX96 Touch (Hercules, CA, USA) using the following PCR conditions: initial denaturing at 95 °C for 30 s, 40 cycles of denaturing at 95 °C for 15 s, various annealing temperatures according to Integrated DNA Technologies (IDT) for 30 s and elongating at 60 °C for 30 s. The data on the expression levels of the genes were obtained as Cq values based on the "second derivative maximum" (=automated method) as computed by the software. For each of the four genes, the reactions were run in duplicate. All assays were quantified by including a standard curve in the real-time qPCR analysis. The next four points of the standard curve were prepared by a 1:10 dilution. Each point of the standard curve was included in duplicate. A graph of Cq vs. log (10) concentrations was produced by the software and the efficiencies were calculated as 10 [1/slope]. The specificity of the amplified real-time RT-PCR products was verified by melting curve analysis (60–95 °C) after 40 cycles, resulting in a number of different specific products, each with a specific melting temperature. Real-time RT-PCR efficiency (E) values for the four genes were as follows: DMT-1, 0.988; DcytB, 1.046; Ferroportin, 1.109; 18S rRNA, 0.934.

2.17. Collection of Microbial Samples and DNA Isolation of Intestinal Contents

The cecum was aseptically (500 mg) removed and placed into a sterile 50 mL tube containing 9 mL of sterile PBS and homogenized by vortexing with glass beads (3 mm diameter) for 3 min. Debris was removed by centrifugation at 700 *g* for 1 min, and the supernatant was collected and centrifuged at 12,000 *g* for 5 min. The pellet was washed twice with 1 × Phosphate Buffered Saline (BP399-1; Fisher Scientific, Inc., Hampton, NH, USA) and stored at −20 °C until DNA extraction. For DNA purification, the pellet was re-suspended in 50 mM Ethylenediaminetetraacetic acid (EDTA) and treated with lysozyme (Sigma Aldrich Co., St. Louis, MO, USA; final concentration of 10 mg/mL for 45 min at 37 °C. The bacterial genomic DNA was isolated using a Wizard® Genomic DNA purification kit (Promega Corp., Madison, WI, USA).

2.18. Primers Design and PCR Amplification of Bacterial 16S rRNA

Primers for Bifidobacterium, Lactobacillus, E. coli and Clostridium were designed according to previously published data [45]. To evaluate the relative proportion of each bacterium, all targeted primers were normalized to the reference gene of the universal primer product 16S rRNA. PCR products were separated by electrophoresis on 2% agarose gel, stained with ethidium bromide, and quantified using the Quantity One 1-D analysis software (Bio-Rad, Hercules, CA, USA).

2.19. Statistical Analysis

All statistical analyses were conducted using IBM SPSS Statistics 25 (IBM Analytics, Armonk, NY, USA). The normality of residuals for each parameter was evaluated using the Kolmogorov-Smirnov test. Equality of variance for each parameter was determined using the Bartlett's test. Measured parameters were found to have a normal distribution and equal variance, and were, therefore, acceptable for ANOVA without additional data transformation steps. Mean separations for measured parameters were determined using ANOVA with the model including dietary treatment (5 levels) as fixed effects; followed by a Duncan *post hoc* test. Differences with p values of ≤ 0.05 were considered statistically significant. Graphs were prepared using GraphPad Prism7 (GraphPad Software, La Jolla, CA, USA).

3. Results

3.1. Cooking Times and Seed Iron-Phytate Concentrations

Table 1 shows the cooking times of the yellow and kidney beans prior to diet formulation. Significant ($p \leq 0.05$) differences in cooking times were measured among the pre-soaked beans, ranging from 15 min for Ervilha to 37 min for Red Hawk (Table 1). Significantly ($p \leq 0.05$) faster cooking times were measured in the yellow beans when compared to the white and dark red kidney bean varieties (Table 1). Iron concentrations of each ingredient after cooking, lyophilizing, and milling are show in Table 2. Differences in seed iron concentrations between the cooked beans were significant ($p \leq 0.05$), ranging from 75 µg/g in Snowdon to 85 µg/g in PI527538 (Table 2). Phytate concentrations and phytate molar ratios of each ingredient used to formulate the bean based diets are shown in Table S2. Significant ($p \leq 0.05$) differences in phytate concentrations were measured between the cooked yellow and kidney beans, ranging from 12.8 mg/g in Red Hawk to 13.7 mg/g in Ervilha (Table S2). Phytate to iron molar ratios also varied significantly ($p \leq 0.05$), ranging from a ratio of 13.4 in Red Hawk and PI527538 to a ratio of 15.3 in Snowdon (Table S2).

3.2. Protein and Fiber Concentrations of Cooked Beans

Table 3 shows the total crude protein concentrations of yellow and kidney beans after cooking. Significant differences ($p \leq 0.05$) in protein concentrations were measured between the cooked beans, ranging from 21 g/100 g in Snowdon to 26 g/100 g in PI527538 (Table 3). The concentrations of insoluble, soluble, and total fiber for each of the cooked beans are also shown in Table 3. Significant differences ($p \leq 0.05$) in each of the fiber fractions were measured among the yellow and kidney beans. The lowest concentrations of the insoluble and total fiber were detected in the fastest cooking yellow bean Ervilha (Table 3). Significantly ($p \leq 0.05$) higher concentrations of all three fiber fractions were in measured in each of the kidney beans, when compared to the yellow beans Ervilha and PI527538 after cooking (Table 3).

Table 3. Protein and Fiber Concentrations (g/100 g) of Cooked Beans Used to Formulate Bean Based Diets. [1]

Cooked Bean	Total Protein	Insoluble Fiber	Soluble Fiber	Total Fiber
Ervilha (*Manteca*)	25.02 ± 0.02 [b]	17.42 ± 1.20 [c]	1.99 ± 0.28 [b]	19.41 ± 1.48 [c]
Uyole 98 (*Amarillo*)	22.30 ± 0.10 [c]	19.95 ± 0.32 [ab]	2.52 ± 0.36 [ab]	22.47 ± 0.04 [ab]
PI527538 (*Njano*)	26.05 ± 0.12 [a]	18.75 ± 0.44 [bc]	2.09 ± 0.21 [b]	20.83 ± 0.22 [bc]
Snowdon (*white kidney*)	21.07 ± 0.14 [d]	20.71 ± 0.49 [a]	2.66 ± 0.01 [a]	23.37 ± 0.50 [a]
Red Hawk (*red kidney*)	22.83 ± 0.13 [c]	21.32 ± 0.64 [a]	2.92 ± 0.45 [a]	24.24 ± 0.19 [a]

[1] Values are means ± SEM (n = 3 replicates). Means sharing the same letter in each column are not significantly different at $p \leq 0.05$.

3.3. Iron-Phytate Analysis of Bean Based Diets

The final composition including the iron concentrations, phytate concentrations, and phytate-iron molar ratios for each of the five bean based diets are shown in Table 2. Iron concentrations between the bean based diets were significantly different ($p \leq 0.05$). Diets formulated from Ervilha, PI527538 and Red Hawk had higher iron concentrations (52–55 µg/g) than diets formulated from Uyole 98 and Snowdon (47 µg/g). Final phytate concentrations also varied between the five diets ranging from 6.91 mg/g in PI527538 to 7.55 mg/g in Ervilha (Table 2). Significant ($p \leq 0.05$) differences in phytate-iron molar ratios were calculated between the bean based diets, ranging from 11.3 mg/g in PI527538 to 13.9 mg/g in Uyole 98 (Table 2).

3.4. Polyphenolic Profile of Beans and Bean Based Diets

The polyphenol concentrations of the yellow and kidney beans after cooking are shown in Table 4. Eleven polyphenols that were previously shown to impact iron bioavailability [5,7] were detected in cooked beans, which included flavonols, phenolic acids, catechins, and procyanidins (precursors to condensed tannins). High concentrations of kaempferol 3-glucoside were measured in each of the yellow beans ranging from 356 nmol/g in Ervilha to 749 nmol/g in Uyole 98. In contrast to the yellow beans, the kidney beans had little to no kaempferol 3-glucoside after cooking (Table 4). The polyphenol profiles of the two fastest cooking yellow beans Ervilha and Uyole 98 were limited to kaempferol, kaempferol 3-glucoside and kaempferol 3-sumbuioside, while the slower cooking yellow bean PI527538 had significantly ($p < 0.05$) higher concentrations of quercetin 3-glucoside, catechins, and procyanidin B1–B2 (Table 4). Red Hawk had the most diverse set of polyphenols after cooking, including higher concentrations of quercetin 3-glucoside, protocatechuic acid, catechin, and procyanidin B1 (Table 4).

Table 4. Polyphenol Concentrations (nmol/g) of Cooked Beans. [1]

Polyphenol	Ervilha (*Manteca*)	Uyole 98 (*Amarillo*)	PI527538 (*Njano*)	Snowdon (*white kidney*)	Red Hawk (*red kidney*)
Kaempferol	74.0 ± 2.3 [a]	42.4 ± 5.8 [b]	40.7 ± 1.5 [b]	-	1.9 ± 0.3 [c]
Kaempferol 3-glucoside	356 ± 25 [c]	749 ± 48 [a]	671 ± 19 [b]	0.9 ± 0.1 [e]	4.7 ± 0.3 [d]
Kaempferol 3-sambuioside	86.4 ± 7.8 [a]	40.8 ± 2.5 [b]	4.4 ± 0.2 [c]	-	3.7 ± 0.1 [d]
Quercetin	2.3 ± 0.1 [c]	-	3.8 ± 0.2 [b]	-	6.2 ± 0.4 [a]
Quercetin 3-glucoside	16.2 ± 0.9 [c]	4.5 ± 0.5 [d]	57.9 ± 1.3 [a]	-	23.4 ± 0.8 [b]
Quercetin 3-rutinoside	-	-	-	-	3.1 ± 0.2
Protocatechuic acid	4.2 ± 0.5 [c]	6.9 ± 0.5 [b]	6.8 ± 0.7 [b]	-	30.6 ± 1.6 [a]
Catechin	-	2.7 ± 0.2 [b]	44.4 ± 2.0 [a]	-	40.0 ± 1.7 [a]
Epicatechin	-	0.4 ± 0.1 [c]	8.5 ± 0.8 [a]	-	5.3 ± 0.3 [b]
Procyanidin B1	-	3.9 ± 0.3 [c]	17.4 ± 0.7 [a]	-	13.7 ± 0.8 [b]
Procyanidin B2	-	-	1.4 ± 0.1 [a]	-	0.8 ± 0.2 [b]

[1] Values are means ± SEM (n = 8 replicates). Means sharing the same letter in each row are not significantly different at $p \leq 0.05$.

The polyphenol concentrations measured in each of the bean based diets are shown in Table 5. The polyphenol profile of each diet reflects the profiles of the cooked beans, with kaempferol 3-glucoside still being the most dominate polyphenol measured in each of the yellow bean diets. When compared to Ervilha and Uyole 98, significantly ($p < 0.05$) higher concentrations of quercetin 3-glucoside, catechins and procyanidins were detected in PI527538 and Red Hawk bean based diets (Table 5).

Table 5. Polyphenol Concentrations (nmol/g) Measured in Bean Based Diets.[1]

Polyphenol	Ervilha (Manteca)	Uyole 98 (Amarillo)	PI527538 (Njano)	Snowdon (white kidney)	Red Hawk (red kidney)
Kaempferol	7.4 ± 0.3 [a]	5.6 ± 0.2 [b]	5.4 ± 0.2 [b]	-	-
Kaempferol 3-glucoside	153 ± 5.1 [c]	327 ± 18 [a]	234 ± 5.9 [b]	0.6 ± 0.1 [e]	1.9 ± 0.1 [d]
Kaempferol 3-sambuioside	37.4 ± 1.6 [a]	17.6 ± 0.3 [b]	1.7 ± 0.1 [c]	-	1.5 ± 0.1 [c]
Quercetin	-	-	-	-	-
Quercetin 3-glucoside	6.6 ± 0.3 [c]	1.8 ± 0.1 [d]	21.4 ± 0.7 [a]	-	8.2 ± 0.5 [b]
Quercetin 3-rutinoside	-	-	-	-	3.0 ± 0.2
Protocatechuic acid	2.4 ± 0.4 [c]	4.5 ± 0.6 [b]	4.4 ± 0.4 [b]	-	16.8 ± 1.3 [a]
Catechin	-	0.8 ± 0.1 [b]	10.5 ± 0.4 [a]	-	10.8 ± 0.8 [a]
Epicatechin	-	0.1 ± 0.0 [b]	1.7 ± 0.2 [a]	-	1.3 ± 0.2 [a]
Procyanidin B1	-	0.7 ± 0.1 [b]	2.9 ± 0.3 [a]	-	2.5 ± 0.2 [a]
Procyanidin B2	-	-	0.2 ± 0.0 [a]	-	0.2 ± 0.0 [a]

[1] Values are means ± SEM (n = 8 replicates). Means sharing the same letter in each row are not significantly different at $p \leq 0.05$.

3.5. In Vitro Iron Bioavailability (Caco-2 Cell Ferritin Formation)

The results in Table 6 show significant ($p \leq 0.05$) differences in iron bioavailability between the cooked beans and their corresponding diets using the Caco-2 cell bioassay. The bioassay measures ferritin protein formation in cells following exposure to a digested sample that was prepared from either cooked beans or bean based diets on an equal weight basis. Among the cooked beans, significantly ($p \leq 0.05$) higher iron bioavailability was measured in Ervilha and Snowdon when compared to the Uyole 98, PI527538, and Red Hawk (Table 6). Significantly ($p \leq 0.05$) higher iron bioavailability was also measured in the Ervilha bean based diet when compared to the other four diets (Table 6).

Table 6. Iron Bioavailability of Cooked Beans and Bean Based Diets Using an in vitro Digestion/Caco-2 Cell Bioassay. [1]

Cooked Bean	Caco-2 Cell Ferritin Formation (ng Ferritin/mg Protein)
Ervilha (Manteca)	9.54 ± 0.59 [a]
Uyole 98 (Amarillo)	5.97 ± 0.52 [b,c]
PI527538 (Njano)	5.01 ± 0.15 [c]
Snowdon (white kidney)	8.20 ± 0.50 [a]
Red Hawk (red kidney)	6.92 ± 0.95 [b]
Bean Based Diet	
Ervilha (Manteca)	15.5 ± 1.4 [A]
Uyole 98 (Amarillo)	9.46 ± 0.19 [C]
PI527538 (Njano)	7.98 ± 0.80 [D]
Snowdon (white kidney)	12.2 ± 0.41 [B]
Red Hawk (red kidney)	7.57 ± 0.67 [D]

[1] In vitro iron bioavailability expressed as Caco-2 cell ferritin concentrations (ng ferritin/mg total cell protein) after a 24 h exposure to an in vitro digestion of either lyophilized cooked beans or bean based diets. Values are means ± SEM of six replicates for each sample. Means sharing the same letter in each group are not significantly different at $p \leq 0.05$.

3.6. In Vivo Iron Bioavailability (Gallus gallus Feeding Trial)

3.6.1. Feed and Iron Intakes

By day 14 of the study, significantly ($p \leq 0.05$) higher feed intakes were measured in the groups receiving the yellow bean diets versus the groups receiving the white and dark red kidney diets (Figure 2A). By day 21, the group receiving the Red Hawk diet had significantly ($p \leq 0.05$) lower feed intakes compared to the other four treatment groups (Figure 2A). Iron intake mirrored the cumulative feed intakes over the course of the experiment. Significant ($p \leq 0.05$) differences in iron intakes between the five treatment groups could be detected as early as day 7 (Figure 2B). By the end of the study, cumulative iron intakes ranged from 117 mg in the groups receiving the Ervilha and PI527538 yellow bean diets to 64 mg in the group receiving the Red Hawk diet (Figure 2B). Although cumulative feed intakes were not different between the groups receiving the yellow bean diets (Figure 2A), lower iron concentrations in the Uyole 98 diet (47 µg/g) resulted in a significantly ($p \leq 0.05$) lower iron intake by day 35 of the study-when compared to the groups receiving the Ervilha and PI527538 diets, which had higher iron concentrations (54–55 µg/g; Figure 2B). The specified values for cumulative feed and iron intake are listed with mean separations in Tables S3 and S4.

3.6.2. Growth Rates and Total Body Hemoglobin Iron

Increases in body weights were consistently higher ($p \leq 0.05$) among the three groups receiving the yellow bean diets when compared the groups receiving the white and red kidney bean diets (Figure 2C). By the end of the experiment, the group receiving the Uyole 98 diet had significantly ($p \leq 0.05$) lower body weight versus the two groups receiving the Ervilha and PI527538 diets (Figure 2C). Throughout the experiment, the lowest body weights were measured in the group receiving the Red Hawk diet (Figure 2C). Total body hemoglobin iron (Hb-Fe) varied significantly ($p \leq 0.05$) between the treatment groups throughout the 6 week feeding trial (Figure 2D). By day 21 of the experiment, the group receiving the Ervilha diet had significantly ($p \leq 0.05$) higher Hb-Fe values when compared to the other four dietary treatments (Figure 2D). Starting at day 7 of the experiment, the lowest Hb-Fe values were measured in the group receiving the Red Hawk diet (Figure 2D). Specified values for body weight and total body hemoglobin iron are listed with mean separations in Tables S5 and S6.

3.6.3. Hemoglobin and Hemoglobin Maintenance Efficiency (HME)

By day 7 of the experiment, the concentrations of hemoglobin (Hb) varied significantly ($p \leq 0.05$) between the five groups receiving the bean based diets (Figure 2E). From days 14–28 of the experiment, a significant ($p \leq 0.05$) drop in Hb was measured in the group receiving the Red Hawk diet. The concentrations of Hb in the Red Hawk group recovered by day 35 of the experiment, with no significant differences detected between the other four dietary treatments (Figure 2E). At the end of the experiment, the group receiving the Uyole 98 diet had significantly ($p \leq 0.05$) higher Hb concentrations than the group receiving the PI527538 diet (Figure 2E). Significant ($p \leq 0.05$) differences in HME were measured between the five treatment groups starting at day 7 of the experiment (Figure 2F). The group receiving the Ervilha diet had the highest HME percentages throughout the experiment ranging from 25%–33%. The lowest HME percentages (9%–15%) were detected in the group receiving the Red Hawk diet (Figure 2F). Specified values for hemoglobin and hemoglobin maintenance efficiency are listed with mean separations in Tables S7 and S8.

3.6.4. Liver Iron and Ferritin Concentrations

The concentrations of liver iron and ferritin measured at the end of the feeding trial are shown in Table 7. Significant ($p \leq 0.05$) differences in liver iron were detected among the five treatment groups with concentrations ranging from 64 µg/g in the group receiving the Ervilha diet to 49–51 µg/g in the groups receiving the PI527538 and Red Hawk diets. Significant ($p \leq 0.05$) differences in liver ferritin concentrations were also measured between the five dietary treatment groups (Table 7). Liver ferritin mirrored liver iron concentrations, ranging from a high of 341 µg/g in the group receiving the Ervilha diet to a low of 110 µg/g in the group receiving the Red Hawk diet. The liver iron and ferritin concentrations between the different treatment groups also mirror the ferritin formation results of the Caco-2 bioassay (Table 6).

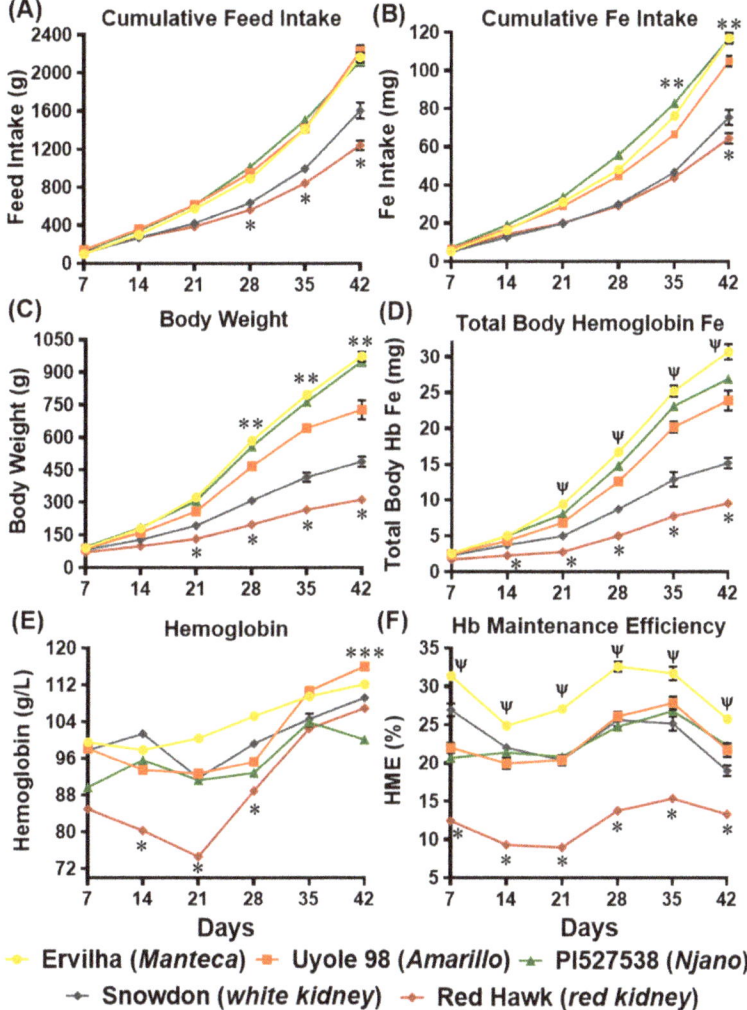

Figure 2. Cumulative feed intake (**A**), Fe intake (**B**), body weight (**C**), total body hemoglobin Fe (**D**), hemoglobin concentration (**E**) and hemoglobin maintenance efficiency (HME); (**F**) during the 6 weeks of consuming bean based diets. Values are means ± SEM (n = 10–13 animals per treatment group). * Significantly ($p \leq 0.05$) lower values measured in the group receiving the Red Hawk diet. ** Significantly ($p \leq 0.05$) higher cumulative Fe intakes and higher body weights measured in the groups receiving the Ervilha and PI527538 diets. *** Significantly ($p \leq 0.05$) higher hemoglobin measured at day 42 in the group receiving the Uyole 98 diet versus the group receiving the PI527538 diet. Ψ Significantly ($p \leq 0.05$) higher total body hemoglobin Fe and HME values measured in the group receiving the Ervilha diet versus the other four treatment groups.

Table 7. Liver Iron and Ferritin Protein Concentrations After 6 Weeks of Consuming Bean Based Diets. [1]

Bean Based Diet	Liver Iron (µg/g)	Liver Ferritin (µg/g)
Ervilha (*Manteca*)	64.3 ± 3.7 [a]	341 ± 14 [a]
Uyole 98 (*Amarillo*)	54.8 ± 3.4 [a,b]	243 ± 34 [b]
PI527538 (*Njano*)	48.6 ± 3.7 [b]	163 ± 28 [c]
Snowdon (*white kidney*)	59.1 ± 1.7 [a,b]	325 ± 4.7 [a]
Red Hawk (*red kidney*)	51.1 ± 2.3 [b]	110 ± 18 [c]

[1] Values are means ± SEM (n = 10–13 animals per treatment group). Means sharing the same letter in each column are not significantly different at $p \leq 0.05$. Total iron and ferritin protein concentrations measured as micrograms per gram of liver tissue (wet weight).

3.6.5. Gene Expression of Iron Import and Export Proteins in the Duodenum

Duodenum gene expression of DMT-1, DcytB and ferroportin relative to 18S rRNA is shown in Figure 3. Significant ($p \leq 0.05$) differences in the expression of DMT-1 and DcytB were detected, but no significant differences in ferroportin were observed between the five treatment groups (Figure 3). The highest expression levels of DMT-1 and DcytB were detected in the group receiving the Uyole 98 diet (Figure 3).

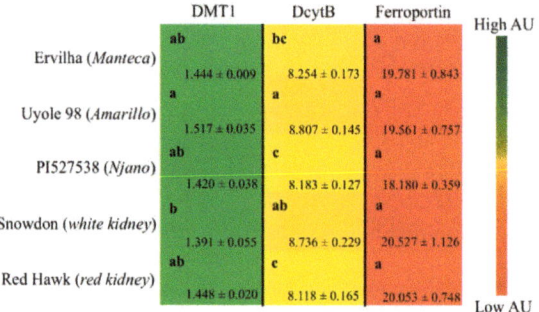

Figure 3. Gene expression of iron proteins in the duodenum after 6 weeks of consuming bean based diets. Values are means ± SEM (*n* = 5 per treatment group). Means sharing the same letter in each column are not significantly different at $p \leq 0.05$. DMT-1, Divalent Metal Transporter-1; DcytB, Duodenal cytochrome b.

3.6.6. Bacterial Populations in the Cecum

Significant ($p \leq 0.05$) differences in the relative abundance of all four bacterial populations (Bifidobacterium, Lactobacillus, E. coli, Clostridium) were measured between each of the groups receiving the bean based diets (Figure 4). Low levels of abundance for Bifidobacterium and Lactobacillus were detected in the group receiving the Snowdon diet, when compared to the other treatment groups (Figure 4). Significantly ($p \leq 0.05$) higher levels of abundance for all four bacterial populations were measured in the group receiving the Red Hawk diet (Figure 4).

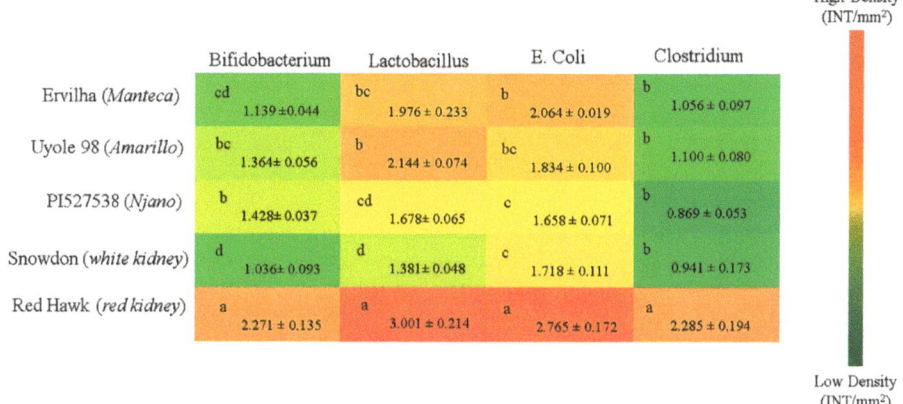

Figure 4. Genera and species-level bacterial populations (AU) from cecal contents after 6 weeks of consuming bean based diets. Values are means ± SEM (n = 6 per treatment group). Means sharing the same letter in each column are not significantly different at $p \leq 0.05$.

4. Discussion

4.1. Assessing the Iron Bioavailability of African Yellow Beans

Three yellow beans were selected from market classes that would be recognized by consumers in Sub-Saharan Africa [23–25]. Two non-yellow bean varieties were also included in this study, each representing a white and red kidney bean produced for commercial food manufacturing. Red beans, such as the dark red kidney, are preferred seed types in many regions of Sub-Saharan Africa and are often marketed alongside yellow beans [23,24]. The white kidney, Snowdon, was included in the study to represent a bean variety with no seed coat polyphenols. Snowdon and Red Hawk are from the same Andean gene pool as the three Africa yellow beans. Snowdon and Red Hawk also share many of the same genetic and agronomic characteristics [30,31]. Previous in vitro and in vivo studies have demonstrated that the iron absorption properties between white and red beans are very different from one another, which creates an ideal frame of reference for comparing the iron bioavailability properties of yellow beans [25,42]. Relative to the each of the yellow beans in this study, both the white and red kidney bean varieties have longer cooking times in boiling water. The overall nutritional value, as well as the iron bioavailability of dry beans is greatly impacted by the conditions in which they are grown, stored, and processed to become edible [25,46–48]. To limit these factors, beans were grown under the same field conditions, stored in a controlled environment, and their cooking time was standardized for each genotype to avoid over-or-under processing before diet formulation.

As previously demonstrated, the Caco-2 bioassay coupled with the *Gallus gallus* in vivo feeding model is an effective two-step system for evaluating the iron bioavailability of staple foods, such as beans [6,38,40–42,49]. The Caco-2 bioassay is an initial assessment used to compare varieties and to identify factors in food crops that could potentially impact the absorption of iron in vivo [38,39]. For this study, the bioassay shows that iron uptake (via ferritin formation) in Caco-2 cells was negatively impacted when diets were formulated with the darker colored yellow and red beans (Table 6). The results of the Caco-2 bioassay also matched the same patterns of liver iron and liver ferritin concentrations in each group of animals after the feeding trial (Table 7). Additionally, the bioassay revealed that diets prepared from the Manteca yellow bean produced a higher iron uptake in Caco-2 cells when compared to the other yellow, white and red bean based diets. The bioassay, however, did not predict the precise patterns of iron absorption between Uyole 98, PI527538 and the kidney beans over the course of the in vivo feeding trial. This exemplifies the need for the *Gallus gallus* model to be coupled with the Caco-2 bioassay because total body hemoglobin iron (Hb-Fe) and hemoglobin maintenance efficiency (HME) are two physiological markers that take into consideration an animal's growth rate, food consumption and adaptation to the bean based diet during the course of a feeding trial [6,40,42,49].

The *Gallus gallus* model can also be used to gain insight into the mechanism(s) of iron bioavailability by measuring the hematological, molecular (gene expression) and microbial changes in response to carefully formulated test diets [14,38,40–42,50]. Similar to humans, the gene expression of iron absorption proteins and the microbiota profiles of *Gallus gallus* are impacted by dietary iron intake [50,51]. The *Gallus gallus* shares >85% homology with the human gene sequences of the dietary iron import/export proteins DMT-1, DcytB, and ferroportin [52]. In addition, the phylum levels of gut microbiota between *Gallus gallus* and humans are similar, each being dominated by Bacteroidetes, Firmicutes, Proteobacteria and Actinobacteria [14,53,54]. The *Gallus gallus* is the first in vivo model to assess the iron nutrition of yellow beans, and this current study represents the first approach to predict the iron bioavailability of yellow beans in humans [38].

The *Gallus gallus* is a useful animal model for testing cooked beans that are combined into diets as either the main ingredient or formulated into a complex meal plan [40–42]. For this study, cooked yellow and kidney beans were the main ingredient of bean based diets, contributing to >60% of the total dietary iron in each diet. Bean based diets were formulated with the complementary foods of potato, rice, and cabbage in combinations similar to previous in vivo experiments that have successfully compared the iron bioavailability of different bean varieties in vivo [14,41]. Although the combination of diet ingredients used in this study would be quite common in Sub-Saharan Africa, future studies can be designed to evaluate the iron bioavailability of yellows beans within a multiple ingredient meal plan (the food basket approach), which is more precisely tailored to specific regions where yellow beans are already familiar to consumers [14,41,55].

4.2. The Iron Bioavailability of African Yellow Beans

Of the three African yellow beans tested in this study, the fastest cooking Manteca yellow bean (Ervilha) delivered the most absorbable iron for growth and hemoglobin production during the six week feeding trial. The Manteca is a pale-yellow bean native to Chile, characterized by its gray-black hilum ring. Higher prices at the market and anecdotal claims of 'low-flatulence' inspired scientists to examine the Manteca seed type's biochemistry [20,56,57]. They found the Manteca has a different fiber profile with more digestible starch and protein when compared to other black and red beans [57–59]. More importantly, they discovered the Manteca carries a recessive allele that closes off the production of procyanidin (condensed tannin) synthesis in the polyphenol pathway [20,56,60].

In addition to producing a darker seed coat color, condensed tannin concentrations influence the cooking time, as well as the digestibility of dry beans [59,61,62]. Although diets formulated with the Ervilha and PI527538 had similar iron concentrations and phytate-iron molar ratios (Table 2), the results of this experiment indicate that the slowest cooking Njano yellow bean PI527538 did not deliver as much iron as the fastest cooking Manteca yellow bean Ervilha. These results are in agreement with the current and past Caco-2 cell culture experiments, which show how Ervilha and PI528537 have distinct iron bioavailability that is independent of their iron concentrations after cooking [25]. The same polyphenols in black and red beans that were previously shown to inhibit the absorption of iron in vitro (quercetin 3-glucoside, procyanidin B1, procyanidin B2) were also detected in PI527538 after cooking [5–8]. These results provide evidence that the fast cooking Manteca is biochemically unique to other yellow beans, and demonstrates how altering the downstream production of polyphenols to prevent the synthesis of condensed tannins could be a useful mechanism to improve the iron bioavailability of dry beans [5–8,25].

Unlike previous investigations that have only compared the iron bioavailability of non-biofortified and biofortified beans in the same market class [6,14,40,41,55], the results of this study demonstrate that the iron bioavailability of yellow beans after cooking is not dependent on seed iron concentrations alone. For example, total dietary iron concentrations (Table 2) and cumulative iron intakes (Figure 2B) were lower for animals receiving the Amarillo yellow bean Uyole 98 diet, yet they were able to maintain their hemoglobin, Hb-Fe, and HME values, as well as their liver iron concentrations just as effectively as the animals receiving the slower cooking PI527538 yellow bean diet. The up-regulation of the iron import genes DMT-1 and DcytB in the animals receiving the Uyole 98 diet indicates there was a physiological adaptation to the lower dietary iron concentrations [6,40,41]. Despite the changes in the gene expression of iron import proteins, animals receiving the Uyole 98 diet were still unable to maintain their growth and hemoglobin production as efficiently as the animals receiving the fastest cooking Ervilha bean based diet. Interestingly, Uyole 98 had the highest concentrations of kaempferol 3-glucoside, but small amounts of the precursors to condensed tannins (catechin, epicatechin, procyanidin B1) were also detected in Uyole 98 bean based diets. There is evidence to suggest that these compounds may be more potent inhibitors of dietary iron than kaempferol 3-glucoside is a promotor of iron in vitro [5–7].

The contrast between Ervilha, Uyole 98, and PI527538 serves as a good example that not all yellow beans will have the same iron bioavailability. Demonstrating that there is phenotypic diversity in iron bioavailability between the different market classes of yellow beans, however, is important for dry bean breeders to identify targets traits that can lead to genetic improvement, while, at the same time, complementing the biofortification efforts that are currently underway to increase raw bean seed iron concentrations in yellow beans [4,63]. This study is the first to show that differences in polyphenols and dietary fiber concentrations between Ervilha, Uyole 98 and PI527538 can also play a role in determining the microbiota populations of the lower intestine (Figure 4). For example, the population densities of Bifidobacterium and E. Coli in the cecum were significantly different between animals fed the Ervilha and PI527538 yellow bean diets. This is an important finding because the polyphenols and fiber (prebiotics) found in dry beans are implicated in maintaining the health of the digestive system by influencing bacterial (probiotic) populations in the lower intestine [9–14]. While the measurements of microbiota at the species level is too broad of an interpretation to make any specific health recommendations about yellow beans, a more detailed study is currently being conducted to examine the microbial diversity and compositional changes of gut microbiota at the Phylum and Genus levels in animals fed the yellow and kidney bean based diets.

4.3. Iron Bioavailability of the White and Red Kidney Beans

Animals receiving the white and red kidney bean diets had low feed intakes and slower growth rates, which prevented these animals from accumulating the Hb-Fe values that were achieved by the animals receiving yellow bean diets (Figure 2). With the exception of Uyole 98, the white and red kidney beans tested in this study had significantly more dietary fiber and less protein than the African yellow beans (Table 3). There is evidence to support that increases in dietary fiber from habitual pulse consumption increase perceived satiety and reduce food intake, while intervention studies show that pulse consumption leads to reductions in body weight with or without energy restriction [64,65]. The differences in soluble and insoluble fiber concentrations between the two seed types are also indicative of differences in seed coat thickness and cotyledon cell wall composition, which are additional factors that need to be considered when comparing the digestibility and iron bioavailability of yellow and kidney beans [66].

The large differences in Hb-Fe between the animals receiving the white kidney Snowdon diet and the yellow Uyole 98 diet, which had the same iron concentrations, phytate-iron molar ratios, and fiber concentrations, suggest that kaempferol 3-glucoside may facilitate the absorption of dietary iron [5–8]. The overall digestibility and iron nutrition of African yellow beans with kaempferol 3-glucoside as their most abundant polyphenol appears to be far superior to that of white and red kidney beans-with polyphenol profiles that contain little to no kaempferol compounds. The large differences in growth rates and feed intakes between the two groups receiving the yellow and kidney bean diets, however, makes it difficult to pin-point kaempferol 3-glucoside as the only contributor of improved iron bioavailability among the three African yellow beans. Future investigations are needed to understand kaempferol 3-glucoside's full potential as a dietary promoter of iron bioavailability in dry beans, as well as in other world food crops that also contain kaempferol compounds, such as the yellow potato or yellow cassava [15].

Comparing the two kidney beans to each other revealed the iron bioavailability of Red Hawk, with a diverse array of polyphenols detected in its dark red seed coat, was significantly lower than Snowdon, which had little to no polyphenols in its white seed coat (Table 4). Animals receiving the Red Hawk diet could not absorb enough iron from the diet to maintain hemoglobin production during the first 2–3 weeks of the feeding trial (Figure 2E). An interesting adaptation in animals receiving the Red Hawk diet, however, was evident between weeks 3 and 4 of the experiment as hemoglobin production began to improve. Of the five beans tested in this study, the highest concentrations of insoluble and soluble fiber were measured in Red Hawk, which is an important observation because a more diverse collection of polyphenols, and more dietary fiber (prebiotics) are important factors that promote the diversity of microbiota populations in the lower intestine [9–14]. All four bacterial populations in the cecum at the end of the feeding trial were significantly elevated in the animals receiving the Red Hawk diet, when compared to the animals receiving the white and yellow bean diets (Figure 4). The probiotic microbial activity and fermentation of fiber in the intestinal lumen produce small chain fatty acids (SCFA) that include acetate, propionate, and butyrate [67–69]. These molecules are important to the metabolism and health of the digestive system because they promote intestinal cell proliferation and serve as an energy source for colonic epithelial cells [67–69]. The recovery of hemoglobin production in the animals receiving the Red Hawk diet by the end of the feeding trial, in conjunction with increased levels of bacteria populations in the cecum, indicates that the microbial composition of the lower intestine can be a contributing factor in the iron status of the host. These results are consistent with previous animal studies that show how dietary fiber can remodel the microbiota in the lower intestine; which in turn, can improve the morphometric parameters of the upper intestine by stimulating the proliferation of enterocytes and the height of duodenal villi [12–14,67,69]. These findings continue to support the idea that breeding for specific traits that promote the health and diversity of bacterial populations in the digestive system is an additional strategy that biofortification programs can use to improve the efficacy of biofortified food crops [14,70,71].

5. Conclusions

The comparisons between the different market classes of yellow and kidney beans tested in this study provide evidence that the iron bioavailability of yellow beans is unique from other bean color classes, and the important quality traits that distinguish yellows from other seed types at the market place, such as seed coat color and cooking time, are key factors in determining the iron benefits of yellow beans. The yellow bean's unique bio-delivery of iron provides a new phenotype breeding programs can utilize to improve the iron quality of new biofortified bean varieties, beyond just increasing raw seed iron concentrations [72]. Introducing traits similar to those found in the Manteca yellow bean that reduces the content of procyanidins (condensed tannins), while maintaining the yellow bean's abundance of kaempferol 3-glucoside, may have a profound impact on dry bean iron bioavailability.

Supplementary Materials: The following are available online at http://www.mdpi.com/2072-6643/11/8/1768/s1, Table S1, Sequences of Forward and Reverse Primers used for PCR Reactions to Measure Gene Expression of Iron Transporter Proteins in the Proximal Duodenum. Table S2, Phytate Concentrations of Each Dietary Component in Bean Based Diets. Table S3, Cumulative Feed Intake During the 6 Weeks of Consuming Bean Based Diets. Table S4, Cumulative Iron Intake During the 6 Weeks of Consuming Bean Based Diets. Table S5, Body Weights During the 6 Weeks of Consuming Bean Based Diets. Table S6, Total Body Hemoglobin Iron (Hb-Fe) During the 6 Weeks of Consuming Bean Based Diets. Table S7, Hemoglobin (Hb) Concentrations. Table S8, Hemoglobin Maintenance Efficacy (HME) During the 6 Weeks of Consuming Bean Based Diets.

Author Contributions: E.T., R.P.G., and K.A.C. led the research. All authors contributed to the conception and design of the experiments. J.A.W., N.K., and J.J.H. collected and analyzed the data. J.A.W. wrote the manuscript. R.P.G., K.A.C., N.K., J.J.H., and E.T. critically reviewed and edited the final draft of the manuscript.

Funding: This research was funded by the USDA-NIFA AFRI Grant # 2016-09666 and by the U.S. Department of Agriculture, Agricultural Research Service Projects 5050-21430-01000D (K.A.C.) and 8062-52000-001-00-D (R.P.G., E.T.).

Acknowledgments: We thank Desirre Morais Dias, Mary Bodis, Yongpei Chang, Shree Giri, and Scott Shaw for their technical expertise and assistance with sample preparation and analyses.

Conflicts of Interest: The authors declare no conflicts of interest. The contents of this publication do not necessarily reflect the views or policies of the U.S. Department of Agriculture, nor does the mention of trade names, commercial products, or organizations imply endorsement by the U.S. government.

Abbreviations

P. vulgaris	Phaseolus vulgaris L.
Hb-Fe	total body hemoglobin iron
Hb	hemoglobin
HME	hemoglobin maintenance efficiency
DMT-1	divalent metal transporter-1
DcytB	duodenal cytochrome B

References

1. Broughton, W.; Hernández, G.; Blair, M.; Beebe, S.; Gepts, P.; Vanderleyden, J. Beans (*Phaseolus* spp.)—Model food legumes. *Plant Soil* **2003**, *252*, 55–128. [CrossRef]
2. Connorton, J.; Balk, J.; Rodríguez-Celma, J. Iron homeostasis in plants—A brief overview. *Metallomics* **2017**, *9*, 813–823. [CrossRef] [PubMed]
3. Blair, M.; Izquierdo, P. Use of the advanced backcross-QTL method to transfer seed mineral accumulation nutrition traits from wild to Andean cultivated common beans. *Theor. Appl. Genet.* **2012**, *125*, 1015–1031. [CrossRef] [PubMed]
4. Petry, N.; Boy, E.; Wirth, J.; Hurrell, R. Review: The potential of the common bean (*Phaseolus vulgaris*) as a vehicle for iron biofortification. *Nutrients* **2015**, *7*, 1144–1173. [CrossRef] [PubMed]
5. Hart, J.; Tako, E.; Kochian, L.; Glahn, R. Identification of black bean (*Phaseolus vulgaris* L.) polyphenols that inhibit and promote iron uptake by Caco-2 cells. *J. Agric. Food Chem.* **2015**, *63*, 5950–5956. [CrossRef] [PubMed]
6. Tako, E.; Beebe, S.; Reed, S.; Hart, J.; Glahn, R. Polyphenolic compounds appear to limit the nutritional benefit of biofortified higher iron black bean (*Phaseolus vulgaris* L.). *Nutr. J.* **2014**, *13*, 28. [CrossRef]
7. Hart, J.; Tako, E.; Glahn, R. Characterization of polyphenol effects on inhibition and promotion of iron uptake by Caco-2 cells. *J. Agric. Food Chem.* **2017**, *65*, 3285–3294. [CrossRef]
8. Petry, N.; Egli, I.; Zeder, C.; Walczyk, T.; Hurrell, R. Polyphenols and phytic acid contribute to the low iron bioavailability from common beans in young women. *J. Nutr.* **2010**, *140*, 1977–1982. [CrossRef]
9. Larrosa, M.; Luceri, C.; Vivoli, E.; Pagliuca, C.; Lodovici, M.; Moneti, G.; Dolara, P. Polyphenol metabolites from colonic microbiota exert anti-inflammatory activity on different inflammation models. *Mol. Nutr. Food Res.* **2009**, *53*, 1044–1054. [CrossRef]
10. Chen, T.; Kim, C.; Kaur, A.; Lamothe, L.; Shaikh, M.; Keshavarzian, A.; Hamaker, B. Dietary fibre-based SCFA mixtures promote both protection and repair of intestinal epithelial barrier function in a Caco-2 cell model. *Food Funct.* **2017**, *8*, 1166–1173. [CrossRef]
11. Duda-Chodak, A.; Tarko, T.; Satora, P.; Sroka, P. Interaction of dietary compounds, especially polyphenols, with the intestinal microbiota: A review. *Eur. J. Nutr.* **2015**, *54*, 325–341. [CrossRef] [PubMed]
12. Pacifici, S.; Song, J.; Zhang, C.; Wang, Q.; Glahn, R.; Kolba, N.; Tako, E. Intra amniotic administration of raffinose and stachyose affects the intestinal brush border functionality and alters gut microflora populations. *Nutrients* **2017**, *9*, 304. [CrossRef] [PubMed]
13. Cardona, F.; Andrés-Lacueva, C.; Tulipani, S.; Tinahones, F.; Queipo-Ortuño, M. Benefits of polyphenols on gut microbiota and implications in human health. *J. Nutr. Biochem.* **2013**, *24*, 1415–1422. [CrossRef] [PubMed]
14. Dias, D.; Kolba, N.; Binyamin, D.; Ziv, O.; Regini Nutti, M.; Martino, H.; Glahn, R.; Koren, O.; Tako, E. Iron biofortified carioca bean (*Phaseolus vulgaris* L.)—Based Brazilian diet delivers more absorbable iron and affects the gut microbiota in vivo (*Gallus gallus*). *Nutrients* **2018**, *10*, 1970. [CrossRef] [PubMed]
15. Ganesan, K.; Xu, B. Polyphenol-rich dry common beans (*Phaseolus vulgaris* L.) and their health benefits. *Int. J. Mol. Sci.* **2017**, *18*, 2331. [CrossRef]

16. Lin, L.; Harnly, J.; Pastor-Corrales, M.; Luthria, D. The polyphenolic profiles of common beans (*Phaseolus vulgaris* L.). *Food Chem.* **2008**, *107*, 399–410. [CrossRef] [PubMed]
17. Beninger, C.; Hosfield, G.; Bassett, M. Flavonoid composition of three genotypes of dry bean (*Phaseolus vulgaris*) differing in seed coat color. *J. Am. Soc. Hortic. Sci.* **1999**, *124*, 514–518. [CrossRef]
18. Beninger, C.; Hosfield, G. Antioxidant activity of extracts, condensed tannin fractions, and pure flavonoids from *Phaseolus vulgaris* L. seed coat color genotypes. *J. Agric. Food Chem.* **2003**, *51*, 7879–7883. [CrossRef]
19. Bassett, M.; Lee, R.; Otto, C.; McClean, P. Classical and molecular genetic studies of the strong greenish yellow seedcoat color in 'Wagenaar' and 'Enola' common bean. *J. Am. Soc. Hortic. Sci.* **2002**, *127*, 50–55. [CrossRef]
20. Bassett, M. The seedcoat color genotype of 'Prim' and the Manteca and Coscorrón market classes of common bean. *HortScience* **1999**, *34*, 336–337. [CrossRef]
21. Harlan, J. *Crops and Man*; Foundations for Modern Corp Science; American Society of Agronomy, Inc.: Madison, WI, USA, 1975.
22. Voysest, O. *Yellow beans in Latin America*; Report 0084-7747; Centro Internacional de Agricultura Tropical (CIAT): Cali, Colombia, 2012.
23. Sichilima, T.; Mapemba, L.; Tembo, G. Drivers of dry common beans trade in Lusaka, Zambia: A trader's perspective. *Sustain. Agric. Res.* **2016**, *5*, 15–26. [CrossRef]
24. United Nations. *A Value Chain Analysis of the Dry Bean Sub-Sector in Uganda: Development of Inclusive Markets in Agriculture and Trade (DIMAT) Project*; United Nations Development Programme Uganda Issuing Body: Kampala, Uganda, 2012.
25. Wiesinger, J.; Cichy, K.; Tako, E.; Glahn, R. The fast cooking and enhanced iron bioavailability properties of the Manteca yellow bean (*Phaseolus vulgaris* L.). *Nutrients* **2018**, *10*, 1609. [CrossRef] [PubMed]
26. Palmer, S.; Winham, D.; Oberhauser, A.; Litchfield, R. Socio-ecological barriers to dry grain pulse consumption among low-income women: A mixed methods approach. *Nutrients* **2018**, *10*, 1108. [CrossRef] [PubMed]
27. Brouwer, I.; Hoorweg, J.; van Liere, M. When households run out of fuel: Responses of rural households to decreasing fuelwood availability, Ntcheu District, Malawi. *World Dev.* **1997**, *25*, 255–266. [CrossRef]
28. Hillocks, R.; Madata, C.; Chirwa, R.; Minja, E.; Msolla, S. Phaseolus bean improvement in Tanzania, 1959–2005. *Euphytica* **2006**, *150*, 215–231. [CrossRef]
29. Sones, D. Soya Njano is the bean for home consumption. In *Our Blog: The Inside Story*; Africa Soil Health Consortium: Nairobi, Kenya, 2015; Available online: http//africasoilhealth.cabi.org/2015/09/29/soya-njano-is-the-bean-for-home-consumption/ (accessed on 28 July 2017).
30. Kelly, J.; Varner, G.; Cichy, K.; Wright, E. Registration of 'Snowdon' white kidney bean. *J. Plant Regist.* **2012**, *6*, 238–242. [CrossRef]
31. Kelly, J.; Hosfield, G.; Varner, G.; Uebersax, M.; Long, R.; Taylor, J. Registration of 'Red Hawk' dark red kidney bean. *Crop Sci.* **1998**, *38*, 280–281. [CrossRef]
32. Morris, H.; Wood, E. Influence of moisture content on keeping quality of dry beans. *Food Technol.* **1956**, *10*, 225–229.
33. Wang, N.; Daun, J. Determination of cooking times of pulses using an automated Mattson cooker apparatus. *J. Sci. Food Agric.* **2005**, *85*, 1631–1635. [CrossRef]
34. AOAC. *Official Methods of Analysis of AOAC International*, 17th ed.; Association of Official Analytical Chemists: Rockville, MD, USA, 2000.
35. Jones, D. *Factors for Converting Percentages of Nitrogen in Foods and Feeds into Percentages of Proteins*; USDA: Washington, DC, USA, 1931.
36. AOAC. *Official Methods of Analysis of AOAC International*, 16th ed.; Association of Official Analytical Chemists International: Gaithersburg, MD, USA, 1997; Volume 2.
37. Glahn, R.; Lee, O.; Yeung, A.; Goldman, M.; Miller, D. Caco-2 cell ferritin formation predicts nonradiolabeled food iron availability in an in vitro digestion/Caco-2 cell culture model. *J. Nutr.* **1998**, *128*, 1555–1561. [CrossRef]
38. Tako, E.; Bar, H.; Glahn, R. The combined application of the Caco-2 cell bioassay coupled with in vivo (*Gallus gallus*) feeding trial represents an effective approach to predicting Fe bioavailability in humans. *Nutrients* **2016**, *8*, 732. [CrossRef]
39. Glahn, R.; Tako, E.; Hart, J.; Haas, J.; Lung'aho, M.; Beebe, S. Iron bioavailability studies of the first generation of iron-biofortified beans released in Rwanda. *Nutrients* **2017**, *9*, 787. [CrossRef]

40. Tako, E.; Blair, M.; Glahn, R. Biofortified red mottled beans (*Phaseolus vulgaris* L.) in a maize and bean diet provide more bioavailable iron than standard red mottled beans: Studies in poultry (*Gallus gallus*) and an in vitro digestion/Caco-2 model. *Nutr. J.* **2011**, *10*, 113. [CrossRef]
41. Tako, E.; Reed, S.; Anandaraman, A.; Beebe, S.; Hart, J.; Glahn, R. Studies of cream seeded carioca beans (*Phaseolus vulgaris* L.) from a Rwandan efficacy trial: In vitro and in vivo screening tools reflect human studies and predict beneficial results from iron biofortified beans. *PLoS ONE* **2015**, *10*, e0138479. [CrossRef]
42. Tako, E.; Glahn, R. White beans provide more bioavailable iron than red beans: Studies in poultry (*Gallus gallus*) and an in vitro digestion/Caco-2 model. *Int. J. Vitam. Nutr. Res.* **2010**, *80*, 416–429. [CrossRef]
43. Mete, A.; van Zeeland, Y.; Vaandrager, A.; Van Dijk, J.; Marx, J.; Dorrestein, G. Partial purification and characterization of ferritin from the liver and intestinal mucosa of chickens, turtledoves and mynahs. *Avian Pathol.* **2005**, *34*, 430–434. [CrossRef]
44. Passaniti, A.; Roth, T. Purification of chicken liver ferritin by two novel methods and structural comparison with horse spleen ferritin. *Biochem. J.* **1989**, *258*, 413–419. [CrossRef]
45. Zhu, X.; Zhong, T.; Pandya, Y.; Joerger, R. 16S rRNA-based analysis of microbiota from the cecum of broiler chickens. *Appl. Environ. Microbiol.* **2002**, *68*, 124–137. [CrossRef]
46. Barampama, Z.; Simard, R. Oligosaccharides, antinutritional factors and protein digestibility of dry beans as affected by processing. *J. Food Sci.* **1994**, *59*, 833–838. [CrossRef]
47. McClean, P.; Moghaddam, S.; Lopéz-Millán, A.; Brick, M.; Kelly, J.; Miklas, P.; Osorno, J.; Porch, T.; Urrea, C.; Soltani, A.; et al. Phenotypic diversity for seed mineral concentration in North American dry bean germplasm of Middle American ancestry. *Crop Sci.* **2017**, *57*, 3129–3144. [CrossRef]
48. Wiesinger, J.; Cichy, K.; Glahn, R.; Grusak, M.; Brick, M.; Thompson, H.; Tako, E. Demonstrating a nutritional advantage to the fast-cooking dry bean (*Phaseolus vulgaris* L.). *J. Agric. Food Chem.* **2016**, *64*, 8592–8603. [CrossRef]
49. Tako, E.; Rutzke, M.; Glahn, R. Using the domestic chicken (*Gallus gallus*) as an in vivo model for iron bioavailability. *Poult. Sci.* **2010**, *89*, 514–521. [CrossRef]
50. Reed, S.; Neuman, H.; Glahn, R.; Koren, O.; Tako, E. Characterizing the gut (*Gallus gallus*) microbiota following the consumption of an iron biofortified Rwandan cream seeded carioca (*Phaseolus Vulgaris* L.) bean-based diet. *PLoS ONE* **2017**, *12*, e0182431. [CrossRef]
51. Yegani, M.; Korver, D. Factors affecting intestinal health in poultry. *Poult. Sci.* **2008**, *87*, 2052–2063. [CrossRef]
52. International Chicken Genome Sequencing Consortium. Sequence and comparative analysis of the chicken genome provide unique perspectives on vertebrate evolution. *Nature* **2004**, *432*, 695–716. [CrossRef]
53. Backhed, F. Host-bacterial mutualism in the human intestine. *Science* **2005**, *307*, 1915–1920. [CrossRef]
54. Qin, J.; Li, R.; Raes, J.; Arumugam, M.; Burgdorf, K.; Manichanh, C.; Nielsen, T.; Pons, N.; Levenez, F.; Yamada, T.; et al. A human gut microbial gene catalogue established by metagenomic sequencing. *Nature* **2010**, *464*, 59–65. [CrossRef]
55. Haas, J.; Luna, S.; Lung'aho, M.; Wenger, M.; Murray-Kolb, L.; Beebe, S.; Gahutu, J.; Egli, I. Consuming iron biofortified beans increases iron status in Rwandan women after 128 days in a randomized controlled feeding trial. *J. Nutr.* **2016**, *146*, 1586–1592. [CrossRef]
56. Beninger, C.; Hosfield, G. Flavonol glycosides from the seed coat of a new Manteca-type dry bean (*Phaseolus vulgaris* L.). *J. Agric. Food Chem.* **1998**, *46*, 2906–2910. [CrossRef]
57. Leakey, C.; Hosfield, G.; Dubois, A. Mantecas, a new class of beans (*Phaseolus vulgaris*) of enhanced digestibility. In Proceedings of the 3rd European Conference on Grain Legumes, Valladolid, Spain, 14–19 November 1998; pp. 336–337.
58. Hooper, S.; Wiesinger, J.; Echeverria, D.; Thompson, H.; Brick, M.; Nchimbi-Msolla, S.; Cichy, K. Carbohydrate profile of a dry bean (*Phaseolus vulgaris* L.) panel encompassing broad genetic variability for cooking time. *Cereal Chem. J.* **2017**, *94*, 135–141. [CrossRef]
59. Hosfield, G.; Bennink, M.; Beninger, C.; Engleright, R.; Ospina, M. Variability for starch digestibility in dry bean (*Phaseolus vulgaris* L.). *HortScience* **1998**, *33*, 472. [CrossRef]
60. Leakey, C. Breeding on the C and J and B loci for modification of bean seed coat flavonoids with the objective of improving food acceptability. *Annu. Rep. Bean Improv. Coop.* **1992**, *35*, 13–17.
61. Elia, F.; Hosfield, G.; Kelly, J.; Uebersax, M. Genetic analysis and interrelationships between traits for cooking time, water absorption, and protein and tannin content of Andean dry beans. *J. Am. Soc. Hortic. Sci.* **1997**, *122*, 512–518. [CrossRef]

62. Ozdal, T.; Capanoglu, E.; Altay, F. A review on protein—Phenolic interactions and associated changes. *Food Res. Int.* **2013**, *51*, 954–970. [CrossRef]
63. Murgia, I.; Arosio, P.; Tarantino, D.; Soave, C. Biofortification for combating 'hidden hunger' for iron. *Trends Plant Sci.* **2012**, *17*, 47–55. [CrossRef]
64. Clark, S.; Duncan, A. The role of pulses in satiety, food intake and body weight management. *J. Funct. Food* **2017**, *38*, 612–623. [CrossRef]
65. Adam, C.; Williams, P.; Garden, K.; Thomson, L.; Ross, A. Dose-dependent effects of a soluble dietary fibre (pectin) on food intake, adiposity, gut hypertrophy and gut satiety hormone secretion in rats. *PLoS ONE* **2015**, *10*, e0115438. [CrossRef]
66. Glahn, R.; Tako, E.; Cichy, K.; Wiesinger, J. The cotyledon cell wall and intracellular matrix are factors that limit iron bioavailability of the common bean (*Phaseolus vulgaris*). *Food Funct.* **2016**, *7*, 3193–3200. [CrossRef]
67. Ding, X.; Li, D.; Bai, S.; Wang, J.; Zeng, Q.; Su, Z.; Xuan, Y.; Zhang, K. Effect of dietary xylooligosaccharides on intestinal characteristics, gut microbiota, cecal short-chain fatty acids, and plasma immune parameters of laying hens. *Poult. Sci.* **2018**, *97*, 874–881. [CrossRef]
68. Tan, J.; McKenzie, C.; Potamitis, M.; Thorburn, A.; Mackay, C.; Macia, L. The role of short-chain fatty acids in health and disease. In *Advances in Immunology*; Elsevier: Amsterdam, The Netherlands, 2014; Volume 121, pp. 91–119.
69. Sakata, T. Stimulatory effect of short-chain fatty acids on epithelial cell proliferation in the rat intestine: A possible explanation for trophic effects of fermentable fibre, gut microbes and luminal trophic factors. *Brit. J. Nutr.* **1987**, *58*, 95–103. [CrossRef]
70. Yeung, C.; Glahn, R.; Welch, R.; Miller, D. Prebiotics and iron bioavailability-is there a connection? *J. Food Sci.* **2005**, *70*, R88–R92. [CrossRef]
71. Welch, R.M. *Biofortification Progress Briefs: Breeding for Improved Micronutrient Bioavailability and Gut Health*; HarvestPlus, c/o IFPRI: Washington, DC, USA, 2014; pp. 53–54.
72. Vasconcelos, M.; Gruissem, W.; Bhullar, N. Iron biofortification in the 21st century: Setting realistic targets, overcoming obstacles, and new strategies for healthy nutrition. *Curr. Opin. Biotechnol.* **2017**, *44*, 8–15. [CrossRef]

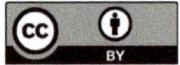 © 2019 by the authors. Licensee MDPI, Basel, Switzerland. This article is an open access article distributed under the terms and conditions of the Creative Commons Attribution (CC BY) license (http://creativecommons.org/licenses/by/4.0/).

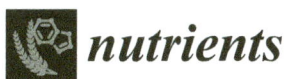

Article

Investigation of Nicotianamine and 2′ Deoxymugineic Acid as Enhancers of Iron Bioavailability in Caco-2 Cells

Jesse T. Beasley [1,*], Jonathan J. Hart [2], Elad Tako [2], Raymond P. Glahn [2] and Alexander A. T. Johnson [1]

1. School of BioSciences, The University of Melbourne, Victoria 3010, Australia
2. Robert W. Holley Center for Agriculture and Health, USDA-ARS, Ithaca, NY 14853, USA
* Correspondence: jesse.beasley@unimelb.edu.au; Tel.: +61-8344-7463

Received: 1 June 2019; Accepted: 28 June 2019; Published: 30 June 2019

Abstract: Nicotianamine (NA) is a low-molecular weight metal chelator in plants with high affinity for ferrous iron (Fe^{2+}) and other divalent metal cations. In graminaceous plant species, NA serves as the biosynthetic precursor to 2′ deoxymugineic acid (DMA), a root-secreted mugineic acid family phytosiderophore that chelates ferric iron (Fe^{3+}) in the rhizosphere for subsequent uptake by the plant. Previous studies have flagged NA and/or DMA as enhancers of Fe bioavailability in cereal grain although the extent of this promotion has not been quantified. In this study, we utilized the Caco-2 cell system to compare NA and DMA to two known enhancers of Fe bioavailability—epicatechin (Epi) and ascorbic acid (AsA)—and found that both NA and DMA are stronger enhancers of Fe bioavailability than Epi, and NA is a stronger enhancer of Fe bioavailability than AsA. Furthermore, NA reversed Fe uptake inhibition by Myricetin (Myr) more than Epi, highlighting NA as an important target for biofortification strategies aimed at improving Fe bioavailability in staple plant foods.

Keywords: biofortification; iron deficiency anemia; iron absorption; ferritin; ascorbic acid; epicatechin

---

1. Introduction

Iron (Fe) possesses unique redox properties that are critical to fundamental biological processes such as cellular respiration and photosynthesis [1]. Although abundant in soil, Fe is largely unavailable for plant uptake under aerobic or calcisol (high pH) conditions (representing ~30% of arable land), due to the formation of insoluble ferric (Fe^{3+}) ion precipitates [2]. As well as negatively impacting on plant growth, inadequate plant Fe uptake translates to human Fe deficiency, as plants provide a major gateway for Fe into human food systems [3]. Plants have evolved sophisticated mechanisms to absorb Fe from the rhizosphere through reduction and/or chelation of Fe^{3+} [2]. Non-graminaceous plants such as common bean (*Phaseolus vulgaris* L.) reduce soil Fe^{3+} ions to the more soluble ferrous (Fe^{2+}) form for uptake into plant roots [4]. By contrast, graminaceous plants such as bread wheat (*Triticum aestivum* L.) secrete mugineic acid phytosiderophores, the most common of which is 2′deoxymugineic acid (DMA), into soil to chelate Fe^{3+} for plant uptake [5]. Some plant species such as rice (*Oryza sativa* L.) utilize aspects of both strategies to maximize Fe uptake under a variety of soil and pH conditions [2].

Within the plant cell, Fe is complexed to chelating agents or is sequestered into plant vacuoles to avoid cellular damage caused by Fe^{2+} oxidation and reactive oxygen species (ROS) formation [3]. Low-molecular weight compounds like citrate, malate, nicotianamine (NA) and the oligopeptide transporter family protein (OPT3) are major chelators of phloem/xylem Fe within all higher plants while DMA is an additional chelator in graminaceous plants. Citrate, NA, DMA and OPT3 all function in the transport of Fe from source tissues (i.e., root, leaf) to sink tissues (i.e., leaf, seed) for Fe storage and/or utilization [4]. Within the leaf, most Fe is bound in a phytoferritin complex within the chloroplast [6]. Leaf Fe is liberated from the phytoferritin complex during senescence and chelated by citrate, NA and/or DMA for transport to the developing seed [4]. Once in the seed of non-graminaceous plants, the proportion of Fe stored in embryonic, seed coat, and provascular tissues is heavily influenced by species, genotype and environment [7,8]. The Fe within embryonic tissue is primarily bound to phytoferritin and represents between 18% to 42% of total seed iron in soybeans (*Glycine max* L.) and peas (*Pisum sativum* L.), respectively [9]. The Fe within the seed coat of common bean ranges between 4% and 26% of total seed iron and is bound primarily to polyphenolic compounds, such as flavonoids and tannins [8,10,11]. The majority of seed Fe therefore accumulates in cotyledonary tissues and is likely bound to inositol hexakisphosphate (also known as phytate) within cell vacuoles, or to small metal chelators like NA in the cytoplasm [7,12]. Certain leguminous plants like soybean and chickpea (*Cicer arietinum* L.) accumulate seed NA to very high concentrations (up to a 1:2 molar ratio with Fe), suggesting that a large proportion of seed Fe is cytoplasmic in these species [13,14]. Graminaceous plant seeds (i.e., grain) store the majority of Fe (~80% of total grain Fe) as phytate complexes in vacuolar regions of the outer aleurone layer [3,15,16]. The remaining Fe within the sub-aleurone and endosperm regions (~20% of total grain Fe) is bound to phytate in intracellular phytin-globoids or chelated to NA and/or DMA (1:0.1 molar ratio with Fe) within the cytoplasm [17–20].

The absorption of dietary Fe in humans (bioavailability) depends on several factors apart from Fe concentration alone. The Fe within plant-based foods is mostly comprised of low-molecular weight (i.e., phytate, NA) and high-molecular weight (i.e., ferritin) compounds and is collectively referred to as non-heme Fe [6]. Non-heme Fe bioavailability is generally low (5–12%) and influenced by the concentration of inhibitors (phytate, polyphenols, calcium, etc.) and enhancers, like ascorbic acid (AsA), in the diet [21,22]. Phytate is the major inhibitor of Fe bioavailability in whole-grain foods, although certain polyphenolic compounds such as myricetin (Myr) and quercetin exhibit a greater inhibitory effect in bean-based diets [10,21,22]. Both phytate and Myr form high affinity complexes with Fe^{3+} that are poorly absorbed across the human intestinal surface [23–25]. Other polyphenolic flavanoids present in wheat embryonic and bean seed coat tissues are widely presumed to inhibit Fe bioavailability through pro-oxidation of Fe^{2+} and/or chelation of Fe^{3+} [21,26,27]. Enhancers of Fe bioavailability such as AsA (the strongest enhancer identified to date) are typically antioxidants that reduce Fe^{3+} and prevent polyphenols binding to newly formed Fe^{2+} ions that are highly bioavailable [22]. Some polyphenols such as epicatechin (Epi) are also thought to reduce Fe^{3+} to Fe^{2+} and can therefore act as potent Fe bioavailability enhancers [21]. Another mechanism of promoting Fe bioavailability is thought to be through direct chelation of Fe^{2+} for uptake in the human small intestine such as that proposed for glycosaminoglycans and proteoglycans [22,28,29]. Nicotianamine has been suggested to enhance Fe bioavailability in Fe biofortified polished rice grains and Fe biofortified white wheat flour, although the extent of this promotion is unclear [17,18,30–32]. Whether DMA, also enhances or inhibits Fe bioavailability is unknown and increased knowledge regarding NA and DMA promotion of Fe bioavailability is needed. Identification of enhancers and inhibitors of Fe bioavailability has traditionally relied on manipulation of dietary components in lengthy human or animal feeding trials [33]. By contrast, the Caco-2 cell bioassay allows rapid investigation of diverse dietary components and accurate estimation of Fe uptake by human intestinal epithelial cells [21,34–36].

Due in large part to high consumption of cereal-based diets that are low in bioavailable Fe, human Fe deficiency is the most common nutritional disorder worldwide and is particularly widespread in less-developed countries [37]. Severe Fe deficiency causes iron-deficiency anemia (IDA), a condition that impairs cognitive development and increases maternal and child mortality, affecting over 40% of pregnant women and preschool-age children worldwide [38–40]. Biofortification efforts aimed at increasing micronutrient intake from staple food consumption represent a key component of alleviating global human IDA, yet there is heavy bias towards increased micronutrient concentration with less regard for bioavailability [41,42]. Recent biofortification studies in rice and wheat have increased NA and/or DMA biosynthesis to enhance both Fe concentration and bioavailability [17,20,28,29,43,44]. Increasing NA/DMA biosynthesis in wheat results in higher Fe accumulation in grain endosperm and increased Fe bioavailability in white flour that is highly correlated with NA and DMA concentration [17]. Understanding the extent to which NA and/or DMA enhance Fe bioavailability is therefore critical to determining the effectiveness of these Fe biofortification programs. Here we utilize modifications of the Caco-2 cell bioassay to characterize NA and DMA as enhancers of *in vitro* Fe bioavailability through comparison to known enhancers (Epi and AsA) and in a competitive assay with the inhibitor Myr.

2. Materials and Methods

2.1. Chemicals

Epicatechin, Myr, dimethyl sulfoxide (DMSO), glucose, hydrocortisone, insulin, selenium, triiodothyronine, and epidermal growth factor were purchased from Sigma-Aldrich (St. Louis, MO, USA). Nicotianamine and DMA were purchased from Toronto Research Chemicals Inc. (Toronto, Canada). Sodium bicarbonate and piperazine-N,N'-bis[2-ethanesulfonic acid] (PIPES) were purchased from Fisher Scientific (Waltham, MA, USA). Iron standard (1000 µg/mL in 2% HCl) was from High-Purity Standards (Charleston, SC, USA). Modified Eagle's medium (MEM), Dulbecco's modified Eagle's medium (DMEM), and 1% antibiotic–antimycotic solution were purchased from Gibco (Grand Island, NY, USA).

2.2. Preparation of Metabolite and Fe solutions

Epicatechin and Myr were dissolved in DMSO (100%) to a concentration of 1.6 mM and NA and DMA were dissolved in DMSO (50%) and 18 MΩ H2O (50%) to a concentration of 0.8 mM. All solutions were diluted with pH 2 saline solution (140 mM NaCl, 5 mM KCl, adjusted to pH 2 with HCl) to achieve 400 µM stock solutions and subsequently diluted with pH 2 saline solution to appropriate concentrations for use in Caco-2 assays. To minimize toxicity to Caco-2 cells, the maximum DMSO concentration in 30 µM Epi/Myr treatments was 1.9% (2.5% in 40 µM polyphenol treatments). Fe stock solutions were prepared from 1000 mg/mL Fe standard in pH 2 saline solution. A 50 µL aliquot of Fe^{2+} stock solution of appropriate concentration was added to 150 µL of prepared metabolite solutions to achieve the desired Fe/metabolite concentration.

2.3. Caco-2 Assays

The Caco-2 cell assays were performed as previously described [21]. Briefly, cells were cultured in 24-well plates (Corning Costar 24 Well Clear TC-Treated Multiple Well Plates) coated with collagen and maintained in supplemented DMEM [3.7 g/L sodium bicarbonate, 25 mM HEPES (pH 7.2), 10% fetal bovine serum] for 12 days postseeding. Twenty-four hours prior to experiments, DMEM was replaced with iron-free supplemented MEM as previously described [36]. The Fe/metabolite solution (200 µL) was incubated (~22 °C, 15 min) and combined with 1 mL of MEM before an aliquot (500 µL) was directly applied to Caco-2 cell monolayers. After overnight incubation (37 °C), cells were washed twice with a buffered saline solution (130 mM NaCl, 5 mM KCl, 5 mM PIPES (pH 6.7)) and lysed by the addition of 0.5 mL 18 MΩ H2O. In an aliquot of the lysed Caco-2 cell solution, ferritin content was determined using an immunoradiometric assay (FER-IRON II Ferritin Assay, Ramco Laboratories, Houston, TX) and total protein content was determined using a colorimetric assay (Bio-Rad DC Protein Assay, Bio-Rad, Hercules, CA) as previously described [36]. As Caco-2 cells synthesize ferritin in response to intracellular Fe, we used the proportion of ferritin/total cell protein (expressed as ng ferritin/mg protein) as an index of cellular Fe uptake and refer to this as 'Fe uptake' throughout the manuscript.

2.4. Graphical Representation and Statistical Analysis

Each figure includes three control treatments as indicated by the white, grey and black bars on the right side of each panel. The first control treatment, "cell baseline", represents ferritin formation in Caco-2 cells in the absence of any metabolite or Fe. The second control treatment, either "+ 4 µM Fe" or "+ 40 µM Fe", represents ferritin formation in the presence of 4 µM Fe (typical Fe concentration for Caco-2 cell assays) or 40 µM Fe alone, respectively. A dotted line between both y-axes is provided to easily compare treatments to this control. The third control treatment, either "+ 80 µM AsA" or "+ 800 µM AsA", represents ferritin formation in the presence of 4 µM Fe with 80 µM AsA or 40 µM Fe with 800 µM AsA (i.e., an Fe:AsA ratio of 1:20), respectively. In Figures 1–3, triangular data points represent a fourth control treatment of ferritin formation in Caco-2 cells in the presence of NA, DMA, Epi or AsA solutions without Fe, and displayed values equivalent to the Cell Baseline. Data represent ng ferritin/mg protein in Caco-2 assays and were generated using SigmaPlot software (v.13.0, Systat Software, San Jose, CA, USA). Statistical differences between means were analyzed by unpaired Student's t-test, and differences among means were assessed using one-way analysis of variance (ANOVA) with Tukey or Hsu's MCB post-hoc tests, using Minitab software (v 18.0, Minitab, State College, PA, USA).

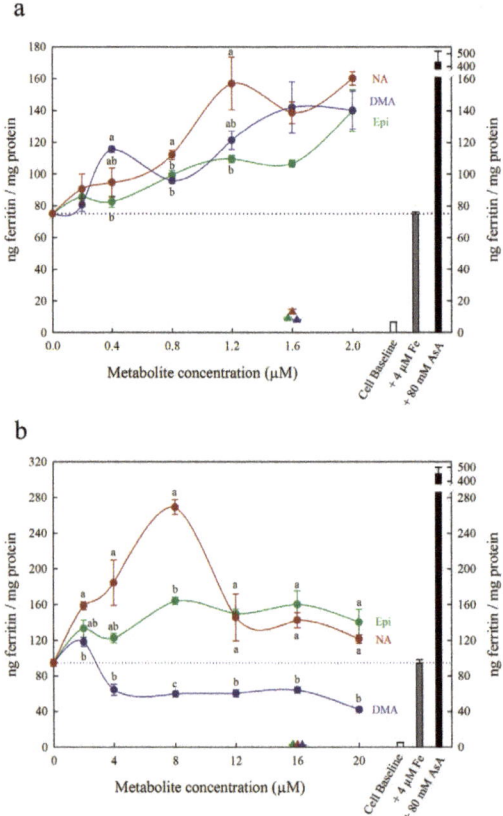

Figure 1. Ferritin formation in Caco-2 cells in response to nicotianamine (NA, red), 2' deoxymugineic acid (DMA, blue) and epicatechin (Epi, green) at concentrations varying between (**a**) 0 and 2.0 µM and (**b**) 0 and 20 µM in solution with Fe (4 µM). Triangles indicate ferritin formation at metabolite solutions (1.6 µM or 16 µM) without Fe. Dotted line indicates ferritin response to 4 µM Fe alone and is extended to both y axes to facilitate comparison with other treatments. Error bars represent standard error of the mean of three replicates. Different letters indicate significantly different ferritin formation between metabolites of the same concentration as analyzed by one-way ANOVA with Tukey post-hoc test ($p < 0.05$).

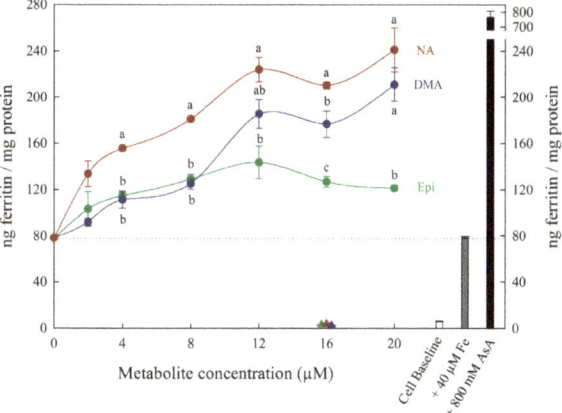

Figure 2. Ferritin formation in Caco-2 cells in response to varying concentrations (0–20 µM) of nicotianamine (NA, red), 2′ deoxymugineic acid (DMA, blue) and epicatechin (Epi, green) at concentrations varying between 0–20 µM in solution with Fe (40 µM). Triangles indicate ferritin formation in metabolite solutions (16 µM) without Fe. Dotted line indicates ferritin response to 40 µM Fe alone and is extended to both y axes to facilitate comparison with other treatments. Error bars represent standard error of the mean of three replicates. Different letters indicate significantly different ferritin formation between metabolites of the same concentration as analyzed by one-way ANOVA with Tukey post-hoc test ($p < 0.05$).

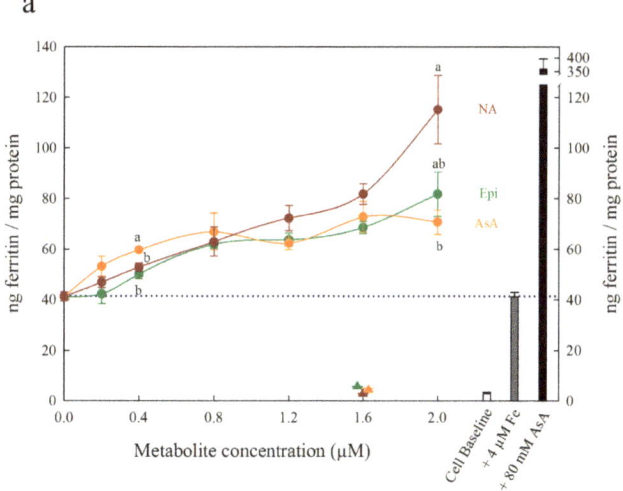

Figure 3. *Cont.*

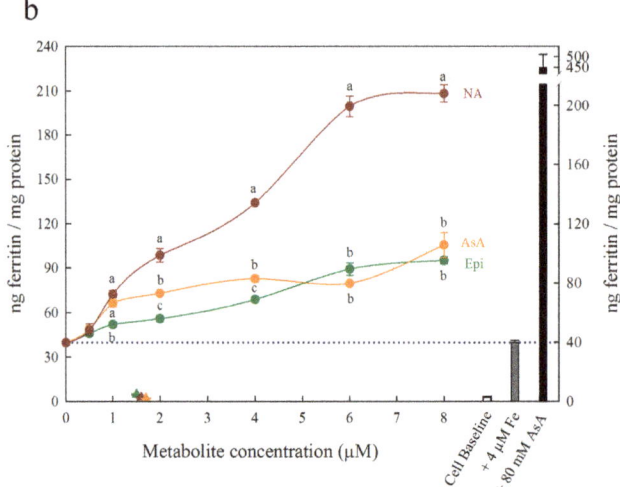

Figure 3. Ferritin formation in Caco-2 cells in response to nicotianamine (NA, red), ascorbic acid (AsA, orange) and epicatechin (Epi, green) at concentrations varying between (**a**) 0–2.0 µM and (**b**) 0–8 µM in solution with Fe (4 µM). Triangles indicate ferritin formation in metabolite solutions (1.6 µM) without Fe. Dotted line indicates ferritin response to 4 µM Fe alone and is extended to both y axes to facilitate comparison with other treatments. Error bars represent standard error of the mean of three replicates. Different letters indicate significantly different ferritin formation between metabolites of the same concentration as analyzed by one-way ANOVA with Tukey post-hoc test ($p < 0.05$).

3. Results

All low concentrations (≤2 µM) of NA, DMA and Epi enhanced Fe uptake into Caco-2 cells, with NA and DMA promoting ferritin formation more than Epi (Figure 1a). Higher concentrations (between 2–20 µM) of NA and Epi enhanced Fe uptake, and higher concentrations of DMA inhibited Fe uptake (Figure 1b). Between concentrations of 2 and 8 µM, NA enhanced Fe uptake more significantly than Epi with peak ferritin formation at 8 µM (i.e., a 1:2 molar ratio with Fe). At Fe molar ratios of 1:3, 1:4 and 1:5, NA and Epi promoted ferritin formation at the same level (Figure 1b and Table S1). At a higher concentration of Fe (40 µM), NA enhanced Fe uptake significantly more than Epi at all concentrations apart from 2 µM, and DMA enhanced Fe uptake significantly more than Epi at 16 and 20 µM (Figure 2). Together, these results demonstrate that NA > DMA > Epi in the promotion of Fe uptake into Caco-2 cells. As the stronger enhancer, NA was compared in subsequent assays alongside Epi and AsA. All low concentrations (<2 µM) of NA, Epi and AsA enhanced Fe uptake into Caco-2 cells at similar levels, with NA showing significantly higher ferritin formation at 2 µM (Figure 3a). Above 2 µM, NA enhanced Fe uptake significantly more than both Epi and AsA with peak ferritin formation at 8 µM, demonstrating that NA > AsA > Epi in the promotion of Fe uptake into Caco-2 cells (Figure 3b). Across all experiments with Fe:metabolite molar ratios ≤ 1:2, the fold increase in ferritin formation over the Fe control was significantly higher in Caco-2 cells exposed to NA compared to AsA, Epi or DMA (Figure 4). To further characterize NA as a strong enhancer of Fe bioavailability, ferritin formation was measured in response to the Fe uptake inhibitor Myr in combination with NA (NA:Myr) or Epi (Epi:Myr). At 4 µM, total metabolite concentration, all NA:Myr solutions enhanced Fe uptake significantly more than Epi:Myr, and a NA:Myr solution of ratio 30:70 increased ferritin formation more than the Fe control (Figure 5a). At 30 µM total metabolite concentration, NA:Myr solutions of ratio 70:30, 80:20 and 90:10 enhanced Fe uptake significantly more than Epi:Myr, and a NA:Myr solution of ratio 90:10 increased ferritin formation more than the Fe control (Figure 5b).

Together these results demonstrate that NA is stronger than Epi in counteracting the inhibitory effect of Myr and enhancing Fe uptake into Caco-2 cells.

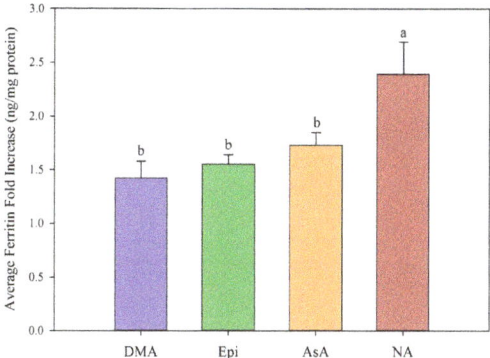

Figure 4. Average fold increase in Caco-2 cell ferritin formation in response to 2′ deoxymugineic acid (DMA, blue), epicatechin (Epi, green), ascorbic acid (AsA, orange), and nicotianamine (NA, red) at Fe:metabolite molar ratios ≤ 1:2 compared to ferritin formation in the presence of Fe alone. Error bars represent standard error of the mean of at least eight replicates. Different letters indicate significant differences between mean fold increase in ferritin formation between metabolites as analyzed by one-way ANOVA with Hsu's MCB post-hoc test ($p < 0.05$).

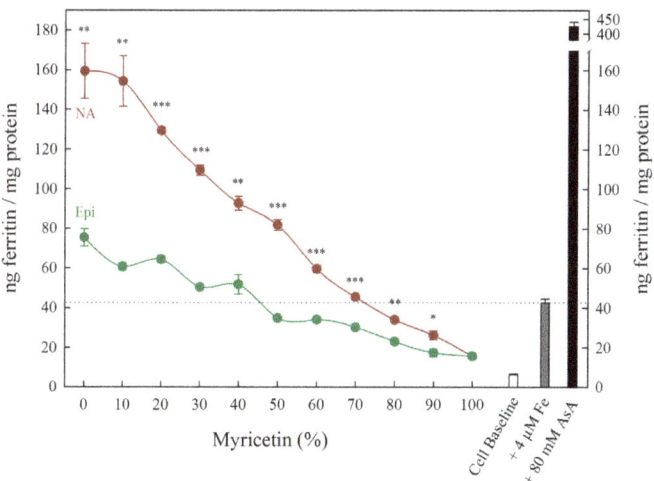

Figure 5. *Cont.*

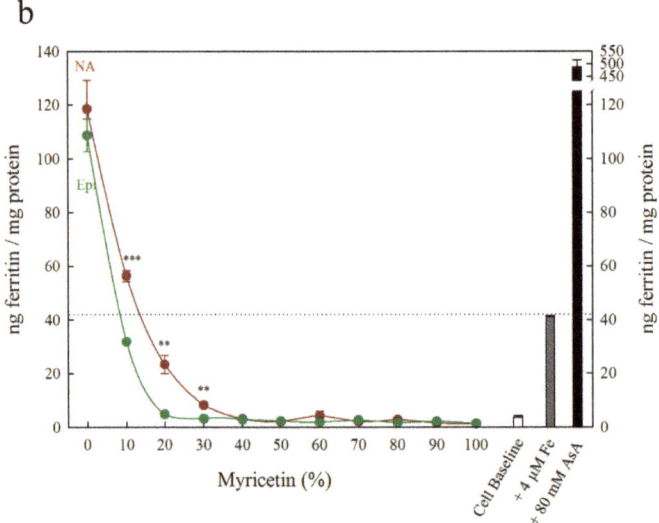

Figure 5. Ferritin formation in Caco-2 cells in response to various molar ratios of nicotianamine:myricetin (NA, red) and epicatechin:myricetin (Epi, green). Total metabolite concentration at each data point was (a) 4 µM and (b) 30 µM. Dotted line indicates ferritin response to 4 µM Fe alone and is extended to both y axes to facilitate comparison with other treatments. Error bars represent standard error of the mean of three replicates. Asterisks denote the significance between NA and Epi at each molar ratio for $p < 0.05$ (*), $p \leq 0.01$ (**), $p \leq 0.001$ (***) as determined by Student's t-test.

4. Discussion

At low ($\leq$1:2) Fe:metabolite molar ratios, NA and DMA enhanced Caco-2 cell ferritin formation more than Epi. Interestingly, the level of promotion was more pronounced at 40 µM Fe concentration compared to 4 µM Fe, despite maintaining the same Fe:metabolite molar ratios (Figures 1a and 2). As ferritin formation was similar in the 'Fe control' at both 4 µM and 40 µM, it is likely that maximum Fe solubility is exceeded somewhere between 4 µM and 40 µM Fe in the absence of any Fe bioavailability enhancer (Figures 1 and 2). Although we provide strong evidence to support NA and DMA as enhancers of Fe bioavailability, the exact mechanism of how NA and DMA facilitate Fe uptake into Caco-2 cells remains unknown and is likely dependent on the proportion of readily bioavailable ferrous Fe^{2+} ions in solution [21]. Both NA and DMA form high affinity 1:1 complexes with Fe^{3+} ions, however only NA is thought to be capable of binding Fe^{2+} [45,46]. Here we demonstrate that DMA promotes ferritin formation at Fe:DMA molar ratios less than 1:1, suggesting that DMA is capable of binding Fe^{2+} and/or reducing Fe^{3+} ions to some degree and requires further investigation. The decreased ferritin formation after exposure to Fe:DMA solutions with molar ratio > 1:1 (Figure 1b) could be due to oxidation of Fe^{2+} ions in solution and excess formation of Fe^{3+}–DMA complexes that have low bioavailability for Caco-2 cell Fe uptake [45]. Some polyphenol compounds capable of complexing Fe^{3+} (e.g., delphinidin and delphinidin 3-glucoside) also demonstrate this biphasic pattern of promoting Fe uptake at molar ratios < 1:1 and inhibiting Fe uptake at molar ratios > 1:1 [21].

Nicotianamine promoted Caco-2 cell Fe uptake at all molar ratios observed, likely due to the formation of stable Fe^{2+}–NA complexes and facilitation of Fe^{2+} uptake. As Fe is provided in a reduced Fe^{2+} state when preparing the assay, Fe^{2+}–NA complexes rapidly form after NA addition and maintain the reduced Fe^{2+} state during exposure to Caco-2 cells. Certain polyphenols are also suggested to promote Caco-2 cell Fe uptake via a similar mechanism of binding Fe^{2+} and slowing the oxidation of Fe^{2+} to Fe^{3+} [21]. The reduced ferritin formation at Fe:NA molar ratios over 1:2 may be due to excess binding of Fe^{2+} by NA, preventing the release of Fe^{2+} for Caco-2 cell uptake, and suggests that an Fe:NA molar ratio less than 1:2 is optimal for promoting Fe bioavailability (Figure 1b, Table S1). Alternatively, NA could enhance Fe bioavailability via direct uptake of Fe^{2+}-NA in a similar mechanism to that proposed for glycosaminoglycans and proteoglycans and exploring this mechanism will be the subject of future research [28,29].

Ascorbic acid promotes Fe uptake into Caco-2 cells through *de novo* reduction of Fe^{3+} ions and maintenance of the Fe^{2+} ions in solution [9,21,22]. Here we demonstrate that at Fe:metabolite molar ratios less than 1:2, NA enhances Caco-2 cell ferritin formation significantly more than AsA and is the strongest enhancer of *in vitro* Fe bioavailability identified to date (Figures 3b and 4). Together, these results suggest that the ability to bind Fe^{2+} ions is critical to enhancing Fe uptake into human intestinal cells. At an Fe:AsA molar ratio of 1:20, complete *de novo* reduction of Fe^{3+} ions in solution (without Fe^{2+} binding) leads to an ~8-fold increase in Caco-2 cell ferritin levels compared to Fe alone (Table S1). An Fe:NA molar ratio of 1:20 was not tested as this ratio does not occur naturally in plant foods, although it is unlikely to show high ferritin formation given the effect of ratios greater than 1:2 (Table S1). Instead, molar ratios less than 1:2 capture the highest ratio of Fe:NA measured to date in conventional plants foods (Fe:NA ratio of 1:1.6 in biofortified soybean) and provide realistic targets for plant breeders to improve Fe bioavailability [13].

To rule out the possibility that NA, DMA, Epi or AsA were promoting Caco-2 cell ferritin formation independent of Fe, Caco-2 cells were exposed to these metabolites alone in concentrations equal to 1.6 µM or 16 µM (Figures 1–3). There was no sign that the metabolite presence alone significantly increased Caco-2 ferritin formation relative to the cell baseline or disrupted the Caco-2 cell monolayer at harvest. Thus, the increased ferritin formation observed in Caco-2 cells exposed to Fe:metabolite solutions is due to the Fe uptake promoting properties of these metabolites.

Although Myr is a potent antioxidant with Fe-reducing properties (normally characteristic of Fe uptake enhancers), it strongly inhibits Caco-2 cell Fe uptake as it forms highly stable Fe–Myr complexes with low Fe bioavailability [47,48]. Nicotianamine increased ferritin formation compared to Epi at all 4 µM solutions and at 30 µM solutions containing over 70% NA or Epi, demonstrating that NA is stronger than Epi at preventing Fe uptake inhibition by Myr (Figure 5). At 30 µM, ferritin formation was equivalent to cell baseline for solutions containing less than 70% NA or 90% Epi, demonstrating that Myr inhibits Fe uptake more effectively than NA/Epi promotes Fe uptake (Figure 5b). At 4 µM (the equivalent of a 1:1 molar ratio with Fe), 30% NA combined with 70% Myr promoted ferritin formation above the Fe control, suggesting that NA can outcompete Myr and form Fe^{2+}–NA complexes with high bioavailability (Figure 5a). An additional assay at 10 µM demonstrated an intermediate response, with low ferritin formation at 20% Myr due to improper Caco-2 cell growth (Figure S1).

Whether NA would enhance Fe bioavailability in the presence of several enhancers and inhibitors (i.e., a bean-based food sample) is unclear. To date, increased NA has not overcome the inhibitory effect of polyphenols/phytate to enhance *in vitro* Fe bioavailability within biofortified whole wheat grain [17]. To further address this question, future studies should explore NA biofortification within plant foods that contain high endogenous NA levels and low Fe:polyphenol molar ratios (e.g., 1:2 in carioca beans) [21]. Nonetheless, plant species with inherently low polyphenol levels (i.e., wheat) serve as ideal candidates for enhanced Fe bioavailability through the overproduction of NA [26,49]. The additional role of NA in the biosynthesis of DMA (itself an enhancer of Fe bioavailability) further reinforces increased NA biosynthesis as an effective cereal biofortification strategy to improve global human Fe nutrition.

5. Conclusions

We utilized a modified Caco-2 cell bioassay to characterize two low-molecular-weight plant metal chelators – NA and DMA – as strong enhancers of Fe bioavailability and demonstrate that NA is also capable of reversing Fe uptake inhibition by Myr. In doing so we highlight NA and DMA as important targets for biofortification strategies aimed at improving Fe bioavailability in cereals. Although we suspect that NA and DMA promote Fe bioavailability in Caco-2 cells by maintaining Fe^{2+} ions in solution, uncovering the exact mechanism by which these metal chelators promote Fe absorption will be the subject of future research studies.

Supplementary Materials: The following are available online http://www.mdpi.com/2072-6643/11/7/1502/s1; Figure S1: Ferritin formation in Caco-2 cells in response to various molar ratios of nicotianamine:myricetin (NA, red) and epicatechin:myricetin (Epi, green), Table S1: Fold increases in Caco-2 cell ferritin formation in response to different molar ratios of 2' deoxymugineic acid (DMA, blue), epicatechin (Epi, green), ascorbic acid (AsA, orange), and nicotianamine (NA, red) compared to ferritin formation in the presence of Fe alone.

Author Contributions: Conceptualization, J.T.B., J.J.H., E.T., R.P.G., and A.A.T.J.; Data curation, J.T.B. and J.J.H.; Formal analysis, J.T.B.; Funding acquisition, R.P.G. and A.A.T.J.; Investigation, J.T.B. and J.J.H.; Methodology, J.T.B. and J.J.H.; Project administration, R.P.G.; Resources, R.P.G. and A.A.T.J.; Supervision, A.A.T.J.; Validation, J.T.B.; Visualization, J.T.B. and J.J.H.; Writing—original draft, J.T.B.; Writing—review & editing, .T.B., J.J.H., E.T., R.P.G., and A.A.T.J. All authors have read and approve the final manuscript.

Funding: Funding was provided by the United States Department of Agriculture, Agricultural Research Service to R.P.G. and the Harvest Plus Challenge program to A.A.T.J.

Acknowledgments: The authors wish to acknowledge Yongpei Chang and Mary Bodis for their excellent technical assistance throughout the study, and Julien Bonneau for advice during manuscript writing. The authors have not received funds for covering the costs to publish in open access.

Conflicts of Interest: The authors declare no conflict of interest.

References

1. Briat, J.F.; Curie, C.; Gaymard, F. Iron utilization and metabolism in plants. *Curr. Opin. Plant Biol.* **2007**, *10*, 276–282. [CrossRef]
2. Kobayashi, T.; Nozoye, T.; Nishizawa, N.K. Iron transport and its regulation in plants. *Free Radic. Biol. Med.* **2018**, *133*, 11–20. [CrossRef] [PubMed]
3. Andresen, E.; Peiter, E.; Küpper, H. Trace metal metabolism in plants. *J. Exp. Bot.* **2018**, *69*, 909–954. [CrossRef] [PubMed]
4. Connorton, J.M.; Balk, J.; Rodríguez-Celma, J. Iron homeostasis in plants-a brief overview. *Metallomics* **2017**, *9*, 813–823. [CrossRef] [PubMed]
5. Beasley, J.T.; Bonneau, J.P.; Johnson, A.A.T. Characterisation of the nicotianamine aminotransferase and deoxymugineic acid synthase genes essential to Strategy II iron uptake in bread wheat (*Triticum aestivum* L.). *PLoS ONE* **2017**, *12*, 1–18. [CrossRef] [PubMed]
6. Zielińska-Dawidziak, M. Plant ferritin—A source of iron to prevent its deficiency. *Nutrients* **2015**, *7*, 1184–1201. [CrossRef] [PubMed]
7. Cvitanich, C.; Przybyłowicz, W.J.; Urbanski, D.F.; Jurkiewicz, A.M.; Mesjasz-Przybyłowicz, J.; Blair, M.W.; Astudillo, C.; Jensen, E.Ø.; Stougaard, J. Iron and ferritin accumulate in separate cellular locations in Phaseolus seeds. *BMC Plant Biol.* **2010**, *10*, 26. [CrossRef] [PubMed]
8. Ariza-Nieto, M.; Blair, M.W.; Welch, R.M.; Glahn, R.P. Screening of iron bioavailability patterns in eight bean (*Phaseolus vulgaris* L.) genotypes using the Caco-2 cell *in vitro* model. *J. Agric. Food Chem.* **2007**, *55*, 7950–7956. [CrossRef]
9. Hoppler, M.; Schönbächler, A.; Meile, L.; Hurrell, R.F.; Walczyk, T. Ferritin-Iron Is Released during Boiling and *In Vitro* Gastric Digestion. *J. Nutr.* **2008**, *138*, 878–884. [CrossRef]
10. Gillooly, M.; Charlton, R.W.; Mills, W.; MacPhail, A.P.; Mayet, F.; Bezwoda, W.R.; Bothwell, T.H.; Torrance, J.D.; Derman, D.P. The effects of organic acids, phytates and polyphenols on the absorption of iron from vegetables. *Br. J. Nutr.* **1983**, *49*, 331. [CrossRef]
11. Blair, M.W.; Izquierdo, P.; Astudillo, C.; Grusak, M.A. A legume biofortification quandary: variability and genetic control of seed coat micronutrient accumulation in common beans. *Front. Plant Sci.* **2013**, *4*, 1–14. [CrossRef] [PubMed]
12. Kim, S.A.; Punshon, T.; Lanzirotti, A.; Li, L.; Alonso, J.M.; Ecker, J.R.; Kaplan, J.; Guerinot, M.L. Localization of Iron in Arabidopsis Seed Requires the Vacuolar Membrane Transporter VIT1. *Science* **2006**, *314*, 1295–1298. [CrossRef] [PubMed]
13. Nozoye, T.; Kim, S.; Kakei, Y.; Takahashi, M.; Nakanishi, H.; Nishizawa, N.K. Enhanced levels of nicotianamine promote iron accumulation and tolerance to calcareous soil in soybean. *Biosci. Biotechnol. Biochem.* **2014**, *78*, 1677–1684. [CrossRef] [PubMed]

14. Tan, G.Z.H.; Das Bhowmik, S.S.; Hoang, T.M.L.; Karbaschi, M.R.; Long, H.; Cheng, A.; Bonneau, J.P.; Beasley, J.T.; Johnson, A.A.T.; Williams, B.; et al. Investigation of Baseline Iron Levels in Australian Chickpea and Evaluation of a Transgenic Biofortification Approach. *Front. Plant Sci.* **2018**, *9*. [CrossRef] [PubMed]
15. Balk, J.; Connorton, J.M.; Wan, Y.; Lovegrove, A.; Moore, K.L.; Uauy, C.; Sharp, P.A.; Shewry, P.R. Improving wheat as a source of iron and zinc for global nutrition. *Nutr. Bull.* **2019**, *44*, 53–59. [CrossRef] [PubMed]
16. De Brier, N.; Gomand, S.V.; Donner, E.; Paterson, D.; Smolders, E.; Delcour, J.A.; Lombi, E. Element distribution and iron speciation in mature wheat grains (Triticum aestivum L.) using synchrotron X-ray fluorescence microscopy mapping and X-ray absorption near-edge structure (XANES) imaging. *Plant. Cell Environ.* **2016**, *39*, 1835–1847. [CrossRef] [PubMed]
17. Beasley, J.T.; Bonneau, J.P.; Sánchez-Palacios, J.T.; Moreno-Moyano, L.T.; Callahan, D.L.; Tako, E.; Glahn, R.P.; Lombi, E.; Johnson, A.A.T. Metabolic engineering of bread wheat improves grain iron concentration and bioavailability. *Plant Biotechnol. J.* **2019**, 1–13. [CrossRef]
18. Eagling, T.; Wawer, A.A.; Shewry, P.R.; Zhao, F.; Fairweather-Tait, S.J. Iron Bioavailability in Two Commercial Cultivars of Wheat: Comparison between Wholegrain and White Flour and the Effects of Nicotianamine and 2′-Deoxymugineic Acid on Iron Uptake into Caco-2 Cells. *J. Agric. Food Chem.* **2014**, *62*, 10320–10325. [CrossRef]
19. Kyriacou, B.; Moore, K.L.; Paterson, D.; de Jonge, M.D.; Howard, D.L.; Stangoulis, J.; Tester, M.; Lombi, E.; Johnson, A.A.T. Localization of iron in rice grain using synchrotron X-ray fluorescence microscopy and high resolution secondary ion mass spectrometry. *J. Cereal Sci.* **2014**, *59*, 173–180. [CrossRef]
20. Johnson, A.A.T.; Kyriacou, B.; Callahan, D.L.; Carruthers, L.; Stangoulis, J.; Lombi, E.; Tester, M. Constitutive overexpression of the *OsNAS* gene family reveals single-gene strategies for effective iron- and zinc-biofortification of rice endosperm. *PLoS ONE* **2011**, *6*, e24476. [CrossRef]
21. Hart, J.J.; Tako, E.; Glahn, R.P. Characterization of Polyphenol Effects on Inhibition and Promotion of Iron Uptake by Caco-2 Cells. *J. Agric. Food Chem.* **2017**, *65*, 3285–3294. [CrossRef] [PubMed]
22. Hurrell, R.; Egli, I. Iron bioavailability and dietary reference values. *Am. J. Clin. Nutr.* **2010**, *91*, 1461–1467. [CrossRef] [PubMed]
23. Schlemmer, U.; Frølich, W.; Prieto, R.M.; Grases, F. Phytate in foods and significance for humans: Food sources, intake, processing, bioavailability, protective role and analysis. *Mol. Nutr. Food Res.* **2009**, *53*, 330–375. [CrossRef] [PubMed]
24. Semwal, D.K.; Semwal, R.B.; Combrinck, S.; Viljoen, A. Myricetin: A dietary molecule with diverse biological activities. *Nutrients* **2016**, *8*, 90. [CrossRef] [PubMed]
25. Sungur, Ş.; Uzar, A. Investigation of complexes tannic acid and myricetin with Fe(III). *Spectrochim. Acta - Part A Mol. Biomol. Spectrosc.* **2008**, *69*, 225–229. [CrossRef] [PubMed]
26. Asenstorfer, R.E.; Wang, Y.; Mares, D.J. Chemical structure of flavonoid compounds in wheat (*Triticum aestivum* L.) flour that contribute to the yellow colour of Asian alkaline noodles. *J. Cereal Sci.* **2006**, *43*, 108–119. [CrossRef]
27. Perron, N.R.; Brumaghim, J.L. A review of the antioxidant mechanisms of polyphenol compounds related to iron binding. *Cell Biochem. Biophys.* **2009**, *53*, 75–100. [CrossRef] [PubMed]
28. Laparra, J.M.; Tako, E.; Glahn, R.P.; Miller, D.D. Isolated Glycosaminoglycans from Cooked Haddock Enhance Nonheme Iron Uptake by Caco-2 Cells. *J. Agric. Food Chem.* **2008**, *56*, 10346–10351. [CrossRef]
29. Huh, E.C.; Hotchkiss, A.; Brouillette, J.; Glahn, R.P. Carbohydrate Fractions from Cooked Fish Promote Iron Uptake by Caco-2 Cells. *J. Nutr.* **2004**, *134*, 1681–1689. [CrossRef]
30. Lee, S.; Kim, Y.S.; Jeon, U.S.; Kim, Y.K.; Schjoerring, J.K.; An, G. Activation of rice nicotianamine synthase 2 (OsNAS2) enhances iron availability for biofortification. *Mol. Cells* **2012**, *33*, 269–275. [CrossRef]
31. Trijatmiko, K.R.; Dueñas, C.; Tsakirpaloglou, N.; Torrizo, L.; Arines, F.M.; Adeva, C.; Balindong, J.; Oliva, N.; Sapasap, M.V.; Borrero, J.; et al. Biofortified indica rice attains iron and zinc nutrition dietary targets in the field. *Sci. Rep.* **2016**, *6*, 1–13. [CrossRef] [PubMed]
32. Zheng, L.; Cheng, Z.; Ai, C.; Jiang, X.; Bei, X.; Zheng, Y.; Glahn, R.P.; Welch, R.M.; Miller, D.D.; Lei, X.G.; et al. Nicotianamine, a Novel Enhancer of Rice Iron Bioavailability to Humans. *PLoS ONE* **2010**, *5*, e10190. [CrossRef] [PubMed]
33. Glahn, R.; Tako, E.; Hart, J.; Haas, J.; Lung'aho, M.; Beebe, S. Iron Bioavailability Studies of the First Generation of Iron-Biofortified Beans Released in Rwanda. *Nutrients* **2017**, *9*, 787. [CrossRef] [PubMed]

34. Glahn, R.P.; Lee, O.A.; Yeung, A.; Goldman, M.I.; Miller, D.D. Caco-2 cell ferritin formation predicts nonradiolabeled food iron availability in an *in vitro* digestion/Caco-2 cell culture model. *J. Nutr.* **1998**, *128*, 1555–1561. [CrossRef] [PubMed]
35. Hu, Y.; Cheng, Z.; Heller, L.I.; Krasnoff, S.B.; Glahn, R.P.; Welch, R.M. Kaempferol in red and pinto bean seed (*Phaseolus vulgaris* L.) coats inhibits iron bioavailability using an *in vitro* digestion/human Caco-2 cell model. *J. Agric. Food Chem.* **2006**, *54*, 9254–9261. [CrossRef] [PubMed]
36. Hart, J.J.; Tako, E.; Kochian, L.V.; Glahn, R.P. Identification of Black Bean (*Phaseolus vulgaris* L.) Polyphenols That Inhibit and Promote Iron Uptake by Caco-2 Cells. *J. Agric. Food Chem.* **2015**, *63*, 5950–5956. [CrossRef] [PubMed]
37. Tako, E.; Bar, H.; Glahn, R.P. The combined application of the Caco-2 cell bioassay coupled with *in vivo* (*Gallus gallus*) feeding trial represents an effective approach to predicting Fe bioavailability in humans. *Nutrients* **2016**, *8*, 732. [CrossRef]
38. McLean, E.; Cogswell, M.; Egli, I.; Wojdyla, D.; de Benoist, B. Worldwide prevalence of anaemia, WHO Vitamin and Mineral Nutrition Information System, 1993-2005. *Public Heal. Nutr.* **2009**, *12*, 444–454. [CrossRef]
39. Kassebaum, N.J.; Jasrasaria, R.; Naghavi, M.; Wulf, S.K.; Johns, N.; Lozano, R.; Regan, M.; Weatherall, D.; Chou, D.P.; Eisele, T.P.; et al. A systematic analysis of global anemia burden from 1990 to 2010. *Blood J.* **2014**, *123*, 615–625. [CrossRef]
40. Lopez, A.; Cacoub, P.; Macdougall, I.C.; Peyrin-Biroulet, L. Iron deficiency anaemia. *Lancet* **2016**, *387*, 907–916. [CrossRef]
41. Bechoff, A.; Dhuique-Mayer, C. Factors influencing micronutrient bioavailability in biofortified crops. *Ann. N. Y. Acad. Sci.* **2017**, *1390*, 74–87. [CrossRef] [PubMed]
42. Bouis, H.E.; Saltzman, A. Improving nutrition through biofortification: A review of evidence from HarvestPlus, 2003 through 2016. *Glob. Food Sec.* **2017**, *12*, 49–58. [CrossRef] [PubMed]
43. Masuda, H.; Usuda, K.; Kobayashi, T.; Ishimaru, Y.; Kakei, Y.; Takahashi, M.; Higuchi, K.; Nakanishi, H.; Mori, S.; Nishizawa, N.K. Overexpression of the barley nicotianamine synthase gene *HvNAS1* increases iron and zinc concentrations in rice grains. *Rice* **2009**, *2*, 155–166. [CrossRef]
44. Singh, S.P.; Keller, B.; Gruissem, W.; Bhullar, N.K. Rice NICOTIANAMINE SYNTHASE 2 expression improves dietary iron and zinc levels in wheat. *Theor. Appl. Genet.* **2017**, *130*, 283–292. [CrossRef] [PubMed]
45. Von Wirén, N.; Klair, S.; Bansal, S.; Briat, J.-F.; Khodr, H.; Shioiri, T.; Leigh, R.A.; Hider, R.C. Nicotianamine Chelates Both Fe^{III} and Fe^{II}. Implications for Metal Transport in Plants1. *Plant Physiol.* **1999**, *119*, 1107–1114. [CrossRef] [PubMed]
46. Tsednee, M.; Huang, Y.C.; Chen, Y.R.; Yeh, K.C. Identification of metal species by ESI-MS/MS through release of free metals from the corresponding metal-ligand complexes. *Sci. Rep.* **2016**, *6*, 1–13. [CrossRef] [PubMed]
47. Ong, K.C.; Khoo, H.-E. Biological Effects of Myricetin. *Gen. Pharmac.* **1997**, *29*, 508–527. [CrossRef]
48. Mira, L.; Fernandez, M.T.; Santos, M.; Rocha, R.; Florêncio, M.H.; Jennings, K.R. Interactions of flavonoids with iron and copper ions: A mechanism for their antioxidant activity. *Free Radic. Res.* **2002**, *36*, 1199–1208. [CrossRef]
49. Carcea, M.; Narducci, V.; Turfani, V.; Giannini, V. Polyphenols in Raw and Cooked Cereals/Pseudocereals/Legume Pasta and Couscous. *Foods* **2017**, *6*, 80. [CrossRef]

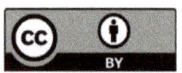

© 2019 by the authors. Licensee MDPI, Basel, Switzerland. This article is an open access article distributed under the terms and conditions of the Creative Commons Attribution (CC BY) license (http://creativecommons.org/licenses/by/4.0/).

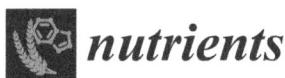

Article

Bioelectrical Impedance Vector Analysis and Phase Angle on Different Oral Zinc Supplementation in Eutrophic Children: Randomized Triple-Blind Study

Karina M. Vermeulen [1], Márcia Marília G. D. Lopes [2], Camila X. Alves [2], Naira J. N. Brito [3], Maria das Graças Almeida [4], Lucia Leite-Lais [2], Sancha Helena L. Vale [2,*] and José Brandão-Neto [5,*]

1. Post-graduate Program in Health Sciences, Federal University of Rio Grande do Norte, CEP 59012-570 Natal, RN, Brazil; karinavermeulen@hotmail.com
2. Department of Nutrition, Federal University of Rio Grande do Norte, CEP 59078-970 Natal, RN, Brazil; mariliagdantas@hotmail.com (M.M.G.D.L.); camila_xavieralves@yahoo.com.br (C.X.A.); ludl10@hotmail.com (L.L.-L.)
3. Department of Pharmacy, University of Cuiabá, CEP 78850-000 Cuiabá, MT, Brazil; nairabrito@yahoo.com.br
4. Department of Clinical and Toxicological Analysis, Federal University of Rio Grande do Norte, CEP 59012-570 Natal, RN, Brazil; mgalmeida84@gmail.com
5. Department of Internal Medicine, Federal University of Rio Grande do Norte, CEP 59012-570 Natal, RN, Brazil
* Correspondence: sanchahelena@hotmail.com (S.H.L.V.); brandao-neto@live.com (J.B.-N.); Tel.: +55-84-3342-2291 (S.H.L.V.)

Received: 31 March 2019; Accepted: 7 May 2019; Published: 28 May 2019

Abstract: The parameters derived from bioelectrical impedance, phase angle (PA) and bioelectrical impedance vector analysis (BIVA) have been associated with cell membrane integrity and body cell mass. Zinc is a micronutrient that exerts important structural functions and acts in maintaining cellular functionality. To evaluate cell integrity and body cell mass, PA and BIVA were evaluated in children orally supplemented with zinc at different concentrations. Anthropometric, bioelectrical (resistance and reactance) and serum zinc variables were collected from two randomized, triple-blind, controlled clinical trials. Sampling was composed of 71 children consisting of three groups: a control group who received a placebo and two experimental groups who received oral supplementation of 5 or 10 mg-Zn/day for three months. The three groups presented increases ($p < 0.001$) in the linear height and weight. In the group supplemented with 10 mg-Zn/day, there was an increase in reactance values ($p = 0.036$) and PA ($p = 0.002$), in addition to vector displacement ($p < 0.001$) in relation to the confidence ellipses. An increase in serum zinc concentration was found ($p < 0.001$) in all three groups. Whit this, the supplementation with 10 mg-Zn/day promotes changes in the integrity of the cell membrane associated with the increase in the cellular mass of healthy children.

Keywords: body composition; cell membrane; bioimpedance

1. Introduction

Bioelectrical impedance (BIA) has been widely used in clinical practice to evaluate the body composition of adults and children. Compared with other methods for this purpose, the BIA has advantages, including safety, low cost, easy-to-use, portability and practicality [1]. The BIA has based on the principle that body tissues behave as an electric circuit in steady state equilibrium, offering opposition to the electric current when it is applied to the circuit. The impedance (Z), the name assigned to this opposition, presents two vectors: resistance (R) and reactance (Xc). R reflects the quantity of intra- and extracellular fluids, and Xc, the quantity of cell mass, the structure and cell membranes functionality. From these vectors, it is possible to calculate the phase angle (PA) and perform the bioelectrical impedance vector analysis (BIVA) [2,3].

PA is related to cell integrity and functionality, being important both in healthy people assessment and in prognosis of diseases because it reflects different electrical properties of the body tissues. It also indicates nutritional status and hydration. Its evaluation is superior to other nutritional, anthropometric and serum indicators in different populations [4–8].

BIVA is useful for clinical purposes because it detects changes in hydration or body composition, as demonstrated by Carrasco-Marginet et al. [9] and Koury et al. [10]. Using BIVA, it is possible to evaluate the patient by direct vector impedance measurements because this method does not depend on equations or models; it is a graphical method with R and Xc corrected for height, which can generate three analyses: individual, follow-up, and groups [3].

The plasma membrane has three main functions: coating, protection and selective permeability [11]. Zinc is involved in the integrity, stabilization of structural membranes, protection and cellular functionality, and exerting structural, catalytic and regulatory functions. Thus, zinc acts as a cofactor of several metabolic pathways [12,13]. Studies show that zinc deficiency increases erythrocyte membrane fragility, and compromises platelet aggregation and osmotic protection [11,14,15].

The participation of zinc in membrane stability is described in the literature through three mechanisms. First, zinc promotes the association between membrane proteins and cytoskeleton proteins. Second, zinc stabilizes the reduced form of sulfhydryl groups, contributing to the antioxidant protection against the effects of membrane rupture caused by lipid and protein oxidation. Third, zinc preserves the integrity of ion channels, thus acting as an antagonist to the adverse effect of free Ca^{+2} [10,16]. However, to the best of our knowledge, no studies evaluate the influence of different zinc concentrations on cell integrity and functionality using PA and BIVA as the evaluation method. This study aimed to evaluate changes in PA and BIVA in healthy children orally supplemented with zinc at different concentrations.

2. Materials and Methods

2.1. Study Design and Population

A database search of two clinical trials, randomized, controlled, triple-blind and non-probabilistic was conducted, had as main objective the supplementation of zinc in apparently healthy children. The partial results of these studies were previously published [17–19]. These studies were approved by the Ethics Committee of the University Hospital Onofre Lopes (HUOL) by the Federal University of Rio Grande do Norte (UFRN) (protocol numbers 323/09 and 542/11).

The tests were carried out with different oral zinc supplementations in apparently healthy children (stage of sexual maturation suitable for the age, without acute, chronic, infectious or inflammatory diseases), aged between six and nine years. The children were recruited at four municipal schools located in the east and west of the city of Natal, Rio Grande do Norte, Brazil.

Exclusion criteria were children in pubarche, thelarche or menarche, who had undergone surgery of any kind, or who used vitamin or mineral supplements. An endocrinologist performed these clinical evaluations.

Among the children who comprised this study's sample, only those eutrophic were included, considering body mass index for age Z-score (BAZ) (Z-scores between −2 and +1) [20]. In addition, children with incomplete information for BIVA implementation were excluded. The values of age (years), weight (kg), height (cm), resistance (Ω), reactance (Ω) and serum zinc (µg/mL) were measured immediately before the beginning of zinc supplementation (T0) and immediately after three months of supplementation (T1). Recruitment, inclusion, and exclusion procedures are described in Figure 1.

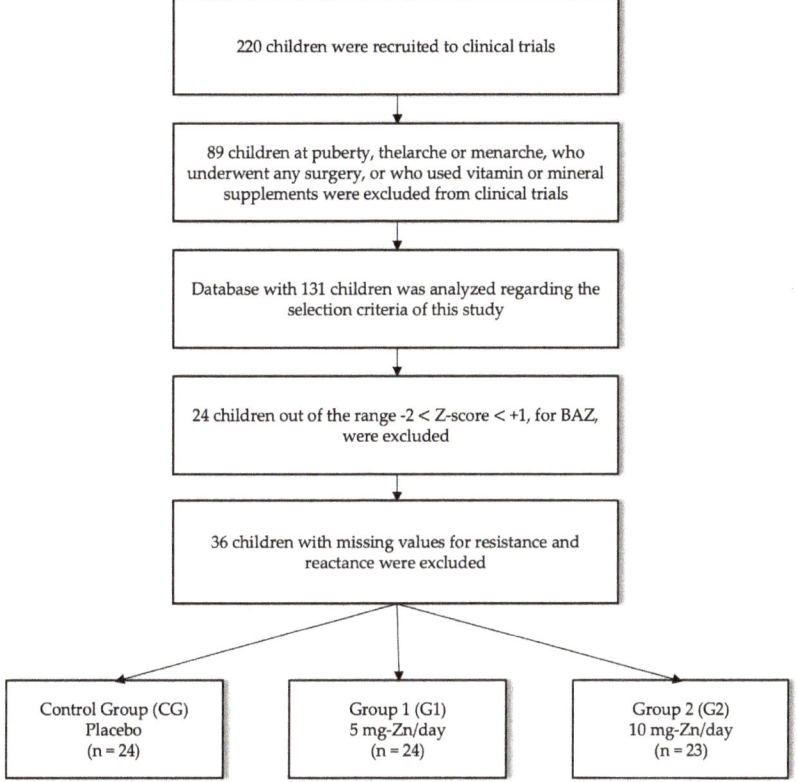

Figure 1. Recruitment flowchart with inclusion and exclusion procedures.

2.2. Standardization of Clinical Trials

Both clinical trials were performed by the same research group and had the same methodology for data collection and analysis with standardized protocols.

2.2.1. Oral Zinc Supplementation

Stratification of the sample according to the oral zinc supplementation resulted in the formation of three groups: the control group (CG) received a placebo (10% sorbitol, the same vehicle used in the zinc solution); Group 1 (G1) received 5 mg-Zn/day; and Group 2 (G2) received 10 mg-Zn/day. The supplementation period was three months. Zinc was supplied in the form of zinc sulfate heptahydrate ($ZnSO_4 \cdot 7H_2O$; Merck, Darmstadt, Germany). Each drop of the supplement contained 1 mg of the zinc element. Zinc sulfate heptahydrate acquisition and the oral zinc solution preparation were performed as described by Brito et al. [19]. Those responsible for the children were instructed to add the supplement to water, milk or juice at breakfast.

2.2.2. Assessment of Serum Zinc

Serum zinc was determined by atomic absorption spectrophotometry (SpectrAA-200, Varian, Victoria, Australia). Four milliliters of blood were collected for serum zinc analyses. All processes related to the collection, separation, dilution, and storage of blood for the serum zinc dosage, as well as the calibration of the apparatus, standard serum control, and zinc measurements, were performed as described by Brito et al. [19]. Zinc sensitivity was 0.01 µg/mL, intra-assay coefficient was 2.09% and reference values was 0.7–1.2 µg/mL, according our laboratory evaluation. The clinical examination found no signs or symptoms of zinc deficiency.

2.2.3. Anthropometric Assessment

The weight and height of the children participating in the trials were measured using an electronic scale (Balmak, BK50F, São Paulo, Brazil) and stadiometer (Sanny, São Paulo, Brazil), respectively. BMI (kg/m^2) was calculated as the ratio between body weight and height squared. The weight-for-age (WAZ), height-for-age (HAZ) Z-scores and BAZ were calculated using AnthroPlus software v1.0.4 (available at www.who.int/growthref/en/) and ranked according to the growth curves of the World Health Organization for healthy children aged 5–19 years [20]. Trained nutritionists performed anthropometric assessments.

2.2.4. Bioelectric Impedance

The bioelectrical impedance parameters, R (Ω) and Xc (Ω), were obtained using the Quantum II® body composition analyzer (RJL Systems, Clinton Township, MI, USA) with a single, safe and painless electrical frequency (50 kHz). This tetrapolar method was applied with the subject lying supinated. Four self-adhesive spot electrodes were placed: two on the dorsal surface of the right hand and two on the dorsal surface of the right foot, as described by Lukaski et al. [21]. With the parameters obtained by the bioelectric impedance, the percentage of fat-free mass (%FFM) was calculated using the equation proposed by Houtkooper [22], then the PA and BIVA were performed.

2.3. Bioelectrical Impedance Vector Analysis

R and Xc data were subsequently used to determine PA and BIVA. The PA was calculated with the formula PA = arc tang (Xc/R) × 180/π [23]. The BIVA results were based on the analysis of normalized R and Xc values for children's height measurements (R/H and Xc/H in Ω/m).

BIVA charts directly measure the vectors R and Xc. According to the RXc chart, children's standardized impedance measurements are represented as bivariate vectors with their confidence and tolerance intervals, which are ellipses in the RXc plane. These vectors do not depend on equations. To investigate the differences between groups, we plotted the 95% confidence intervals for the mean impedance difference of the bivariate vectors measured under two conditions for each group [24].

The position and length of the vector provide information on the hydration status, cell mass, and cell integrity. It is an upward or downward displacement of the main axis associated with more or less soft tissue cell mass, respectively. A significant value for the T2 statistic is evidence that the mean vectors of each group are different [24].

2.4. Statistical Analysis

Statistical analysis was performed by observing the data distribution using the Shapiro–Wilk test. All quantitative variables presented normal distribution and were expressed as mean (standard deviation), except the age that presented non-normal distribution and was expressed as median (Q1; Q3). Intragroup comparisons were performed using Student's t-test.

For BIVA, all analyses were performed using the BIVA software [24]. The mean differences between the impedance vectors in the different supplemented groups were determined using the Hoteling T2 test. Statistical tests were considered significant at 5% ($p \leq 0.05$).

3. Results

With the methodology described, data were collected from 71 children aged 6.2–9.9 years. The sex distribution in each group were: 50% both sexes of the CG; and 58% and 39% female in G1 and G2, respectively.

Concerning serum zinc concentrations, we observed that the children had no apparent zinc deficiency before the intervention (Table 1). There was a significant increase ($p < 0.001$) in serum zinc concentrations in all groups, regardless of supplementation (Figure 2).

Table 1. Group characterization before oral zinc supplementation with different concentrations (CG = placebo; G1 = 5 mg-Zn/day; G2 = 10 mg-Zn/day).

Group	CG	G1	G2	p^1
n	24	24	23	–
Age (years)	8.4 (0.5)	8.1 (1.0)	9.1 (0.5)	<0.001
Serum zinc (µg/mL)	0.92 (0.13)	1.01 (0.12)	0.90 (0.11)	0.007
WAZ	−0.15 (0.79)	−0.85 (0.82)	−0.43 (1.05)	0.031
HAZ	0.26 (0.98)	−0.64 (0.82)	−0.39 (1.19)	0.008
BAZ	−0.47 (0.74)	−0.70 (0.68)	−0.27 (0.75)	0.142
Resistance (Ω)	773 (41)	807 (65)	748 (91)	0.017
R/H (Ω/cm)	590.1 (41.7)	654.4 (73.3)	576.0 (87.8)	0.001
Reactance (Ω)	71 (8)	75 (9)	68 (6)	0.008
Xc/H (Ω/cm)	54.3 (7.2)	60.8 (7.9)	52.2 (6.4)	<0.001
Phase angle (°)	5.28 (0.68)	5.34 (0.61)	5.25 (0.64)	0.879
FFM (%)	79.8 (2.8)	78.7 (4.2)	78.8 (3.7)	0.524

WAZ, weight-for-age Z-score; HAZ, height-for-age Z-score; BAZ, Body mass index-for-age Z-score; R/H, Resistance/Height; Xc, Reactance/Height; FFM, fat-free mass. Continuous variables are presented as the means (standard deviations). [1] One-way ANOVA.

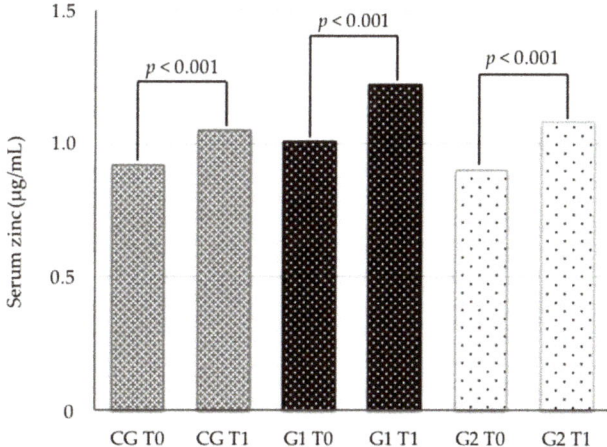

Figure 2. Intragroup comparison of serum zinc before (T0) and after (T1) three months of intervention with different oral supplementation of zinc in eutrophic children.

Table 2 shows that regardless of the zinc concentration offered, the three groups improved ($p < 0.001$) the linear height and weight, but only the group that received a concentration of 10 mg-Zn/day had an improvement in the values of Xc ($p = 0.036$) and the PA ($p = 0.002$).

Regarding the BIVA (Figure 3), only the concentration of 10 mg-Zn/day was enough to promote significant displacement ($p < 0.001$) in relation to the confidence ellipses, indicating a possible increase in the cellular mass in these children.

Table 2. Anthropometric characteristics and bioelectric parameters before and after oral supplementation with different concentrations of zinc.

Anthropometrics	Control Group Before	Control Group After	p^1	Group 1 Before	Group 1 After	p^1	Group 2 Before	Group 2 After	p^1
Weight (Kg)	27.4 (3.3)	27.2 (3.9)	<0.001	22.8 (3.4)	23.4 (3.8)	<0.001	27.1 (4.4)	28.0 (4.5)	<0.001
Height (cm)	131.2 (6.4)	132.6 (6.4)	<0.001	123.8 (6.9)	125.1 (7.0)	<0.001	130.6 (6.8)	132.1 (6.9)	<0.001
BMI (Kg/m^2)	15.3 (1.1)	15.4 (1.3)	0.141	14.8 (1.1)	14.9 (1.2)	0.334	15.8 (1.2)	15.9 (1.3)	0.053
WAZ	−0.15 (0.79)	−0.15 (0.89)	0.980	−0.85 (0.82)	−0.85 (0.88)	0.938	−0.47 (1.08)	−0.43 (1.07)	0.152
HAZ	0.26 (0.98)	0.24 (0.99)	0.339	−0.64 (0.82)	−0.65 (0.80)	0.574	−0.39 (1.19)	−0.37 (1.18)	0.316
BAZ	−0.47 (0.74)	−0.46 (0.87)	0.809	−0.70 (0.68)	−0.69 (0.75)	0.970	−0.27 (0.75)	−0.24 (0.75)	0.500
Bioelectrical	**Before**	**After**	p^1	**Before**	**After**	p^1	**Before**	**After**	p^1
R (Ω)	772.8 (41.3)	777.7 (50.7)	0.559	806.7 (65.1)	800.0 (71.6)	0.370	748.3 (91.1)	747.2 (101.6)	0.835
R/H (Ω/cm)	590.1 (41.7)	588.3 (56.5)	0.782	654.4 (73.3)	642.9 (83.7)	0.079	576.0 (87.8)	568.6 (93.0)	0.089
Xc (Ω)	71.0 (7.7)	71.9 (9.3)	0.579	75.0 (8.6)	75.0 (6.6)	0.955	67.9 (6.2)	70.0 (7.5)	0.036
Xc/H (Ω/cm)	54.3 (7.2)	54.5 (9.0)	0.863	60.8 (7.9)	60.3 (7.9)	0.737	52.2 (6.4)	53.3 (7.3)	0.163
PA (Ω)	5.28 (0.68)	5.30 (0.58)	0.882	5.34 (0.61)	5.40 (0.49)	0.537	5.25 (0.64)	5.43 (0.68)	0.002
FFM (%)	79.8 (2.8)	79.2 (3.3)	0.065	78.7 (4.2)	78.9 (4.2)	0.478	78.8 (3.7)	78.7 (3.2)	0.558

WAZ, weight-for-age Z-score; HAZ, height-for-age Z-score; BAZ, Body mass index-for-age Z-score; R, resistance; Xc, reactance; H, height; FFM, Fat-free mass. Variables are presented as mean (standard deviation). ^{1} Student's t-test.

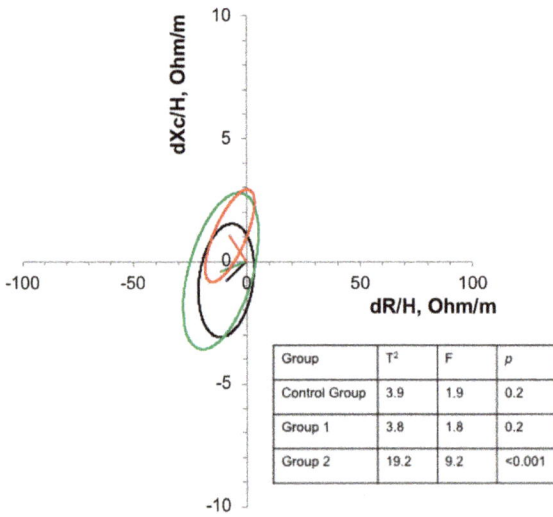

Figure 3. Confidence ellipses of 95% of impedance vectors measured before (T0) and after (T1) three months of intervention with oral supplementation with different concentrations of zinc in eutrophic children. Black ellipse = control group; Green ellipse = Group 1; Red ellipse = Group 2. An upward or downward displacement of the main axis is associated with more or less soft tissue cell mass, respectively.

4. Discussion

Our results show that zinc supplementation modified intrinsic factors related to body composition, such as cell integrity and cell mass, even before changes in serum zinc or anthropometric indicators can be detected, as discussed below.

In the population studied, there was an increase in serum zinc over time in all groups, with no differences between them. This study was conducted in a city located on the Atlantic coast, where the supply of food sources rich in zinc is vast. In the study developed by Alves et al. (2016), consumption of energy, protein, fat, carbohydrates, iron and zinc were adequate according to dietary reference intakes by age and sex. Mean zinc intake in these population was 6.00 ± 1.01 mg/day [25].

Recently, zinc supplementation studies with concentrations ranging from 5 to 50 mg-Zn/day in different infant populations to assess the influence on growth and development have been conducted [26–29]. In a systematic review, Liu et al. [30] described that zinc supplementation improves growth parameters with potentially stronger effects in children after two years of age.

The children were in a phase that naturally shows changes in growth. In our study, the anthropometric parameters of WAZ and HAZ did not show differences between the supplemented and control groups. Cho et al. [29], when evaluating children who received 5 mg-Zn/day for six months, also did not observe differences in WAZ and HAZ when compared with the control group. It should be emphasized that the population of our study, although classified as having negative scores at T0, neither demonstrated a deficit in height or weight at the beginning of the study, nor indicated zinc deficiency.

Zinc is essential for the integrity and functionality of cell membranes. Its concentration in the cell membrane can be quite high depending on the cell type and is influenced by the nutritional status of zinc in the organism [31]. In the present study, supplementation with 10 mg-Zn/day significantly increased the values of Xc and PA. Increased PA values are associated with improved cell integrity, lean mass, and the relationship between water distribution in the intracellular and extracellular compartments [32].

Koury et al. [10] found higher PA in adolescents with zinc concentrations in the erythrocyte above the median, concluding that bone age and erythrocyte zinc contribute to PA values in young male soccer players. PA has also been described as a sensitive and useful tool to detect changes in nutritional status in addition to being associated with the clinical prognosis of several diseases [4,5]. Pileggi et al. [8] concluded that PA is a useful tool for detecting nutritional risk in children with osteogenesis imperfecta.

In addition to the increase in Xc and PA in the present study, a significant shift to the upper left quadrant was observed in relation to the confidence ellipses in the group that received 10 mg-Zn/day.

The use of bioelectric impedance to estimate body composition is a promising methodology [33]. However, one disadvantage is the need to choose equations validated for each specific population [34], since they can be influenced by biological and clinical factors [35,36].

Piccoli et al. [37] proposed that impedance can be plotted in a cartesian plane as a bivariate vector derived from R and Xc, standardized by the height of the individual. Thus, the displacement up or down of the main axis becomes associated with more or less soft tissue cell mass, respectively [24].

In their study, Meleleo et al. (2017) concluded that BIVA could provide more reliable details about differences in body composition in competitive and noncompetitive adolescents [38]. This method of evaluation can also be used in other clinical conditions, as described by Juarez et al. (2018), who noted that BIVA might be an option for cachexia in patients with rheumatoid arthritis [39]. Therefore, PA and BIVA can be used together to indicate cellular integrity and hydration without requiring predictive equations.

A strength of this study was the early detection of changes in bioelectrical parameters as a result of zinc supplementation. Based on that, we suggest that PA and BIVA can be used together to indicate cellular integrity and hydration status, respectively, without requiring predictive equations. These findings encourage the replication of this study in other populations. On the other hand, the sample size and the disregard of other micronutrients, such iron, were limitations of this study. The exclusion of 24 participants with missing data and the distribution of the children in three different groups reduced the sample size and may have affected the power of the study. Iron and calcium interact with zinc and may influence bioelectrical parameters. Thus, the nutrition status of other micronutrients must be considered in future studies with a similar aim.

5. Conclusions

Oral zinc supplementation with 10 mg/day promoted Xc and PA changes, in addition to a vector shift by BIVA, which was associated with changes in cell membrane integrity and an increase in cell mass in eutrophic children. These original results were observed before changes in serum zinc concentrations or anthropometric indicators.

Author Contributions: Conceptualization, K.M.V. and J.B.-N.; Formal analysis, K.M.V. and M.M.G.D.L.; Funding acquisition, M.d.G.A., S.H.L.V. and J.B.-N.; Investigation, K.M.V., M.M.G.D.L., C.X.A., N.J.N.B., L.L.-L. and S.H.L.V.; Methodology, K.M.V., M.M.G.D.L. and C.X.A.; Project administration, S.H.L.V.; Supervision, J.B.-N.; Writing—original draft, K.M.V.; and Writing—review and editing, M.M.G.D.L., C.X.A., L.L.-L., S.H.L.V and J.B.-N.

Funding: Vermeulen's work on this article was supported by a scholarship from National Council for Scientific and Technological Development (CNPq) to the Federal University of Rio Grande do Norte.

Acknowledgments: The BIVA software was kindly provided by Antonio Piccoli (Institute of Internal Medicine, Division of Nephrology and Unit of Clinical Nutrition of the University of Padova, Italy).

Conflicts of Interest: The authors declare no conflict of interest.

References

1. Bera, T.K. Bioelectrical impedance methods for noninvasive health monitoring: A review. *J. Med. Eng.* **2014**, *2014*, 381251. [CrossRef]
2. Gonzalez, M.C.; Barbosa-Silva, T.G.; Bielemann, R.M.; Gallagher, D.; Heymsfield, S.B. Phase angle and its determinants in healthy subjects: Influence of body composition. *Am. J. Clin. Nutr.* **2016**, *103*, 712–716. [CrossRef]
3. Margutti, A.V.B.; Bustamante, C.R.; Sanches, M.; Padilha, M.; Beraldo, R.A.; Monteiro, J.P.; Camelo, J.S., Jr. Bioelectrical impedance vector analysis (BIVA) in stable preterm newborns. *J. Pediatr.* **2012**, *88*, 253–258. [CrossRef]
4. Berbigier, M.C.; Pasinato, V.F.; Rubin, B.A.; Moraes, R.B.; Perry, I.D.S. Bioelectrical impedance phase angle in septic patients admitted to intensive care units. *Rev. Bras. Ter. Intensiva* **2013**, *25*, 25–31. [CrossRef]
5. Vermeulen, K.M.; Leal, L.L.A.; Furtado, M.C.M.B.; Vale, S.H.L.; Lais, L.L. Phase angle and Onodera's prognostic nutritional index in critically ill patients. *Nutr. Hosp.* **2016**, *33*, 1268–1275. [CrossRef]
6. Norman, K.; Stobäus, N.; Pirlich, M.; Bosy-Westphal, A. Bioelectrical phase angle and impedance vector analysis—Clinical relevance and applicability of impedance parameters. *Clin. Nutr.* **2012**, *31*, 854–861. [CrossRef]
7. Genton, L.; Norman, K.; Spoerri, A.; Pichard, C.; Karsegard, V.L.; Herrmann, F.R.; Graf, C.E. Bioimpedance-derived phase angle and mortality among older people. *Rejuvenation Res.* **2017**, *20*, 118–124. [CrossRef]
8. Pileggi, V.N.; Scalize, A.R.H.; Camelo, J.S., Jr. Phase angle and World Health Organization criteria for the assessment of nutritional status in children with osteogenesis imperfecta. *Rev. Paul. Pediatr.* **2016**, *34*, 484–488. [CrossRef] [PubMed]
9. Carrasco-Marginet, M.; Castizo-Olier, J.; Rodríguez-Zamora, L.; Iglesias, X.; Rodríguez, F.A.; Chaverri, D.; Brotons, D.; Irurtia, A. Bioelectrical impedance vector analysis (BIVA) for measuring the hydration status in young elite synchronized swimmers. *PLoS ONE* **2017**, *12*, e0178819. [CrossRef] [PubMed]
10. Koury, J.C.; Oliveira-Junior, A.V.; Portugal, M.R.C.; Oliveira, K.J.F.; Donangelo, C.M. Bioimpedance parameters in adolescent athletes in relation to bone maturity and biochemical zinc indices. *J. Trace Elem. Med. Biol.* **2018**, *46*, 26–31. [CrossRef] [PubMed]
11. O'Dell, B.L. Role of zinc in plasma membrane function. *J. Nutr.* **2000**, *130*, 1432S–1436S. [CrossRef]

12. Chasapis, C.T.; Loutsidou, A.C.; Spiliopoulou, C.A.; Stefanidou, M.E. Zinc and human health: An update. *Arch. Toxicol.* **2012**, *86*, 521–534. [CrossRef]
13. Oliveira, K.J.F.; Koury, J.C.; Donangelo, C.M. Micronutrients and antioxidant capacity in sedentary adolescents and runners. *Rev. Nutr.* **2007**, *20*, 171–179. [CrossRef]
14. Marreiro, D.; Cruz, K.; Morais, J.; Beserra, J.; Severo, J.; Oliveira, A. Zinc and oxidative stress: Current mechanisms. *Antioxidants* **2017**, *6*, 24. [CrossRef]
15. Lee, S.R. Critical role of zinc as either an antioxidant or a prooxidant in cellular systems. *Oxid. Med. Cell. Longev.* **2018**, *2018*, 9156285. [CrossRef]
16. Wood, R.J. Assessment of marginal zinc status in humans. *J. Nutr.* **2000**, *130*, 1350S–1354S. [CrossRef]
17. Alves, C.X.; Vale, S.H.L.; Dantas, M.M.G.; Maia, A.A.; Franca, M.C.; Marchini, J.S.; Leite, L.D.; Brandao-Neto, J. Positive effects of zinc supplementation on growth, GH, IGF1, and IGFBP3 in eutrophic children. *J. Pediatr. Endocrinol. Metab.* **2012**, *25*, 881–887. [CrossRef]
18. Rocha, É.D.M.; Brito, N.J.N.; Dantas, M.M.G.; Silva, A.A.; Almeida, M.G.; Brandão-Neto, J. Effect of zinc supplementation on GH, IGF1, IGFBP3, OCN, and ALP in non-zinc-deficient children. *J. Am. Coll. Nutr.* **2015**, *34*, 290–299. [CrossRef]
19. Neves, N.J.B.; Rocha, É.D.M.; Silva, A.A.; Costa, J.B.; França, M.C.; Almeida, M.G.; Brandão-Neto, J. Oral zinc supplementation decreases the serum iron concentration in healthy schoolchildren: A pilot study. *Nutrients* **2014**, *6*, 3460–3473. [CrossRef]
20. WHO Multicentre Growth Reference Study Group. *WHO Child Growth Standards: Length/Height-For-Age, Weight-For-Age, Weight-For-Length, Weight-For-Height and Body Mass Index-For-Age: Methods and Development*; World Health Organization: Geneva, Switzerland, 2006; 312p.
21. Lukaski, H.C.; Bolonchuk, W.W.; Hall, C.B.; Siders, W.A. Validation of tetrapolar bioelectrical impedance method to assess human body composition. *J. Appl. Physiol.* **1986**, *60*, 1327–1332. [CrossRef]
22. Houtkooper, L.B.; Going, S.B.; Lohman, T.G.; Roche, A.F.; Van Loan, M. Bioelectrical impedance estimation of fat-free body mass in children and youth: A cross-validation study. *J. Appl. Physiol.* **1992**, *72*, 366–373. [CrossRef] [PubMed]
23. Baumgartner, R.N.; Chumlea, W.C.; Roche, A.F. Bioelectric impedance phase angle and body composition. *Am. J. Clin. Nutr.* **1988**, *48*, 16–23. [CrossRef] [PubMed]
24. Piccoli, A.; Pastori, G. *BIVA Software*; Department of Medical and Surgical Sciences, University of Padova: Padova, Italy, 2002.
25. Alves, C.X.; Brito, N.J.N.; Vermeulen, K.M.; Lopes, M.M.G.D.; França, M.C.; Bruno, S.S.; Almeida, M.G.; Brandão-Neto, J. Serum zinc reference intervals and its relationship with dietary, functional, and biochemical indicators in 6- to 9-year-old healthy children. *Food Nutr. Res.* **2016**, *60*, 30157. [CrossRef]
26. Park, S.G.; Choi, H.N.; Yang, H.R.; Yim, J.E. Effects of zinc supplementation on catch-up growth in children with failure to thrive. *Nutr. Res. Pract.* **2017**, *11*, 487–491. [CrossRef]
27. Chao, H.C.; Chang, Y.J.; Huang, W.L. Cut-off Serum zinc concentration affecting the appetite, growth, and nutrition status of undernourished children supplemented with zinc. *Nutr. Clin. Pract.* **2018**, *33*, 701–710. [CrossRef]
28. Hamza, R.T.; Hamed, A.I.; Sallam, M.T. Effect of zinc supplementation on growth hormone Insulin growth factor axis in short Egyptian children with zinc deficiency. *Ital. J. Pediatr.* **2012**, *38*, 21. [CrossRef] [PubMed]
29. Cho, J.M.; Kim, J.Y.; Yang, H.R. Effects of oral zinc supplementation on zinc status and catch-up growth during the first 2 years of life in children with non-organic failure to thrive born preterm and at term. *Pediatr. Neonatol.* **2018**, 1–9. [CrossRef] [PubMed]
30. Liu, E.; Pimpin, L.; Shulkin, M.; Kranz, S.; Duggan, C.; Mozaffarian, D.; Fawzi, W. Effect of zinc supplementation on growth outcomes in children under 5 years of age. *Nutrients* **2018**, *10*, 377. [CrossRef] [PubMed]
31. Koury, J.C.; Donangelo, C.M. Zinc, oxidative stress and physical activity. *Rev. Nutr.* **2003**, *16*, 433–441. [CrossRef]
32. Więch, P.; Dąbrowski, M.; Bazaliński, D.; Sałacińska, I.; Korczowski, B.; Binkowska-Bury, M. Bioelectrical impedance phase angle as an indicator of malnutrition in hospitalized children with diagnosed inflammatory bowel diseases—A case control study. *Nutrients* **2018**, *10*, 499. [CrossRef]

33. Lukaski, H.C. Evolution of bioimpedance: A circuitous journey from estimation of physiological function to assessment of body composition and a return to clinical research. *Eur. J. Clin. Nutr.* **2013**, *67*, S2–S9. [CrossRef] [PubMed]
34. Barbosa-Silva, M.C.G.; Barros, A.J. Bioelectrical impedance analysis in clinical practice: A new perspective on its use beyond body composition equations. *Curr. Opin. Clin. Nutr. Metab. Care* **2005**, *8*, 311–317. [CrossRef] [PubMed]
35. Marra, M.; Sammarco, R.; Filippo, E.; Caldara, A.; Speranza, E.; Scalfi, L.; Contaldo, F.; Pasanisi, F. Prediction of body composition in anorexia nervosa: Results from a retrospective study. *Clin. Nutr.* **2018**, *37*, 1670–1674. [CrossRef]
36. Ward, L.C. Bioelectrical impedance analysis for body composition assessment: Reflections on accuracy, clinical utility, and standardization. *Eur. J. Clin. Nutr.* **2019**, *73*, 194–199. [CrossRef] [PubMed]
37. Piccoli, A.; Nigrelli, S.; Caberlotto, A.; Bottazzo, S.; Rossi, B.; Pillon, L.; Maggiore, Q. Bivariate normal values of the bioelectrical impedance vector in adult and elderly populations. *Am. J. Clin. Nutr.* **1995**, *61*, 269–270. [CrossRef]
38. Meleleo, D.; Bartolomeo, N.; Cassano, L.; Nitti, A.; Susca, G.; Mastrototaro, G.; Armenise, U.; Zito, A.; Devito, F.; Scicchitano, P.; et al. Evaluation of body composition with bioimpedence. A comparison between athletic and non-athletic children. *Eur. J. Sport Sci.* **2017**, *17*, 710–719. [CrossRef]
39. Pineda-Juárez, J.A.; Lozada-Mellado, M.; Ogata-Medel, M.; Hinojosa-Azaola, A.; Santillán-Díaz, C.; Llorente, L.; Orea-Tejeda, A.; Alcocer-Varela, J.; Espinosa-Morales, R.; González-Contreras, M.; et al. Body composition evaluated by body mass index and bioelectrical impedance vector analysis in women with rheumatoid arthritis. *Nutrition* **2018**, *53*, 49–53. [CrossRef]

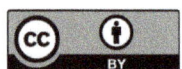

© 2019 by the authors. Licensee MDPI, Basel, Switzerland. This article is an open access article distributed under the terms and conditions of the Creative Commons Attribution (CC BY) license (http://creativecommons.org/licenses/by/4.0/).

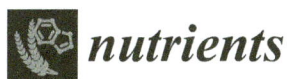

Article
Dietary Silicon and Its Impact on Plasma Silicon Levels in the Polish Population

Anna Prescha *, Katarzyna Zabłocka-Słowińska and Halina Grajeta

Department of Food Science and Dietetics, Wroclaw Medical University, 50-556 Wrocław, Poland; katarzyna.zablocka-slowinska@umed.wroc.pl (K.Z.-S.); halina.grajeta@umed.wroc.pl (H.G.)
* Correspondence: anna.prescha@umed.wroc.pl

Received: 19 March 2019; Accepted: 24 April 2019; Published: 29 April 2019

Abstract: Silicon in nutritional amounts provides benefits for bone health and cognitive function. The relationship between silicon intake from a common daily diet and silicon blood level has been scarcely elucidated, so far. The aim of this study was to analyze the associations between plasma silicon levels and the total and bioavailable silicon intake—along with the contribution of silicon made by food groups—in a healthy adult Polish population. Si intake was evaluated in 185 healthy adults (94 females and 91 males, aged 20–70) using a 3-day dietary recall and a database on the silicon content in foods, which was based on both previously published data and our own research. Fasting plasma silicon levels were measured in 126 consenting subjects, using graphite furnace atomic absorption spectrometry. The silicon intake in the Polish population differed significantly according to sex, amounting to 24.0 mg/day in women and 27.7 mg/day in men. The median plasma silicon level was 152.3 µg/L having no gender dependency but with a negative correlation with age. Significant correlations were found between plasma silicon level and total and bioavailable silicon intake, as well as water intake in the diet ($r = 0.18$, $p = 0.044$; $r = 0.23$, $p = 0.011$; $r = 0.28$, $p = 0.002$, respectively). Silicon intakes from non-alcoholic beverages, cereal foods, and carotene-rich vegetables were also positively associated with plasma silicon levels. These results may help establish dietary silicon recommendations and formulate practical advice on dietary choices to ensure an appropriate supply of silicon. The outcome of this study, however, needs to be confirmed by large-scale epidemiological investigations.

Keywords: silicon; diet; plasma; adults

---

1. Introduction

The essentiality of silicon in human health is supported by a growing body of evidence [1–3]. Epidemiological studies have shown that dietary silicon was favorably related to markers of bone density and turnover. Moreover, Si in nutritional amounts may lower the risk of Alzheimer's disease and may improve photo-damaged skin or hair and nail conditions [4–7].

The silicon level in the blood may be considered as a silicon status indicator. However, only a few reports have been published on silicon concentrations in the blood, and the values reported for fasting serum concentration in healthy adult subjects have ranged from 100 to 310 µg/L. Moreover, the relationship between silicon intake from a common daily diet and silicon blood level has so far been scarcely elucidated [8]. This results partly from the limited number of studies on the silicon content in foods and its intake in the diet.

Dietary silicon has only been assessed in certain populations so far. According to published data, a Western-type diet provides between 19 and 31 mg of Si per day [9,10]. Few studies have been performed on an appropriate dietary silicon level which would ensure beneficial health effects. An adequate intake of between 10 and 25 mg/day has been suggested, but dietary silicon levels approaching 25 mg/day or higher seem to be the most efficacious, at least for maintaining bone health in men and premenopausal women, with no adverse effects [1,5].

Although the data on silicon content in foods are incomplete, it has been assumed that cereals, along with beverages (especially beer) and some vegetables and fruits, contribute the most to the dietary intake of silicon [10–12]. The higher daily silicon intake of men than women which has been reported by some authors has been attributed to the typically higher beer consumption among men [9,11]. The bioavailability of silicon differs between foods: orthosilicic acid and water-soluble silicates from beverages are easily absorbed, whereas phytolytic silica, present in solid plant foods, is less absorbable [9,10,13]. The bioavailability of silicon from foods may have, along with the total silicon intake, an impact on its level in the organism.

The results of our recently published study have indicated that diet composition might be related to plasma silicon level in healthy Polish subjects [8], however no thorough analysis of this relationship has been carried out with regard to bioavailable silicon intake. The aim of this study was, therefore, to assess the relationship between plasma silicon levels and total and bioavailable silicon intake from a typical diet, with respect to the contribution of food groups into the total dietary silicon, in a healthy adult Polish population. To achieve this aim, we assessed the total silicon content in the diet, largely based on data available in the scientific literature on the silicon content of various foods. In order to complete the food silicon database used in this study, the amounts of Si contained in cereal products and beverages purchased on the Polish market were measured. The bioavailable silicon content in the diet was calculated, using previously published data on the bioavailability of this element from individual foods. The contribution of silicon from particular food groups to total silicon intake was also assessed. The plasma silicon levels in the study population were measured and then correlated with the total and bioavailable silicon contents in the diet and with the silicon intake from food groups.

2. Materials and Methods

2.1. Subjects

Two hundred and ten healthy adult subjects were recruited for the study from the Lower Silesia Regional Center of Occupational Medicine in Wrocław, Poland, from public offices and from Wrocław's University of the 3rd Age. The exclusion criteria included serious diseases, metabolic disorders, mental health issues, and declared regular use of medication and/or dietary supplements. Of the participants that were recruited, 25 were excluded from the study because of particular dietary habits and a history of prior medication use. The study group finally consisted of 185 adults aged 20–70. All subjects gave their written informed consent. The study was conducted in accordance with the Declaration of Helsinki, and the protocol was approved by the Wrocław Medical University Ethics Board (consent No. KB-202/2012).

The anthropometric measurements and the assessment of dietary intake and habits were performed by a trained dietician for all subjects. Fasting blood samples were also drawn from 126 consenting subjects on the day of the dietary interview, and plasma samples were collected for the measurement of silicon levels—exclusively using plastic ware to prevent pre-analysis silicon contamination of the samples. Subsequent analyses were performed for the whole population and for men and women separately, considering gender differences between silicon intake and silicon blood levels, as previously reported [9,11,14]. As the silicon level in the blood has been shown to be significantly influenced by age, and because differences in silicon intake might be age-related, according to previously published studies, we decided to analyze silicon intake and serum levels in age groups largely conforming to those applied by the National Food and Nutrition Institute (Warsaw, Poland) when reporting recommended daily intake values for trace elements in adults [15]. However, groups of 66–75 year olds and >75 year olds could not be represented in our study population. Therefore the assessment of study variables was performed in the following age groups: ≤30 years, 31–50 years, and ≥51 years.

2.2. Dietary Intake Assessment

A 3-day dietary recall (2 weekdays and 1 weekend day in the same week) was used to assess energy and macronutrient intake, as well as silicon intake from the diet. Calculations of the composition of foods were performed using Diet v. 6.0 software with an uploaded photo album of products and meals (National Food and Nutrition Institute, Warsaw, Poland, 2019). Amounts of silicon in the diet were calculated using data from analyses of Polish food products performed at the Department of Food Science and Dietetics (Wroclaw Medical University) and from published data on the silicon content of foods originating in Poland, the UK, Belgium, the USA, and South Korea [9,10,16–21]. The following products purchased on the Polish market were analyzed in our laboratory: cereal products, fruit and vegetable juices, and mineral and spring waters. The resulting data on the silicon content of these products were then included into the food silicon database created using previously published data. For multiple data reported on the same foods, the following order of priority was applied: (1) the reliability of the method used for silicon measurement, (2) the degree of representativeness of the data, and (3) the origin of the products analyzed.

Bioavailable silicon in the diet was estimated using published data from human research on excreted silicon after the consumption of various foods with a determined silicon content [9]. In several cases, data on the bioavailability assessed by in vitro experiments were also used [10]. Bioavailable silicon was calculated for foods providing 93.9% ± 3.8% of the total silicon in the diet of the study group, and the percentage of bioavailable silicon in these foods was 36.5% ± 4.0%. This value was used for foods when no data on their bioavailability was available.

In addition to total and bioavailable silicon intake from the diet, the contribution of silicon from particular food groups to the total amount in the diet was assessed and expressed in percentage of total silicon intake. The database used for total silicon intake calculation was also applied for the calculation of silicon in food groups. The silicon intakes from individual foods were added up to obtain the main food groups as well as subgroups of foods relevant in silicon intake. For example, silicon intake from cereal products was calculated in the following groups: refined grain foods, comprising white breads and rolls, foods made from white flour and white flour pasta, whole grain foods comprising wholemeal and wholegrain breads and rolls, cereal flakes, cereal snacks, groats, and wholemeal dishes.

2.3. Food Sampling for Silicon Analysis

Cereal food products: breads, groats, flakes, rice, pasta, and beverages in cartons and plastic bottles, along with bottled mineral and spring waters, were purchased in domestic grocery stores and hypermarkets (Lower Silesia region). In the case of beverages, at least three production batches of each product were collected at least 1 month apart. In total, 486 food products from 99 manufacturers were analyzed for silicon. Solid food samples were finely ground in a mill, then packed in polyethylene bags and stored at room temperature prior to analysis. The samples of bread were dried in a laboratory oven and the dry weight was measured. The juice samples were stored in plastic flasks below −20 °C prior to analysis. Water samples for analysis were taken directly from the original bottles stored at room temperature.

2.4. Silicon Measurement in Foods

The solid food and juice samples were thoroughly blended and then mineralized (0.5 g) with 4 mL 65% HNO_3 (Instra-Analyzed JTBaker, USA) and 1 mL 30% H_2O_2 (Ultrex II JTBaker, USA) in a microwave oven (Milestone 1200 Mega, USA). The mineralization was done according to the manufacturer's recommendations. The blank digests were carried out in the same way. Measurements of the silicon content in the mineralized samples and the bottled water samples were performed on a Perkin Elmer PinAAcle 900 (USA) atomic absorption spectrometer in graphite furnace mode (GF-AAS). The operating parameters of the GF-AAS for the silicon analysis are presented in Supplementary Table S1. Two samples of each food product were measured four times each. The plastic and Teflon utensils were pre-cleaned or rinsed in 10% HNO$_3$ and then rinsed in deionized water. All reagents were prepared using deionized water, with a specific resistivity of 18.2 MΩ cm. The calibration working standard solutions were prepared from a silicon standard solution of 1 mg/L, as (NH$_4$)$_2$SiF$_6$ in H$_2$O (Perkin Elmer, USA), in a silicon concentration ranging from 40 to 120 µg/L. The samples were measured directly, or after appropriate dilution with deionized water. The mean recovery of total silicon obtained for selected spiked samples of food was 101.2%. Accuracy and precision were also assessed by measuring the silicon in certified reference materials: NCS ZC73008 Rice (NACIS, China) and MISSIPPI-03 River Water (Environment Canada, Canada). The agreement with the defined values was 95.2% and 100.5%, respectively.

The resulting data on the silicon content of cereal products and beverages were then included in the food silicon database which was used to assess the silicon intake of the healthy Polish subjects. Data on Si in cereal products that require preparation with water were re-calculated, taking into account the final percentage of water.

2.5. Silicon Measurement in Plasma

The direct measurement of silicon in plasma was performed by GF-AAS (PinAAcle 900, Perkin Elmer, USA) using the method of standard addition calibration described elsewhere [8]. The operating conditions and instrumental parameters for silicon measurement are summarized in Supplementary Table S1.

2.6. Statistical Analyses

Statistical calculations were performed using Statistica StatSoft 13.0. The distribution of continuous variables (dietary intake, food consumption, and plasma silicon concentration) was checked using the Shapiro–Wilk test. Depending on the distribution of variables, either Student's *t*-test or the Mann–Whitney U test were used for gender comparisons (dietary intake, food group consumption and plasma silicon concentration); either Tukey's HDS test or the Kruskal–Wallis test was used for age comparisons (dietary intakes, food group consumption, and plasma silicon concentration). Pearson correlation analysis was used to measure the association between plasma silicon and age, and age-adjusted partial correlation analyses were performed for the determination of associations between plasma silicon level and the dietary variables. The correlation analyses were carried out in the whole study population and in both gender groups. Pearson's χ^2 test was used to assess any differences in age distribution between the gender groups.

3. Results

3.1. Study Population Characteristics, Dietary Intake, and Dietary Habit Assessment

The baseline characteristics of the subjects, as well as the dietary intake of energy and macronutrients are presented in Table 1.

3.2. Silicon Content in Cereal Products and Beverages from the Polish Market

The determination of silicon was performed in cereal products that are generally of local origin in stores, and for which no data on silicon content were available. Silicon content was also measured in beverages, which are mostly manufactured by domestic producers usually from concentrates reconstituted with water. The content of silicon in cereal products on the Polish market varied over a wide range, from 0.94 mg/100 g in Basmati rice to 14.03 mg/100 g in oat bran (Table 2). Refined products contained less silicon than wholemeal products and wholegrain products. There were also differences between grain species, with the highest values found in oat, millet, and barley products. High amounts of silicon were also found in unrefined rice products. The content of silicon in selected beverages—juices and bottled water available on the Polish market—ranged between 0.63 and 1.22 mg/100 (Table 3). The fruit juices we analyzed may provide silicon in amounts similar to vegetable and fruit–vegetable juices. Mineral waters contained 25% more Si on average than spring waters. As the silicon content in beverages was measured in at least three production batches of products, the coefficient of variance (CV) was calculated for each product, in order to assess the variability of silicon levels in beverages available on the market. The highest CV values were obtained for orange juices (Table 3).

Table 1. Characteristics of the study population and dietary intake.

	All Subjects (n = 185)	Female (n = 94)	Male (n = 91)
Characteristics			
Age (years), median (range)	45.1 (20.2–70.2)	45.2 (23.6–68.2) [a]	45.1 (20.2–70.2) [a]
≤30 years, n (%)	49 (26.5)	23 (24.5) [A]	26 (28.6) [A]
31–50 years, n (%)	74 (40.0)	38 (40.4)	36 (39.7)
≥51 years, n (%)	62 (33.5)	33 (35.1)	29 (31.9)
BMI (kg/m2), median (range)	25.6 (18.3–32.0)	24.4 (18.3–32.0) [a]	25.9 (18.8–31.8) [b]
Body weight (kg), median (range)	73.0 (46.5–130.0)	63.0 (46.5–86.0) [a]	78.0 (60.0–130.0) [b]
Dietary intake, median (Q1–Q3)			
Energy (MJ/day)	8.07 (7.19–9.42)	7.57 (6.97–8.12) [a]	9.35 (8.12–10.70) [b]
Nutrients (g/day)			
Protein	76.5 (63.1–92.7)	66.8 (57.9–78.2) [a]	91.3 (74.0–108.2) [b]
Carbohydrates	281.4 (246.1–319.6)	269.3 (236.6–300.5) [a]	304.1 (254.6–350.1) [b]
Fat	58.2 (42.8–77.7)	46.1 (36.6–59.7) [a]	72.7 (54.8–90.7) [b]
Ash	17.7 (14.8–21.3)	16.3 (15.9–13.4–18.6) [a]	20.3 (17.5–23.8) [b]
Fiber	21.9 (17.6–27.7)	21.6 (16.3–25.6) [a]	22.9 (18.3–30.4) [b]
Water	2158 (1715–2634)	2053 (1626–2589) [a]	2269 (1886–2686) [b]
Alcohol	3.0 (0.0–6.4)	0.0 (0.0–5.0) [a]	6.0 (0.0–10.7) [a]

BMI—body mass index; Q1–Q3—range between 25th and 75th percentiles. Values in the same row which do not share the same superscript letter are significantly different ($p < 0.05$). For the variable comparison between female and male groups, lowercase letters were used; for the comparison of age-group distribution in the female and male groups, uppercase letters were used.

Table 2. Silicon content in cereal products (mg/100 g).

Product	n	Mean ± SD
Breads		
Bread, white	15	1.88 ± 0.83
Rolls, white	10	1.59 ± 0.64
Breads, wholemeal & wholegrain	13	2.00 ± 0.63
Rolls, wholemeal & wholegrain	6	1.82 ± 0.48
Crispbread	15	3.97 ± 3.62
Matzo, classic	2	1.50 ± 0.12
Matzo, wholemeal	2	2.45 ± 0.13
Groats		
Couscous	4	2.35 ± 0.78
Buckwheat & Roasted buckwheat	9	1.17 ± 0.59
Millet	5	7.96 ± 0.71
Barley	6	6.64 ± 3.73
Corn	3	1.67 ± 1.71
Flakes		
Corn	5	2.12 ± 0.46
Oat	5	13.89 ± 2.62
Wheat	3	2.49 ± 0.59
Spelt	4	2.42 ± 0.87
Rye	3	2.29 ± 0.40
Muesli (various types)	6	4.58 ± 2.31
Bran		
Oat	3	14.03 ± 7.69
Wheat	4	6.80 ± 2.19
Rice		
Long grain, white	4	3.41 ± 2.62
Jasmine, white	4	1.47 ± 0.28
Basmati, white	4	0.94 ± 0.30
Whole grain, brown	10	9.72 ± 2.57
Chinese, black	3	10.63 ± 7.46

Table 2. *Cont.*

Product	n	Mean ± SD
Wild rice (*Zizania aquatica*)	4	2.99 ± 0.44
Pasta		
Wheat, white	4	1.22 ± 0.31
Wheat, wholemeal	5	5.20 ± 2.82
Spelt	2	2.86 ± 0.64
Rye	2	5.28 ± 1.24
Mixed grain	2	5.63 ± 1.41

SD—standard deviation.

Table 3. Silicon content in beverages (mg/100 g).

Product	n	Mean ± SD	Range of CV Values for Products from a Single Brand (%) *
Juice			
Orange	8	0.87 ± 0.35	32–99
Apple	8	0.90 ± 0.58	7–33
Grapefruit	8	0.63 ± 0.39	11–54
Blackcurrant	3	0.66 ± 0.05	13–32
Multi-fruit	4	1.22 ± 0.29	14–28
Carrot–Fruit	6	1.17 ± 0.48	16–57
Tomato	6	0.75 ± 0.22	11–38
Multi-vegetable	7	0.76 ± 0.26	6–34
Bottled water			
Spring	5	0.77 ± 0.40	3–42
Mineral	17	0.96 ± 0.63	3–50

SD—standard deviation; CV—coefficient of variation, %. * CV assessed by analysis of at least 3 samples, from different production batches, of each shop-bought product.

3.3. Silicon Intake

Total and Bioavailable Silicon in the Diet and Silicon Intake from Food Groups

The total intake of silicon in the study group, the amount and percentage of bioavailable silicon, and the contribution of silicon from particular food groups to total silicon intake are presented in Table 4. It may be noted that men consumed significantly more silicon in their diet than women, however, no differences in total silicon intake were found between the age groups of the study population. Bioavailable silicon comprised 36.5% of total dietary silicon in the study population. In line with total silicon, both the bioavailable silicon content and its percentage in total silicon were higher in men than in women. A higher percentage of bioavailable silicon in the diet was also shown for the younger subjects rather than the older ones. Non-alcoholic beverages in total were found to be a major source of silicon in the diet. These products provided ca. 30% of dietary silicon in the study population, with an equivalent contribution made by hot beverages (tea and coffee) and cold ones. However, women gained more silicon from hot beverages than men, and in the youngest subjects a higher intake of silicon from cold non-alcoholic beverages was noticed in comparison with older age groups. The high contribution of cereal products in total, accounting for 25.8% of the amount of silicon in the diet, was also revealed. Among them, whole grain foods were shown to be more important in providing silicon for women than for men. Fruit and vegetables provided considerable amounts of silicon, whilst the lowest contribution of these products to silicon intake was shown for subjects aged ≤30. Divergent eating patterns influenced the contribution of silicon from meats, eggs, and fats to the total silicon intake in both sexes, as these products provided almost half as much silicon in the diet of women than of men.

Table 4. Total silicon intake, contribution of food groups to silicon intake, bioavailable Si in the diet, and plasma silicon, median (Q1–Q3).

	All Subjects	Female	Male	Age Groups (Years)		
				≤30	31–50	≥51
Silicon Intake (mg/day)	26.1 (22.0–30.3)	24.0 (21.2–29.7) [a]	27.7 (23.4–31.6) [b]	25.2 (22.7–29.0) [α]	26.0 (21.5–30.2) [α]	26.4 (22.7–31.9) [α]
Silicon Intake from Food Groups (% Of Total Si intake)						
Refined grain foods	17.9 (12.2–23.9)	19.3 (12.4–24.7) [a]	17.2 (11.9–21.5) [a]	18.3 (13.6–24.6) [α]	18.0 (11.5–24.4) [α]	17.5 (12.2–20.2) [α]
Whole grain foods	7.9 (1.3–13.0)	10.0 (4.0–14.2) [a]	4.6 (0.0–11.2) [b]	5.5 (1.0–10.8) [α]	5.8 (1.5–13.0) [α]	10.5 (2.6–14.1) [α]
Potatoes and Starches	2.5 (1.3–4.0)	2.3 (1.1–3.3) [a]	3.0 (1.8–5.2) [b]	2.4 (1.2–3.4) [α]	2.5 (1.5–4.0) [α]	2.6 (1.4–4.5) [α]
Vegetables	8.5 (5.9–11.7)	8.3 (5.6–11.6) [a]	8.7 (6.4–11.9) [a]	7.4 (5.2–10.7) [α]	8.9 (7.0–12.9) [β]	8.7 (5.9–12.0) [αβ]
Fruits	10.4 (5.5–15.0)	11.1 (5.6–15.1) [a]	9.6 (5.5–14.4) [a]	6.4 (2.5–12.8) [α]	11.0 (6.0–15.2) [αβ]	11.8 (7.8–15.0) [β]
Cold, n/a beverages	15.1 (7.1–24.1)	14.8 (7.3–25.7) [a]	15.2 (6.9–23.6) [a]	21.9 (13.6–30.5) [α]	11.1 (6.8–19.9) [β]	16.7 (5.4–22.2) [αβ]
Tea & Coffee	15.0 (9.9–21.2)	17.4 (11.5–22.5) [a]	14.0 (9.1–19.8) [b]	14.3 (9.3–20.6) [α]	15.2 (10.3–21.0) [α]	14.4 (8.7–21.0) [α]
Dairy products	1.7 (0.9–2.9)	1.7 (1.0–2.8) [a]	1.8 (0.9–2.9) [a]	1.9 (1.1–3.0) [α]	1.9 (1.2–3.2) [α]	1.1 (0.8–2.3) [α]
Meats & Meat products	4.8 (2.3–9.2)	3.9 (1.8–7.8) [a]	6.5 (2.7–11.2) [b]	4.8 (1.8–8.1) [α]	5.1 (2.9–10.3) [α]	4.5 (2.1–9.2) [α]
Fish & Fish products	0.2 (0.0–1.0)	0.2 (0.0–0.8) [a]	0.4 (0.0–1.3) [a]	0.2 (0.0–1.7) [α]	0.0 (0.0–0.5) [α]	0.4 (0.0–1.5) [α]
Eggs	1.0 (0.3–2.1)	0.8 (0.3–1.6) [a]	1.3 (0.3–2.4) [b]	0.6 (0.1–1.5) [α]	1.3 (0.6–2.2) [α]	0.9 (0.3–2.0) [α]
Fats	1.3 (0.7–2.1)	1.1 (0.6–2.0) [a]	1.5 (0.9–2.3) [b]	1.3 (0.8–2.1) [α]	1.3 (0.8–2.3) [α]	1.4 (0.7–2.0) [α]
Legumes	0.2 (0.0–1.1)	0.3 (0.0–0.5) [a]	1.0 (0.0–1.3) [a]	0.2 (0.0–0.7) [α]	0.5 (0.0–1.5) [α]	0.2 (0.0–0.9) [α]
Nuts & Seeds	0.4 (0.0–0.3)	0.3 (0.0–0.4) [a]	0.5 (0.0–0.2) [a]	0.6 (0.0–1.0) [α]	0.4 (0.0–0.6) [α]	0.4 (0.0–0.9) [α]
Sugar & Sweets	0.3 (0.1–0.7)	0.3 (0.1–0.5) [a]	0.4 (0.1–0.9) [a]	0.4 (0.2–0.9) [α]	0.3 (0.1–0.6) [α]	0.3 (0.1–0.6) [α]
Alcoholic beverages	1.8 (0.0–3.7)	0.0 (0.0–2.9) [a]	4.1 (0.0–6.3) [a]	2.2 (0.0–6.6) [α]	2.0 (0.0–4.2) [α]	0.0 (0.0–4.4) [α]
Others	0.9 (0.6–1.2)	0.9 (0.6–1.1) [a]	1.0 (0.7–1.3) [a]	0.8 (0.6–1.1) [α]	0.9 (0.7–1.2) [α]	0.9 (0.6–1.3) [α]
Bioavailable Dietary Silicon						
(mg/day)	9.4 (7.7–11.5)	8.6 (7.1–11.0) [a]	9.9 (5.5–29.6) [b]	9.7 (8.0–11.0) [α]	9.0 (7.4–11.5) [α]	9.7 (8.0–11.9) [α]
% total silicon in diet	36.5 (33.6–38.9)	36.2 (33.4–38.5) [a]	37.2 (28.5–47.9) [b]	37.5 (35.9–39.5) [α]	36.2 (33.2–38.7) [β]	36.4 (33.4–38.8) [β]
Plasma Silicon						
(µg/L)	152.3 (116.3–195.6)	168.5 (121.2–208.2) [a]	144.8 (114.7–175.0) [a]	197.8 (140.5–224.1) [α]	147.9 (120.8–171.6) [β]	123.6 (94.2–180.1) [β]
(n)	–126	–64	–63	–32	–46	–48

Q1–Q3—range between 25th and 75th percentiles; n/a—non-alcoholic. Values in the same row which do not share the same superscript letter are significantly different. For variable comparisons between female and male groups, Latin lowercase letters were used; for comparisons between age groups, Greek lowercase letters were used.

3.4. Plasma Silicon and Its Relation to Diet

Fasting plasma silicon levels were measured in 126 of the study participants; the median value amounted to 152.3 µg/L, with no significant differences in terms of gender (Table 4). However, an impact of age on plasma silicon level was noted. Subjects younger than 31 years had higher silicon plasma levels than those in the older age groups. This was confirmed by the negative correlation of plasma silicon values with age ($r = -0.40$, $p < 0.000$). Further correlation analyses were performed after adjusting for age and measured anthropometric parameters (body mass index and body weight). In the assessment of dietary impact on plasma silicon, we included the following dietary variables: total and bioavailable silicon intake, macronutrient intakes, and silicon intakes from food groups and subgroups. Animal protein-rich foods (meat and meats products, fish and fish eggs, and milk products) were taken into consideration in total, as the intake of silicon from these products was relatively low. Only the significant correlations are presented in Table 5.

Table 5. Significant partial correlations between plasma silicon level and dietary variables ($n = 126$).

Variable	r [†]	p-Value
Nutrient (intake/day)		
Silicon	0.18	0.044
Bioavailable silicon	0.23	0.011
Water	0.28	0.002
Fat	−0.19	0.036
Animal protein	−0.18	0.045
Silicon from food groups and subgroups (intake/day)		
Cold, non-alcoholic beverages	0.21	0.022
Mineral & Spring water	0.22	0.013
Fruit & Vegetable juices	0.22	0.011
Groats	0.19	0.037 *
White rice	0.2	0.034
Cereal flakes	0.32	0.009 **
Carotene-rich vegetables	0.28	0.002
Animal protein-rich foods	−0.18	0.045

[†] Partial correlation coefficient, adjusted for age, body mass index and body weight. * only in female subjects. ** only in male subjects.

Plasma silicon levels positively correlated with total and bioavailable silicon content in the diet—along with water intake—in the study population. Moreover, a negative correlation with fat and animal protein was noted. The silicon intake from particular food groups was also associated with plasma silicon level. Among them, the consumption of cold, non-alcoholic beverages was shown to be positively related to silicon concentration in the blood. Silicon intake from cereal products in total was not associated with plasma silicon level, although positive correlations were found for selected cereal products. From among vegetable and fruit food groups, a positive correlation with plasma silicon was recorded only for carotene-rich vegetables. A negative relationship found for silicon from animal protein-rich foods supported the negative correlation for animal protein intake.

4. Discussion

In our study, we assessed thoroughly the relationship between silicon intake from a typical diet and fasting plasma silicon level, taking into consideration both total dietary silicon and bioavailable silicon, as well as silicon intake from food groups.

In the assessment of dietary silicon in the Polish population we found it necessary to complete the database on the silicon content of foods, by determining the silicon content of cereals and non-alcoholic beverages available on the Polish market. Cereals greatly contribute to the energy intake of the Polish population, according to the National Multicenter Health Survey (WOBASZ II, 2013–2014), and may provide considerable amounts of silicon in the diet [16,22]. The silicon content of these products on the Polish market, however, had not been measured. Beverages were shown to be important sources of highly absorbable orthosilicic acid [9,10], but there was only a single study published on the silicon content of these products in Poland [19]. Our results confirmed the high silicon content of cereal products found by other authors, though some differences were shown, including a lower silicon content of Polish wholemeal and wholegrain breads [16,17]. In the fruit and vegetable juices analyzed in our study, a lower range of silicon concentration was recorded than the range previously published for Polish products (0.12–2.67 mg/100 g) [23]. This discrepancy might result from the relatively high variation of silicon content in these products, even among different production batches of the same brand. As the juices were not fortified, the differences might result from the variable content of silicon in the raw material or in the water used in the manufacturing process. This indicates that the contribution of juices to silicon intake may vary even if the same product is consistently present in the diet. In the mineral waters and spring waters analyzed, we found higher silicon concentrations than those reported for bottled waters produced in northern Poland [19]. The differences in silicon content might therefore be attributed to the geographic features of the area from which the water is sourced [24].

Self-selected food consumption in the Polish population has translated into a daily intake of silicon which is close to the lower limit (25 mg/day) that is considered beneficial. This finding was also similar to the results obtained from the original Framingham and Framingham Offspring cohorts [9]. Nevertheless, the negative impact of age on total silicon intake found in the Framingham study was not confirmed in our study group. The higher amount of silicon in men observed in our study might not be attributed to higher beer consumption in this gender group—as previously reported [9–11]—because the overall consumption of alcohol in men was low and did not differ significantly from that of women. The distribution of foods contributing to silicon intake in our study population confirmed the significant role of cereals and non-alcoholic beverages in the provision of silicon, and the smaller but still relevant position of fruits and vegetables in silicon intake, as shown elsewhere [9–11].

In our assessment of dietary silicon, we also calculated the proportion of total intake of Si which represented a bioavailable form of silicon. As the data used in these calculations originated from experiments estimating silicon absorption from individual foods [9,10,13], the dietary silicon bioavailability presented in this study should be regarded as the potential bioavailability from the diet not taking account the factors that can influence the uptake of silicon from mixed meals. Some gender and age-related divergences in dietary habits, and therefore in food contributions to total silicon intake, have corresponded with differences in bioavailable silicon amount in the diet. The higher contribution of cold non-alcoholic beverages to silicon intake in subjects aged under 31 translated into a higher percentage of bioavailable silicon in their diet. Meat products—providing more silicon in the diet of male subjects than female ones—were shown to contain available silicon amounting to more than 70% of total silicon [10]. Moreover, despite the low consumption of alcoholic beverages in the study population, men tended to consume more of the products that are known for their high bioavailable silicon content, especially beers. This pattern of consumption resulted in a higher intake of bioavailable silicon in this gender group. The actual bioavailability of silicon from a mixed diet needs to be investigated in order to collect more reliable data.

Silicon content in the diet of the study population was then tested against plasma silicon level. As with results reported for the German population, plasma silicon showed an inverse relationship to age [14]. After adjusting for age and anthropometric parameters, the total silicon content in the diet of healthy adults was shown to be weakly correlated with plasma silicon level. To date, only one study—of an adult Korean population—has investigated the associations between self-selected food consumption and body silicon status, determined by silicon urine excretion [11]. The authors reported that dietary silicon, assessed by the food record method and their own food silicon database, was significantly positively related to diurnal silicon in the urine among males alone. When taking into consideration bioavailable dietary silicon, its relationship to plasma silicon level was slightly more pronounced in the Polish population, indicating that the consumption of a diet rich in bioavailable silicon may be important for the maintenance of body silicon status. The positive relationship between plasma silicon level and silicon intake from non-alcoholic beverages, which was accompanied by a positive correlation with water intake, clearly confirms the substantial role of foods rich in monomeric silicon, such as spring water, mineral water, and fruit and vegetable juices, in providing silicon to the human body [10,13]. This association was not observed for hot beverages (coffee and tea), which may be related to coffee and tea polyphenols affecting the availability of minerals [25]. However, in our recent study we noticed a positive association between plasma silicon and tea and coffee consumption in rheumatoid arthritis patients [8]. As the body silicon status in rheumatoid arthritis seems to be affected, other factors related to the disease may interfere with the associations found. A significant correlation with plasma silicon was also observed for some cereal foods, including groats, which are known to be generally rich in silicon (especially barley and millet, see Table 2). Taking into consideration the high contribution of cereal products to the total silicon intake in Polish populations and in others, their role as a source of dietary silicon and in maintaining silicon levels in the body appears to be significant. Among carotene-rich vegetables, which also positively correlated with plasma silicon, green beans and spinach have been reported to be high-silicon foods [16,23]. This might have an impact on the observed correlation. Despite the high bioavailability of silicon from animal foods, their relationship with plasma silicon level was negative, as in the case of silicon from fats. The influence of the chemical environment created by food components on the absorption and retention of silicon has not yet been recognized, however, the impact of dietary fat on the absorption of trace elements could play a role, among others [26].

The results of this study may be helpful in establishing dietary recommendations on silicon and the formulation of practical advice on dietary choices to ensure its appropriate supply. Further studies are merited in order to explain the mechanisms which interfere with Si absorption and retention in the body.

5. Conclusions

In our study, significant correlations were found between plasma silicon level and the total and bioavailable silicon intake, and the consumption of fluids, cereal foods, and carotene-rich vegetables. However, our findings need to be supported by large-scale epidemiological studies. Moreover, a number of issues concerning dietary silicon interactions with nutrients and metabolic factors must still be elucidated.

Supplementary Materials: The following are available online at http://www.mdpi.com/2072-6643/11/5/980/s1, Table S1: The operating conditions and instrumental parameters for silicon determination in food and plasma samples by graphite furnace atomic absorption spectrometry.

Author Contributions: Conceptualization, A.P.; validation, A.P.; methodology, A.P. and K.Z.-S.; investigation, A.P. and K.Z.-S.; writing—original draft preparation A.P.; formal analysis, A.P. and K.Z.-S.; writing—review and editing, K.Z.-S.; supervision, H.G.; project administration, A.P. and H.G.

Funding: This work was financially supported by the Wrocław Medical University (grant No. ST-846).

Acknowledgments: The authors would like to thank Joanna Kaliszczyk; Anna Burdzy; Justyna Targowska; and Paulina Michalak for their technical support.

Conflicts of Interest: The authors declare no conflict of interest.

References

1. Nielsen, F.H. Update on the possible nutritional importance of silicon. *J. Trace Elem. Med. Biol.* **2014**, *28*, 379–382. [CrossRef] [PubMed]
2. Ratcliffe, S.; Jugdaohsingh, R.; Vivancos, J.; Marron, A.; Deshmukh, R.; Ma, J.F.; Mitani-Ueno, N.; Robertson, J.; Wills, J.; Boekschoten, M.V.; et al. Identification of a mammalian silicon transporter. *Am. J. Physiol. Cell Physiol.* **2017**, *312*, C550–C561. [CrossRef]

3. Garneau, A.P.; Carpentier, G.A.; Marcoux, A.A.; Frenette-Cotton, R.; Simard, C.F.; Rémus-Borel, W.; Caron, L.; Jacob-Wagner, M.; Noël, M.; Powell, J.J.; et al. Aquaporins mediate silicon transport in humans. *PLoS ONE* **2015**, *10*, e0136149. [CrossRef]
4. MacDonald, H.M.; Hardcastle, A.C.; Jugdaohsingh, R.; Fraser, W.D.; Reid, D.M.; Powell, J.J. Dietary silicon interacts with oestrogen to influence bone health: Evidence from the Aberdeen prospective osteoporosis screening study. *Bone* **2012**, *50*, 681–687. [CrossRef] [PubMed]
5. Jugdaohsingh, R.; Tucker, K.L.; Qiao, N.; Cupples, L.A.; Kiel, D.P.; Powell, J.J. Dietary silicon intake is positively associated with bone mineral density in men and premenopausal women of the Framingham Offspring cohort. *J. Bone Min. Res.* **2004**, *19*, 297–307. [CrossRef]
6. Gillette-Guyonnet, S.; Andrieu, S.; Vellas, B. The potential influence of silica present in drinking water on Alzheimer's disease and associated disorders. *J. Nutr. Health Aging* **2007**, *11*, 119.
7. Barel, A.; Calomme, M.; Timchenko, A.; Paepe, K.D.; Demeester, N.; Rogiers, V.; Clarys, D.; Berghe, D.V. Effect of oral intake of choline-stabilized orthosilicic acid on skin, nails and hair in women with photodamaged skin. *Arch. Dermatol. Res.* **2005**, *297*, 147–153. [CrossRef] [PubMed]
8. Prescha, A.; Zabłocka-Słowińska, K.; Płaczkowska, S.; Gorczyca, D.; Łuczak, A.; Grajeta, H. Silicon intake and plasma level and their relationship with systemic redox and inflammatory markers in rheumatoid arthritis patients. *Adv. Clin. Exp. Med.* **2019**, *28*, ahead of print. [CrossRef]
9. Jugdaohsingh, R.; Anderson, S.H.; Tucker, K.L.; Elliott, H.; Kiel, D.P.; Thompson, R.P.; Powell, J.J. Dietary silicon intake and absorption. *Am. J. Clin. Nutr.* **2002**, *75*, 887–893. [CrossRef] [PubMed]
10. Robberecht, H.; Van Cauwenbergh, R.; Van Vlaslaer, V.; Hermans, N. Dietary silicon intake in Belgium: Sources, availability from foods, and human serum levels. *Sci. Total Environ.* **2009**, *407*, 4777–4782. [CrossRef] [PubMed]
11. Kim, Y.Y.; Kim, M.H.; Choi, M.K. Relationship between dietary intake and urinary excretion of silicon in free-living Korean adult men and women. *Biol. Trace. Elem. Res.* **2019**, 1–8. [CrossRef]
12. McNaughton, S.A.; Bolton-Smith, C.; Mishra, G.D.; Jugdaohsingh, R.; Powell, J.J. Dietary silicon intake in post-menopausal women. *Br. J. Nutr.* **2005**, *94*, 813–817. [CrossRef]
13. Sripanyakorn, S.; Jugdaohsingh, R.; Dissayabutr, W.; Anderson, S.H.; Thompson, R.P.; Powell, J.J. The comparative absorption of silicon from different foods and food supplements. *Br. J. Nutr.* **2009**, *102*, 825–834. [CrossRef]
14. Bissé, E.; Epting, T.; Beil, A.; Lininger, G.; Lang, H.; Wieland, H. Reference values for serum silicon in adults. *Anal. Biochem.* **2005**, *337*, 130–135. [CrossRef]
15. Jarosz, M. *Polish Dietary Reference Intakes*; National Food and Nutrition Institute: Warsaw, Poland, 2017; pp. 203–237.
16. Powell, J.J.; McNaughton, S.A.; Jugdaohsingh, R.; Dear, J.; Khot, F.; Mowatt, L.; Gleason, K.L.; Sykes, M.; Thompson, R.P.H.; Bolton-Smith, C.; et al. A provisional database for the silicon content of foods in the United Kingdom. *Br. J. Nutr.* **2005**, *94*, 804–812. [CrossRef]
17. Pennington, J.A.T. Silicon in foods and diets. *Food Addit. Contam.* **1991**, *8*, 97–118. [CrossRef]
18. Prescha, A.; Zabłocka-Słowińska, K.; Hojka, A.; Grajeta, H. Instant food products as a source of silicon. *Food Chem.* **2012**, *135*, 1756–1761. [CrossRef]
19. Mojsiewicz-Pieńkowska, K.; Łukasiak, J. Analytical fractionation of silicon compounds in foodstuffs. *Food Control* **2003**, *14*, 153–162. [CrossRef]
20. Dejneka, W.; Łukasiak, J. Determination of total and bioavailable silicon in selected foodstuffs. *Food Control* **2003**, *14*, 193–196. [CrossRef]
21. Choi, M.K.; Kim, M.H. Dietary silicon intake of Korean young adult males and its relation to their bone status. *Biol. Trace. Elem. Res.* **2017**, *176*, 89–104. [CrossRef]
22. Waśkiewicz, A.; Szcześniewska, D.; Szostak-Węgierek, D.; Stepaniak, U.; Kozakiewicz, K.; Tykarski, A.; Zdrojewski, T.; Zujko, M.E.; Drygas, W. Are dietary habits of the Polish population consistent with the recommendations for prevention of cardiovascular disease?—WOBASZ II project. *Kardiol. Pol.* **2016**, *74*, 969–977. [CrossRef]
23. Montesano, F.F.; D'Imperio, M.; Parente, A.; Cardinali, A.; Renna, M.; Serio, F. Green bean biofortification for Si through soilless cultivation: Plant response and Si bioaccessibility in pods. *Sci. Rep.* **2016**, *6*, 31662. [CrossRef] [PubMed]

24. Giammarioli, S.; Mosca, M.; Sanzini, E. Silicon content of Italian mineral waters and its contribution to daily intake. *J. Food Sci.* **2005**, *70*, s509–s512. [CrossRef]
25. Hussain, S.A.; Jaccob, A.A. Effects of single oral doses of flavonoids on absorption and tissue distribution of orally administered doses of trace elements in rats. *Am. J. Pharmacol. Sci.* **2013**, *1*, 84–89.
26. Finley, J.W.; Davis, C.D. Manganese absorption and retention in rats is affected by the type of dietary fat. *Biol. Trace Elem. Res.* **2001**, *82*, 143–158. [CrossRef]

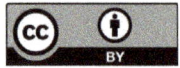

© 2019 by the authors. Licensee MDPI, Basel, Switzerland. This article is an open access article distributed under the terms and conditions of the Creative Commons Attribution (CC BY) license (http://creativecommons.org/licenses/by/4.0/).

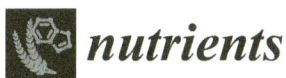

Article

Biotin Is Required for the Zinc Homeostasis in the Skin

Youichi Ogawa *, Manao Kinoshita, Takuya Sato, Shinji Shimada and Tatsuyoshi Kawamura

Department of Dermatology, Faculty of Medicine, University of Yamanashi, Yamanashi 409-3898, Japan; mkinoshita@yamanashi.ac.jp (M.K.); d17sm039@yamanashi.ac.jp (T.S.); sshimada@yamanashi.ac.jp (S.S.); tkawa@yamanashi.ac.jp (T.K.)
* Correspondence: yogawa@yamanashi.ac.jp; Tel./Fax: +81-55-273-6766

Received: 30 March 2019; Accepted: 23 April 2019; Published: 24 April 2019

Abstract: Patients with biotin deficiency present symptoms that are similar to those in patients with acrodermatitis enteropathica (inherent zinc deficiency). However, the association between biotin and zinc deficiency remains unknown. We have previously shown that epidermal keratinocytes of mice fed zinc-deficient (ZD) diets secreted more adenosine triphosphate (ATP) than those of mice fed zinc-adequate (ZA) diets and that epidermal Langerhans cells are absent in ZD mice. Langerhans cells highly express CD39, which potently hydrolyzes ATP into adenosine monophosphate (AMP). Thus, a lack of Langerhans cells in ZD mice leads to non-hydrolysis of ATP, thereby leading to the development of ATP-mediated irritant contact dermatitis. In this study, we examined if biotin-deficient (BD) mice showed the same underlying mechanisms as those in ZD mice. BD mice showed reduced serum zinc levels, disappearance of epidermal Langerhans cells, and enhanced ATP production in the skin. Consequently, irritant contact dermatitis was significantly enhanced and prolonged in BD mice. In conclusion, the findings of our study showed that biotin deficiency leads to zinc deficiency because of which patients with biotin deficiency show similar symptoms as those with acrodermatitis enteropathica.

Keywords: biotin deficiency; zinc deficiency; acrodermatitis enteropathica; Langerhans cells; adenosine triphosphate

1. Introduction

Biotin is a water-soluble vitamin that serves as a co-enzyme for five carboxylases, namely, the covalently bound coenzyme for acetyl-CoA carboxylases 1 and 2, pyruvate carboxylase, propionyl-CoA carboxylase, and 3-methylcrotonyl-CoA carboxylase. These biotin-dependent carboxylases facilitate various metabolic reactions such as gluconeogenesis, fatty acid synthesis, and amino acid synthesis. Mammals cannot synthesize biotin by themselves; they obtain biotin through food and some gut microbiota produce biotin. Biotin deficiency (BnD) rarely occurs in people who consume a normal mixed diet [1,2]. However, genetic deficiency of holocarboxylase synthetase and biotinidase, continuous consumption of raw egg whites, parenteral nutrition, and modified milk without biotin supplementation could result in BnD [1–3]. Patients with BnD [4] are known to develop clinical symptoms that are similar to those in patients with acrodermatitis enteropathica (AE), which is caused by loss-of-function mutations in Zrt-, Irt-like protein (ZIP) 4 [5–7]. The clinical symptoms of AE include characteristic skin lesions, alopecia, and diarrhea.

Patients with AE exhibit severe zinc deficiency (ZnD) because their intestines lack the ability to absorb zinc. The characteristic skin lesions of AE occur in the periorificial, anogenital, and acral regions, which are exposed to the external environment. These lesions were caused by adenosine triphosphate (ATP)-mediated irritant contact dermatitis (ICD) [8–10]. Mice fed zinc-deficient (ZD) diet showed an impaired allergic contact dermatitis (ACD) in response to dinitrofluorobenzene (DNFB) compared to mice fed a zinc-adequate (ZA) diet. ZnD leads to impaired immune responses because of dysfunction in the immune cells. Thus, DNFB-mediated ACD is attenuated in ZD mice. However, ZD mice exhibited a significantly increased and prolonged ICD in response to croton oil (CrO) compared with ZA mice [8–10]. ATP is released from keratinocytes (KCs) in response to various environmental stimuli through lytic and non-lytic mechanisms, which results in ICD [11]. An ex vivo organ culture with CrO showed that the amount of ATP released from the skin of ZD mice was much greater than that released from the skin of ZA mice. Additionally, an injection of apyrase that hydrolyzes ATP into adenosine monophosphate (AMP) restored the increased and prolonged ICD caused by CrO application in ZD mice [8]. These results suggest that the prolonged ICD response in ZD mice was mediated via the excess ATP release by KCs in response to irritants.

Langerhans cells (LCs) are a subset of antigen-presenting cells that are distributed in the epidermis [12]. LCs but not KCs express CD39 (ecto-nucleoside triphosphate diphosphohydrolase 1; ENTPD-1) that potently hydrolyzes ATP into AMP [13–15], thereby assuming approximately 80% of the epidermal ATP hydrolysis [16]. Interestingly, epidermal LCs were absent in the skin lesions of patients with AE and of ZD mice [8–10]. The impaired ATP hydrolysis because of the disappearance of LCs leads to ATP-mediated inflammation in the epidermis, followed by the development of ICD. Therefore, the characteristic skin lesions in patients with AE are developed by aberrant ATP production from ZD–KCs and defective ATP hydrolysis due to loss of CD39-expressing LCs.

Patients with BnD show similar characteristic skin lesions as patients with AE. Thus, we hypothesized that skin lesions in BnD are caused by the same underlying mechanisms as those in ZnD.

2. Materials and Methods

2.1. Study Approval

Murine studies were conducted with the approval of and in accordance with the guidelines for animal experiments of the University of Yamanashi.

2.2. Animals and Diets

Five-week-old female BALB/c mice were purchased from Oriental Yeast Co. Ltd. (Tokyo, Japan). Mice were maintained under specific pathogen-free conditions throughout this study. Biotin-deficient (BD) and zinc-deficient (ZD) diets were purchased from CLEA Japan Inc (Tokyo, Japan). The mice were fed control (biotin-adequate; BA) or BD diet from 5 to 21 weeks of age. BA and BD diets were of almost the same nutritional quality, differing only in terms of biotin content. In another experiment (Figure 1B), the mice were fed ZD or control (zinc-adequate; ZA) diet from 5 to 11 weeks of age.

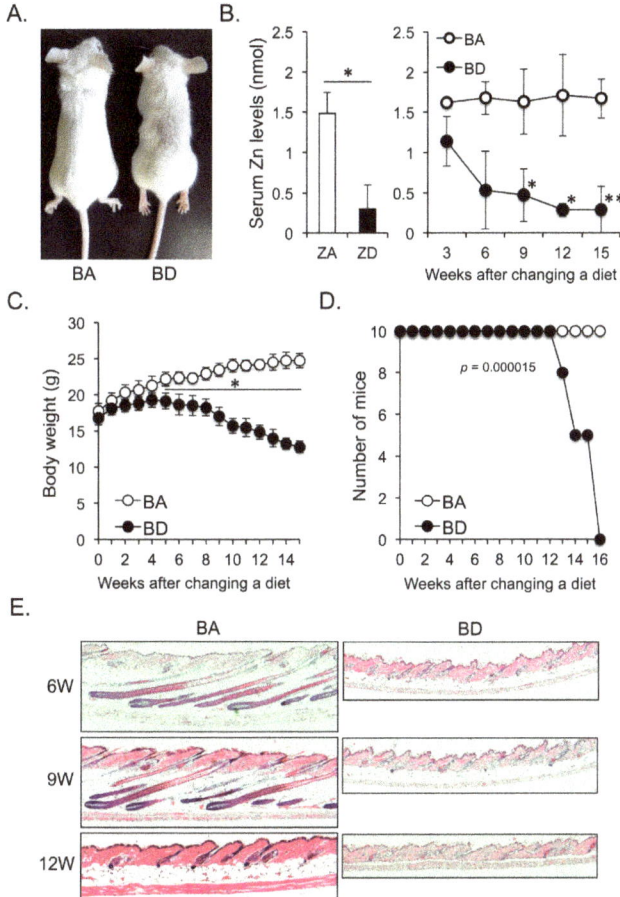

Figure 1. (**A**) Five-week-old female BALB/c mice were fed biotin-adequate (BA) (control diet) or biotin-deficient (BD) diet for 12 weeks. (**B**) Serum zinc levels of zinc-adequate (ZA) and zinc-deficient (ZD) mice after consumption of ZA (control) and ZD diet for seven weeks (left panel). Serum zinc levels of BA and BD mice fed BA (control) and BD diets for the indicated weeks (right panel). Five mice of each group were analyzed. Course of body weight (**C**) and survival rate (**D**) of BA and BD mice. Ten mice of each group were analyzed. (**E**) Change of skin phenotype of BA and BD mice after consumption of BA and BD diets for the indicated weeks (hematoxylin and eosin stain, ×100). Data are representative of three independent experiments. * $p < 0.05$, ** $p < 0.01$.

2.3. Reagents and Antibodies

Dinitrofluorobenzene (DNFB), croton oil (CrO), and bis(2-acrylamidoethyl) disulfide (BAC) were purchased from Sigma-Aldrich (St. Louis, MO, USA). FITC-conjugated anti-mouse IA/IE and PE-conjugated anti-mouse CD45 mAbs were purchased from BioLegend (San Diego, CA, USA).

2.4. Quantification of Zinc Levels in the Serum

Serum zinc levels of BA, BD, ZA, and ZD mice were determined using the Zinc Quantification Kit (abcam, Cambridge, MA, USA) as per the manufacturer's instructions.

2.5. Histological Examination

Skin specimens from the backs (Figure 1E) and ears (Figure 2E,F) of BA or BD mice were surgically removed, fixed in 4% paraformaldehyde overnight at 4 °C, and then dehydrated in 70% ethanol. Samples were embedded in paraffin. Sections were stained with hematoxylin and eosin.

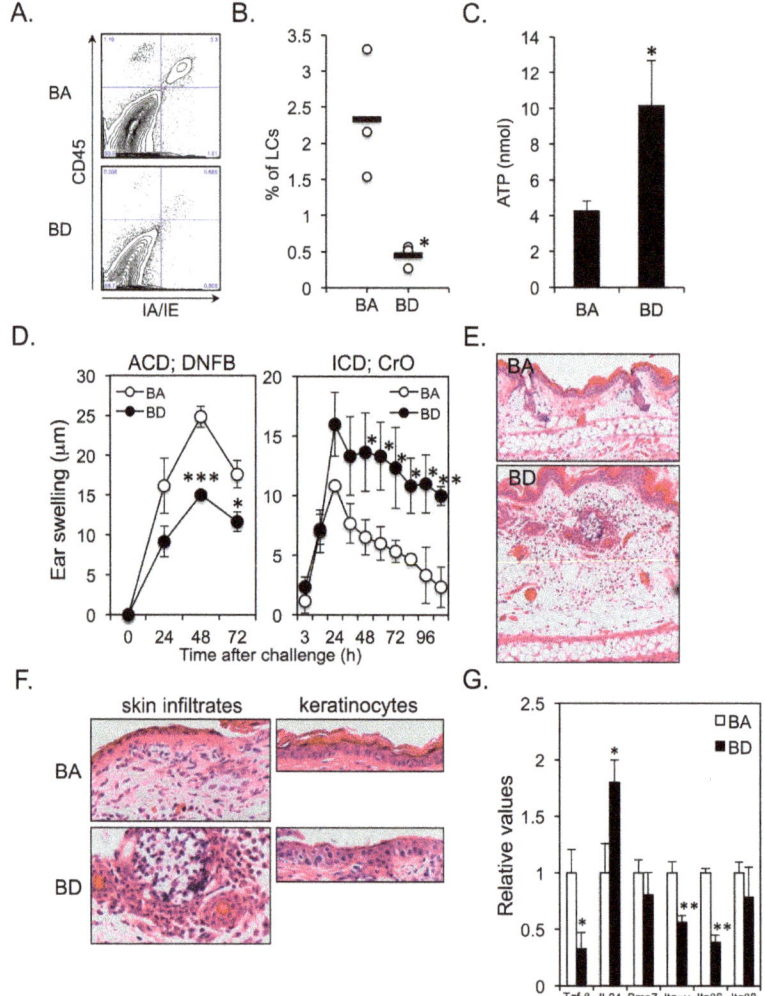

Figure 2. (**A,B**) Five-week-old female BALB/c mice were fed BA (control diet) or BD diet for 12 weeks. Epidermal langerhans cells (LCs) were identified as CD45$^+$IA/IE$^+$ cells. Three mice for each group were analyzed. (**C**) ATP release in response to BAC from the ear skins of BA and BD mice at 12 weeks after the initiation of BA and BD diets. Five mice of each group were analyzed. (**D**) ACD (left panel) and ICD (right panel) in BA and BD mice at 12 weeks after the initiation of BA and BD diets. Five mice of each group were analyzed. (**E,F**) ears of BA and BD mice elicited irritant contact dermatitis (ICD) response at 24 h after CrO application. (**G**) mRNA expression of molecules associated with LC differentiation and survival in KCs. Data are representative of 3 independent experiments. * $p < 0.05$, ** $p < 0.01$, *** $p < 0.001$.

2.6. Preparation of Epidermal Cell Suspensions

The dorsal back skin was removed and incubated with 0.5% solution of trypsin (type XI, Sigma-Aldrich, St. Louis, MO, USA) in PBS for 30 min at 37 °C to separate the epidermis from the underlying dermis. After the removal of the loosened dermis, the epidermal sheets were gently agitated with 0.05% DNase1 (Sigma-Aldrich, St. Louis, MO, USA) in PBS for 10 min, and the resulting epidermal cell suspension was passed through a nylon mesh to remove hair and stratum corneum prior to use.

2.7. Flow Cytometry

Single-cell suspensions (1×10^6) of epidermal sheets from BA and BD mice (3 mice per group) were stained for LCs with FITC-conjugated anti–IA/IE and PE-conjugated anti-CD45 mAbs for 30 min at 4 °C. Live/dead discrimination was performed using propidium iodide (Sigma-Aldrich, St. Louis, MO, USA). After washing, samples were analyzed using a FACSCalibur flow cytometer (BD Biosciences, San Jose, CA, USA).

2.8. Quantification of ATP Release from the Skin

Both ears from all the mice were taken immediately after sacrifice. Ear skins of the dorsal (back) side were used in the experiment. Ear skin explants were prepared by cutting into 8.0 mm circular pieces. The 2 pieces of ear skin were floated with the epidermis side upward in 12-well plates containing 4 mL PBS and incubated on ice for 10 min. Subsequently, 0.1% BAC was added to the culture. After 30 min, ATP concentrations in the supernatants were quantified using the luciferin-luciferase assay.

2.9. ACD and ICD Responses

For chemical induction of allergic contact dermatitis (ACD), all mice were topically treated with 20 µL of 0.5% DNFB dissolved in acetone/olive oil (4:1), which was painted onto the shaved abdomen at days 0 and 1. The ears were then challenged by application of 10 µL of 0.2% DNFB on the right ear and vehicle alone on the left ear on day 5. For chemically induced irritant contact dermatitis (ICD), all mice received topical application of 1% CrO on the right ear and vehicle alone on the left ear. Swelling responses were quantified (right ear thickness minus left ear thickness) by a third experimenter using a micrometer.

2.10. Quantitative Real-Time PCR Analysis

Epidermal Cell Suspensions were prepared from back skins of BA and BD mice. To isolate keratinocytes (KCs), $CD45^+$ cells were eliminated using MACS (Miltenyi Biotec, Bergisch Gladbach, Germany). Total RNA was extracted using QIAzol® Lysis Reagent (Qiagen, Hilden, Germany) and RNeasy® Plus Universal Mini kit (Qiagen, Hilden, Germany) as per the manufacturer's instructions. Reverse transcription reaction was performed using ReverTra Ace® qPCR RT Kit (Toyobo, Osaka, Japan) as per the manufacturer's instructions. mRNA levels were determined using commercially available primer/probe sets (TaqMan® Gene Expression Assay, Applied Biosystems, Foster City, Calif) and the AB7500 real-time PCR system (Applied Biosystems, Foster City, Calif). The amount of target gene mRNA obtained using real-time PCR was normalized against the amount of the housekeeping control gene (β-actin) mRNA. Primers corresponding to murine *TGF-β*, *Il-34*, *Bmp7*, *Itgαv*, *Itg$\beta 6$*, and *Itg$\beta 8$* were designed by Takara (Shiga, Japan).

2.11. Statistics

Significant differences between experimental groups were analyzed by Student's t test. p values less than 0.05 were considered significant. The survival of BA and BD mice was analyzed in the Kaplan–Meier format using log-rank (Mantel–Cox) test (Figure 1D).

3. Results

3.1. Dietary Biotin Deficiency Leads to Zinc Deficiency

After a 12-week biotin-adequate (BA; control) or biotin-deficient (BD) diet, the body size of BD mice was smaller than that of BA mice. Although BD mice did not exhibit apparent alopecia, the hair distribution was apparently sparse (Figure 1A). We next compared serum zinc levels between dietary zinc-deficient (ZD) and BD mice. Mice started to die after 8 weeks of initiation of ZD diet [8]. Accordingly, we measured serum zinc levels of zinc-adequate (ZA; control) and ZD mice at 7 weeks after the initiation of the ZA or ZD diet. Serum zinc levels were significantly impaired in ZD mice compared with ZA mice at this time point (Figure 1B; left panel). We found that BD mice showed a quick reduction in the serum zinc levels after initiation of the BD diet. After 9 weeks of initiation of the BD diet, the serum zinc levels in BD mice were significantly reduced compared with those in BA mice (Figure 1B; right panel), and were almost comparable to those in ZD mice after 7 weeks of initiation of ZD diet (Figure 1B; left and right panels). These data suggest that dietary biotin deficiency (BnD) leads to zinc deficiency (ZnD).

The body weight of BD mice was significantly lesser than that of BA mice after 5 weeks of initiation of BD diet (Figure 1C). Moreover, the survival rate in BD mice was also significantly reduced in BD mice compared with that in BA mice after 13 weeks of initiation of the BD diet (Figure 1D). Akin to ZD mice, BD mice showed strong atrophy of fat tissues and an arrest in the hair cycle (Figure 1E). These data suggest that dietary BnD-mediated ZnD affects skin homeostasis.

3.2. Dietary Biotin Deficiency Leads to the Development of ATP-Mediated Irritant Contact Dermatitis

We found that epidermal LCs ($CD45^+IA/IE^+$ cells) almost disappeared in BD mice (Figure 2A,B), thereby resulting in increased ATP production from the ear skins in response to irritants (Figure 2C). ACD was significantly impaired and ICD was significantly enhanced and prolonged in BD mice (Figure 2D,E). There was a massive neutrophil infiltration in both dermis and epidermis of BD mice compared to that in BA mice (Figure 2F; left panel). Histological examination of ICD lesions in BD mice revealed parakeratosis and cytoplasmic pallor, sub-corneal vacuolization, and ballooning degeneration of KCs (Figure 2F; right panel). These signs are histological features of cutaneous AE lesions in humans [17], whereas no such degeneration of KCs was observed in the ICD lesions of BA mice (Figure 2F; right panel). Several proteins are involved in the maintenance and survival of epidermal LCs, including transforming growth factor (TGF)-β [18], interleukin (IL)-34 [19], bone morphogenetic protein (BMP)-7 [20], integrin (ITG) $\alpha v \beta 6$ [21], and ITG$\alpha v \beta 8$ [22]. We examined if BnD alters the mRNA expression of these molecules in KCs. The expression of TGF-β was significantly downregulated in BD–KCs (Figure 2G). However, the expression of IL-34 was significantly upregulated in BD–KCs (Figure 2G). Interestingly, the expression of ITG$\alpha v \beta 6$, but not ITG$\alpha v \beta 8$, was significantly downregulated in BD–KCs.

4. Discussion

BnD causes abnormalities in the fatty acid composition of skin, such as accumulation of odd-chain fatty acids and abnormal metabolism of long-chain polyunsaturated fatty acids [4,23,24]. In this study, we found that dietary BnD leads to ZnD. However, the decline in the serum zinc levels in BD mice was relatively slower than that in ZD mice [8]. Accordingly, although changes in terms of the body weight and survival rate were similar to those observed in ZD mice, the kinetics in BD mice was slower than that in ZD mice [8]. LCs were found to be almost absent in the epidermis of BD mice, thereby leading to enhanced ATP production in skin, and similar findings were observed for ZD mice. This aberrant ATP accumulation in the skin results in the recruitment of neutrophils [25] and development of characteristic skin lesions in patients with ZnD and BnD. Indeed, decreased serum zinc levels have been reported in some patients with BnD [26–28]. On the other hand, some studies have demonstrated normal serum zinc levels in patients with BnD [29–31]. We speculate that this discrepancy might be attributable for the duration of BnD. Reduced serum biotin and zinc levels have been recently reported in patients with male androgenetic alopecia, suggesting the close association between biotin and zinc [32]. We investigated how dietary BnD led to ZnD but the precise mechanisms could not be elucidated (data not shown). Further analysis is required for elucidating the underlying mechanisms.

Three groups of molecules hydrolyze ATP, namely, ENTPDs, ectonucleotide pyrophosphatase/phosphodiesterases (ENPPs), and alkaline phosphatase (ALP) [33,34]. The latter two molecules are zinc-dependent molecules. Among ENTPDs and ENPPs, ENTPD-1 (CD39), -2, -3, and -8 and ENPP-1, -2, and -3 hydrolyze ATP [33]. LCs strongly express ENTPD-1 (CD39) and weakly express ENTPD-2 and ENPP-1, -2, and -3. KCs weakly express CD39, ENTPD-2 and -3, and ENPP-1 and -2 [16]. Neither LCs nor KCs express ENTPD-8 or ALP. Therefore, although LCs strongly express CD39, other ATP-hydrolyzing molecules are weakly expressed in both LCs and KCs. LCs occupy approximately 3% of the epidermis, whereas KCs occupy approximately 97%. Regardless of this numeric difference between LCs and KCs in the epidermis, LCs perform approximately 80% of epidermal ATP hydrolysis, whereas KCs perform the remaining 20% [16]. Additionally, ZnD impairs the activity of ENPPs [35]. KCs weakly express ENPP-1 and ENPP-2. This explains one underlying mechanism by which ZD–KCs and BD–KCs show increased ATP production.

Both ZnD and BnD result in disappearance of epidermal LCs. TGF-β knock out (KO) mice, Langerin-Cre TGF-β1$^{fl/fl}$ mice, Langerin-Cre TGF-βRI$^{fl/fl}$ mice, and Langerin-Cre TGF-βRII$^{fl/fl}$ mice lack epidermal LCs [36], suggesting that although TGF-β is produced by both LCs and KCs, LC-derived autocrine and/or paracrine TGF-β is critical for LC development and survival. TGF-β is secreted as an inactive latency-associated peptide (LAP)-TGF-β. LAP-TGF-β is processed by integrin (ITG) αvβ6 and/or αvβ8 expressed on KCs but not on LCs, which convert LAP-TGF-β into active TGF-β [36,37]. Thus, ITGαvβ6 or αvβ8 KO mice show substantially reduced number of epidermal LCs [21,22]. In BD–KCs, the mRNA expression levels of TGF-β and ITGαvβ6 were significantly downregulated. As described above, LC-derived, but not KC-derived, TGF-β is critical for LC homeostasis. In this respect, it is unclear how much downregulated TGF-β mRNA expression in BD–KCs is involved in disappearance of epidermal LCs. On the other hand, LAP-TGF-β produced by LCs is not processed into active TGF-β, because of downregulated ITGαvβ6 expression in BD–KCs. This may be one of underlying mechanisms for the loss of epidermal LCs in BD mice.

5. Conclusions

In this study, we found that dietary BnD led to ZnD. BD mice lost epidermal LCs possibly due to impaired ITGαvβ6 expression in KCs, as seen in ZD mice. This resulted in ATP accumulation in the epidermis, thereby leading to the development of ATP-mediated ICD lesions in the skin. We concluded that the characteristic skin lesions in patients with AE and BnD have common underlying mechanisms, and biotin is required for zinc homeostasis in the skin.

Author Contributions: Investigation, Y.O., M.K., and T.S.; formal analysis, Y.O., M.K., and T.S.; conceptualization, Y.O., S.S., and T.K.; writing, Y.O.; supervision, S.S. and T.K. All authors critically reviewed the manuscript and approved the final version.

Funding: None.

Conflicts of Interest: The authors declare no conflict of interest.

References

1. Leon-Del-Rio, A. Biotin in metabolism, gene expression, and human disease. *J. Inherit. Metab. Dis.* **2019**. [CrossRef]
2. Zempleni, J.; Wijeratne, S.S.; Hassan, Y.I. Biotin. *Biofactors* **2009**, *35*, 36–46. [CrossRef]
3. Zempleni, J.; Hassan, Y.I.; Wijeratne, S.S. Biotin and biotinidase deficiency. *Expert Rev. Endocrinol. Metab.* **2008**, *3*, 715–724. [CrossRef] [PubMed]
4. Mock, D.M. Skin manifestations of biotin deficiency. *Semin. Dermatol.* **1991**, *10*, 296–302.

5. Wang, K.; Pugh, E.W.; Griffen, S.; Doheny, K.F.; Mostafa, W.Z.; al-Aboosi, M.M.; el-Shanti, H.; Gitschier, J. Homozygosity mapping places the acrodermatitis enteropathica gene on chromosomal region 8q24.3. *Am. J. Hum. Genet.* **2001**, *68*, 1055–1060. [CrossRef] [PubMed]
6. Wang, K.; Zhou, B.; Kuo, Y.M.; Zemansky, J.; Gitschier, J. A novel member of a zinc transporter family is defective in acrodermatitis enteropathica. *Am. J. Hum. Genet.* **2002**, *71*, 66–73. [CrossRef] [PubMed]
7. Kury, S.; Dreno, B.; Bezieau, S.; Giraudet, S.; Kharfi, M.; Kamoun, R.; Moisan, J.P. Identification of SLC39A4, a gene involved in acrodermatitis enteropathica. *Nat. Genet.* **2002**, *31*, 239–240. [CrossRef]
8. Kawamura, T.; Ogawa, Y.; Nakamura, Y.; Nakamizo, S.; Ohta, Y.; Nakano, H.; Kabashima, K.; Katayama, I.; Koizumi, S.; Kodama, T.; et al. Severe dermatitis with loss of epidermal Langerhans cells in human and mouse zinc deficiency. *J. Clin. Invest.* **2012**, *122*, 722–732. [CrossRef]
9. Ogawa, Y.; Kawamura, T.; Shimada, S. Zinc and skin biology. *Arch. Biochem. Biophys.* **2016**, *611*, 113–119. [CrossRef]
10. Ogawa, Y.; Kinoshita, M.; Shimada, S.; Kawamura, T. Zinc and Skin Disorders. *Nutrients* **2018**, *10*, 199. [CrossRef]
11. Mizumoto, N.; Mummert, M.E.; Shalhevet, D.; Takashima, A. Keratinocyte ATP release assay for testing skin-irritating potentials of structurally diverse chemicals. *J. Invest. Dermatol.* **2003**, *121*, 1066–1072. [CrossRef]
12. Kashem, S.W.; Haniffa, M.; Kaplan, D.H. Antigen-Presenting cells in the skin. *Annu. Rev. Immunol.* **2017**, *35*, 469–499. [CrossRef]
13. Georgiou, J.G.; Skarratt, K.K.; Fuller, S.J.; Martin, C.J.; Christopherson, R.I.; Wiley, J.S.; Sluyter, R. Human epidermal and monocyte-derived langerhans cells express functional P2X receptors. *J. Invest. Dermatol.* **2005**, *125*, 482–490. [CrossRef]
14. Ho, C.L.; Yang, C.Y.; Lin, W.J.; Lin, C.H. Ecto-nucleoside triphosphate diphosphohydrolase 2 modulates local ATP-induced calcium signaling in human HaCaT keratinocytes. *PLoS ONE* **2013**, *8*, e57666. [CrossRef]
15. Mizumoto, N.; Kumamoto, T.; Robson, S.C.; Sevigny, J.; Matsue, H.; Enjyoji, K.; Takashima, A. CD39 is the dominant Langerhans cell-associated ecto-NTPDase: Modulatory roles in inflammation and immune responsiveness. *Nat. Med.* **2002**, *8*, 358–365. [CrossRef] [PubMed]
16. Ogawa, Y.; Kinoshita, M.; Mizumura, N.; Miyazaki, S.; Aoki, R.; Momosawa, A.; Shimada, S.; Kambe, T.; Kawamura, T. Purinergic molecules in the epidermis. *J. Investig. Dermatol.* **2018**, *138*, 2486–2488. [CrossRef] [PubMed]
17. Maverakis, E.; Fung, M.A.; Lynch, P.J.; Draznin, M.; Michael, D.J.; Ruben, B.; Fazel, N. Acrodermatitis enteropathica and an overview of zinc metabolism. *J. Am. Acad. Dermatol.* **2007**, *56*, 116–124. [CrossRef] [PubMed]
18. Borkowski, T.A.; Letterio, J.J.; Farr, A.G.; Udey, M.C. A role for endogenous transforming growth factor beta 1 in Langerhans cell biology: The skin of transforming growth factor beta 1 null mice is devoid of epidermal Langerhans cells. *J. Exp. Med.* **1996**, *184*, 2417–2422. [CrossRef]
19. Wang, Y.; Szretter, K.J.; Vermi, W.; Gilfillan, S.; Rossini, C.; Cella, M.; Barrow, A.D.; Diamond, M.S.; Colonna, M. IL-34 is a tissue-restricted ligand of CSF1R required for the development of Langerhans cells and microglia. *Nat. Immunol.* **2012**, *13*, 753–760. [CrossRef] [PubMed]
20. Yasmin, N.; Bauer, T.; Modak, M.; Wagner, K.; Schuster, C.; Koffel, R.; Seyerl, M.; Stockl, J.; Elbe-Burger, A.; Graf, D.; et al. Identification of bone morphogenetic protein 7 (BMP7) as an instructive factor for human epidermal Langerhans cell differentiation. *J. Exp. Med.* **2013**, *210*, 2597–2610. [CrossRef] [PubMed]
21. Yang, Z.; Mu, Z.; Dabovic, B.; Jurukovski, V.; Yu, D.; Sung, J.; Xiong, X.; Munger, J.S. Absence of integrin-mediated TGFbeta1 activation in vivo recapitulates the phenotype of TGFbeta1-null mice. *J. Cell Biol.* **2007**, *176*, 787–793. [CrossRef] [PubMed]
22. Aluwihare, P.; Mu, Z.; Zhao, Z.; Yu, D.; Weinreb, P.H.; Horan, G.S.; Violette, S.M.; Munger, J.S. Mice that lack activity of alphavbeta6- and alphavbeta8-integrins reproduce the abnormalities of Tgfb1- and Tgfb3-null mice. *J. Cell Sci.* **2009**, *122*, 227–232. [CrossRef] [PubMed]
23. Mock, D.M. Evidence for a pathogenic role of omega 6 polyunsaturated fatty acid in the cutaneous manifestations of biotin deficiency. *J. Pediatr. Gastroenterol. Nutr.* **1990**, *10*, 222–229. [CrossRef]
24. Proud, V.K.; Rizzo, W.B.; Patterson, J.W.; Heard, G.S.; Wolf, B. Fatty acid alterations and carboxylase deficiencies in the skin of biotin-deficient rats. *Am. J. Clin. Nutr.* **1990**, *51*, 853–858. [CrossRef]

25. Da Silva, G.L.; Sperotto, N.D.; Borges, T.J.; Bonorino, C.; Takyia, C.M.; Coutinho-Silva, R.; Campos, M.M.; Zanin, R.F.; Morrone, F.B. P2X7 receptor is required for neutrophil accumulation in a mouse model of irritant contact dermatitis. *Exp. Dermatol.* **2013**, *22*, 184–188. [CrossRef]
26. Matsusue, S.; Kashihara, S.; Takeda, H.; Koizumi, S. Biotin deficiency during total parenteral nutrition: Its clinical manifestation and plasma nonesterified fatty acid level. *JPEN J. Parenter. Enteral. Nutr.* **1985**, *9*, 760–763. [CrossRef]
27. Higuchi, R.; Mizukoshi, M.; Koyama, H.; Kitano, N.; Koike, M. Intractable diaper dermatitis as an early sign of biotin deficiency. *Acta Paediatr.* **1998**, *87*, 228–229. [CrossRef]
28. Lagier, P.; Bimar, P.; Seriat-Gautier, S.; Dejode, J.M.; Brun, T.; Bimar, J. Zinc and biotin deficiency during prolonged parenteral nutrition in the infant. *Presse. Med.* **1987**, *16*, 1795–1797. [PubMed]
29. Khalidi, N.; Wesley, J.R.; Thoene, J.G.; Whitehouse, W.M., Jr.; Baker, W.L. Biotin deficiency in a patient with short bowel syndrome during home parenteral nutrition. *JPEN J. Parenter. Enteral. Nutr.* **1984**, *8*, 311–314. [CrossRef] [PubMed]
30. Higuchi, R.; Noda, E.; Koyama, Y.; Shirai, T.; Horino, A.; Juri, T.; Koike, M. Biotin deficiency in an infant fed with amino acid formula and hypoallergenic rice. *Acta. Paediatr.* **1996**, *85*, 872–874. [CrossRef]
31. Fujimoto, W.; Inaoki, M.; Fukui, T.; Inoue, Y.; Kuhara, T. Biotin deficiency in an infant fed with amino acid formula. *J. Dermatol.* **2005**, *32*, 256–261. [CrossRef] [PubMed]
32. El-Esawy, F.M.; Hussein, M.S.; Ibrahim Mansour, A. Serum biotin and zinc in male androgenetic alopecia. *J. Cosmet. Dermatol.* **2019**. [CrossRef] [PubMed]
33. Yegutkin, G.G. Nucleotide- and nucleoside-converting ectoenzymes: Important modulators of purinergic signalling cascade. *Biochim. Biophys. Acta.* **2008**, *1783*, 673–694. [CrossRef]
34. Zimmermann, H. Extracellular metabolism of ATP and other nucleotides. *Naunyn. Schmiedebergs. Arch. Pharmacol.* **2000**, *362*, 299–309. [CrossRef] [PubMed]
35. Takeda, T.A.; Miyazaki, S.; Kobayashi, M.; Nishino, K.; Goto, T.; Matsunaga, M.; Ooi, M.; Shirakawa, H.; Tani, F.; Kawamura, T.; et al. Zinc deficiency causes delayed ATP clearance and adenosine generation in rats and cell culture models. *Commun. Biol.* **2018**, *1*, 113. [CrossRef]
36. Kaplan, D.H. Ontogeny and function of murine epidermal Langerhans cells. *Nat. Immunol.* **2017**, *18*, 1068–1075. [CrossRef] [PubMed]
37. Mohammed, J.; Beura, L.K.; Bobr, A.; Astry, B.; Chicoine, B.; Kashem, S.W.; Welty, N.E.; Igyarto, B.Z.; Wijeyesinghe, S.; Thompson, E.A.; et al. Stromal cells control the epithelial residence of DCs and memory T cells by regulated activation of TGF-beta. *Nat. Immunol.* **2016**, *17*, 414–421. [CrossRef]

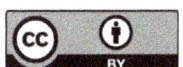

© 2019 by the authors. Licensee MDPI, Basel, Switzerland. This article is an open access article distributed under the terms and conditions of the Creative Commons Attribution (CC BY) license (http://creativecommons.org/licenses/by/4.0/).

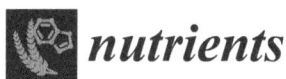

Article

The Germ Fraction Inhibits Iron Bioavailability of Maize: Identification of an Approach to Enhance Maize Nutritional Quality via Processing and Breeding

Raymond Glahn [1,*], Elad Tako [1] and Michael A. Gore [2]

[1] United States Department of Agriculture, Agricultural Research Service, Robert Holley Center for Agriculture and Health, 538 Tower Road, Ithaca, NY 14853, USA; elad.tako@ars.usda.gov
[2] Plant Breeding and Genetics Section, School of Integrative Plant Science, Cornell University, Ithaca, NY 14853, USA; mag87@cornell.edu
* Correspondence: Raymond.Glahn@ars.usda.gov

Received: 1 March 2019; Accepted: 10 April 2019; Published: 12 April 2019

Abstract: Improving the nutritional quality of Fe in maize (*Zea mays*) represents a biofortification strategy to alleviate iron deficiency anemia. Therefore, the present study measured iron content and bioavailability via an established bioassay to characterize Fe quality in parts of the maize kernel. Comparisons of six different varieties of maize demonstrated that the germ fraction is a strong inhibitory component of Fe bioavailability. The germ fraction can contain 27–54% of the total kernel Fe, which is poorly available. In the absence of the germ, Fe in the non-germ components can be highly bioavailable. More specifically, increasing Fe concentration in the non-germ fraction resulted in more bioavailable Fe. Comparison of wet-milled fractions of a commercial maize variety and degerminated corn meal products also demonstrated the inhibitory effect of the germ fraction on Fe bioavailability. When compared to beans (*Phaseolus vulgaris*) containing approximately five times the concentration of Fe, degerminated maize provided more absorbable Fe, indicating substantially higher fractional bioavailability. Overall, the results indicate that degerminated maize may be a better source of Fe than whole maize and some other crops. Increased non-germ Fe density with a weaker inhibitory effect of the germ fraction are desirable qualities to identify and breed for in maize.

Keywords: maize; iron; bioavailability; germ; Caco-2; in vitro digestion; bioassay; biofortification

---

1. Introduction

Biofortification was a term officially coined in 2001 and became a formal strategy for nutritional enhancement of staple crops around 2003. It was at this time that the organization known as HarvestPlus was formed and headquartered at the International Food Policy Research Institute in Washington, DC. Biofortification has its early roots in the United States Department of Agriculture (USDA) research program at centers such as the Plant, Soil and Nutrition Lab in Ithaca, NY (now known as the Robert Holley Center for Agriculture and Health), and in various CGIAR (Consultative Group for International Agricultural Research) Centers worldwide (harvestplus.org). The biofortification research objective is simply to improve human health via enhancement of the nutritional content in staple food crops of the micronutrients vitamin A, zinc (Zn), and iron (Fe). These three micronutrients represent the majority of the "hidden hunger" affecting approximately two billion people worldwide.

Maize (*Zea mays*) is the cereal crop with the highest production worldwide, consistently ranking third or higher as a staple food behind wheat and rice [1]. Biofortification of maize therefore has the potential to have a major impact on human health. Maize biofortifcation efforts have focused primarily on increasing Vitamin A content, with significant advances evidenced by release of enhanced varieties in Nigeria and Zambia [2]. In contrast to Vitamin A, iron biofortification of maize has been explored with limited success using in vitro (Caco-2 cell bioassay) and in vivo (poultry) models for Fe bioavailability [3]. In vitro studies of tropical maize varieties from Nigeria documented relatively small varietal differences in Fe and Zn content, and in Fe bioavailability [4–6]. Although some varieties were identified as promising, they were not pursued further. Additional in vitro studies on lines of superior hybrids from the International Maize and Wheat Improvement Center (CYMMYT) were also conducted [7]. Overall, this study of CYMMT lines was encouraging as it demonstrated that breeding for Fe bioavailability and Fe concentration were distinct and largely unrelated traits; however, the environmental effects were large for both traits, and no follow-up studies were conducted.

Subsequent studies using the combination of Caco-2 cell bioassay and the poultry model developed maize varieties with high Fe bioavailability [8]. This research utilized the Caco-2 cell bioassay to guide identification of quantitative trait loci (QTL) in an established recombinant inbred population, essentially identifying genetic regions important to Fe concentration and Fe bioavailability. Animal feeding trials confirmed the in vitro approach to marker-assisted breeding, demonstrating that Fe bioavailability of maize could be highly enhanced, and that such varieties can be produced in large quantity [9]. However, in a subsequent retraction note [10], the authors point out that the in vitro and in vivo results of that work were indeed valid, and that these lines clearly demonstrated enhanced Fe bioavailability. Retraction of the paper was because the genotypes were not isogenic and homozygous for the genetic regions as originally described. Due to this research setback, regeneration of the enhanced lines has not yet occurred.

It should be noted that in the previously mentioned study, the enhanced lines were equal in Fe content to the controls [9]. Furthermore, the scientists were unable to find specific compounds, such as polyphenolics or lower phytate, in one variety that could explain the difference in bioavailability. Thus, there appears to be some other factor(s) that influences the Fe bioavailability from maize.

The present study therefore seeks to address gaps in knowledge related to Fe concentration and bioavailability in the maize kernel, as such information could shed light on a strategy for Fe biofortification of maize. Two key observations contributed to the design of the present study. First, it is a common observation that diversity populations of maize exhibit significant differences in the amount of floury and horny endosperm present in the seed. Second, a thorough review of the literature also shows that very little has been published on the concentration and relative amounts of Fe in the various parts of the maize kernel; and, there are no reports of Fe bioavailability from the individual components of the maize kernel. Therefore, the objectives of the present study were to determine the relative concentration and bioavailability of Fe in the germ and non-germ fraction of the maize kernel, and to investigate the Fe concentration and bioavailability of fractions generated during commercial wet-milling of maize.

2. Materials and Methods

2.1. Chemicals, Enzymes, and Hormones

All chemicals, enzymes, and hormones were purchased from Sigma Chemical Co. (St. Louis, MO, USA) unless stated otherwise.

2.2. Sample Source and Preparation

A 500 g sample of a commercial maize variety (Pioneer 3245, Iowa State University, Ames, IA, USA) was subjected to a wet-milling process at the Center for Crops Utilization Research, Iowa State University, Ames, Iowa. The diagram presented in Figure 1 illustrates the wet-milling procedure and where fractions were extracted.

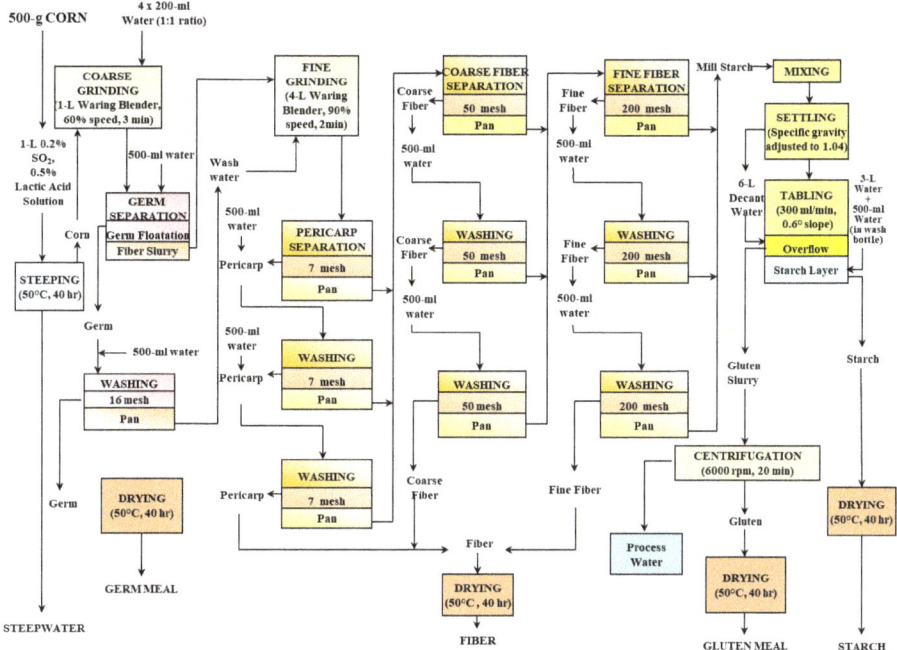

Figure 1. Diagram of the wet-milling process used in the present study. Image courtesy of Mr. Steven Fox, Center for Crops Utilization Research, Iowa State University, Ames, IA.

In 2014, a set of five maize inbred lines (B73, CML333, Ki3, M37W, Tx303) ranging from dent to flint kernel types was evaluated at Cornell University's Musgrave Research Farm in Aurora, NY. These five inbred lines were selected to span a range of whole-kernel Fe concentrations (Gore, unpublished data). Conventional maize cultivation practices for the northeastern United States were used. Self-pollinated ears were hand-harvested at physiological maturity and dried with forced air to 10–15% kernel moisture. The dried ears of each plot were manually shelled and bulked to form a representative sample from which 100 kernels were randomly selected. Whole kernels of the Pioneer 3245 were also obtained from the Iowa facility. For all six varieties mentioned above, a scalpel was used to remove the tip cap from each kernel, followed by a center longitudinal excision, followed by excision of the germ tissue. This was done for each kernel in the sample. The germ and the non-germ fractions (which included the aleurone and pericarp) were weighed for subsequent calculations related to content. As shown in Figure 2, the samples exhibited diversity in kernel size, floury endosperm, and horny endosperm composition.

Maize samples purchased in a local supermarket included the following: "Organic Cornmeal", which is an unfortified ground whole kernel maize flour (19 μg Fe/g); a fortified whole kernel maize flour (65 μg Fe/g); and a degerminated fortified maize flour (44 μg Fe/g). According to the package labels, these products were fortified with "reduced Fe".

Unfortified whole grain wheat flour (37 μg Fe/g) and an unfortified 80% extraction wheat flour (9 μg Fe/g) were also purchased at a local supermarket.

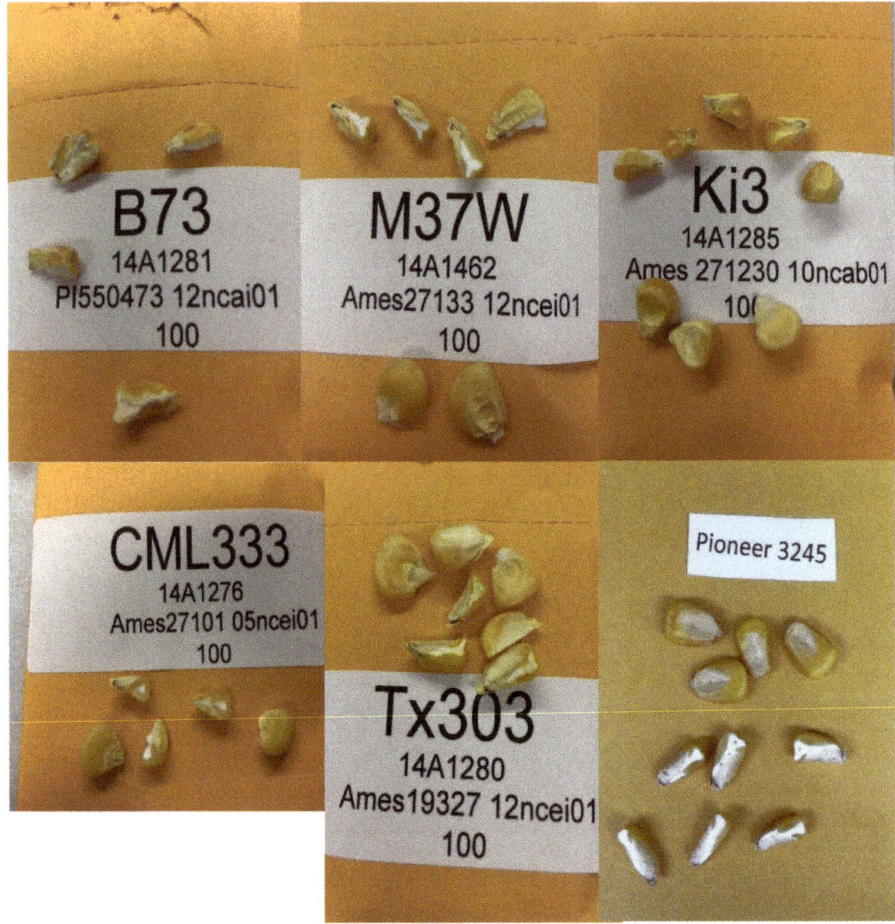

Figure 2. Images of maize kernels analyzed in the present study. Note that some kernels are split longitudinally to expose visual differences between varieties.

For comparison of Fe bioavailability, two commercial white bean samples and one red mottled bean were included in the study. The white beans were Merlin Navy beans and the red mottled variety were PR0737-1. The beans samples were grown in research plots in Montcalm, Michigan in the summer of 2015. The dry weight Fe concentrations of the beans were 76, 82, and 89 µg Fe/g, for the white bean 1, white bean 2, and red mottled bean, respectively.

Due to the small sample sizes available for six varieties of maize, all maize samples were not cooked in this study. The bean samples were cooked by autoclave for 15 min in a 3:1 volume of water:bean, then freeze-dried and ground into powder with a common coffee grinder.

2.3. Mineral Analysis

Dried, ground food samples (0.5 g) were treated with 3.0 mL of a 60:40 HNO_3 and $HClO_4$ mixture in a Pyrex glass tube and left overnight to destroy organic matter. The mixture was then heated to 120 °C for two hours, and 0.25 mL of 40 µg/g Yttrium was added as an internal standard to compensate for any drift during the subsequent inductively coupled plasma atomic emission spectrometer (ICP-AES) analysis. The model of the ICP used was a Thermo iCAP 6500 series (Thermo Jarrell Ash Corp.,

Franklin, MA, USA). The temperature of the heating block was then raised to 145 °C for 2 h. If necessary, more nitric acid (1–2 mL) was added to destroy the brownish color of the organic matter. Then, the temperature of the heating block raised to 190 °C for ten minutes and turned off. The cooled samples in the tubes were then diluted to 20 mL, vortexed, and transferred onto auto sampler tubes to be analyzed via ICP-AES.

2.4. In Vitro Digestion

The in vitro digestion protocol was conducted as per an established, highly validated, in vitro digestion model [11,12]. Briefly, exactly 1 g of each sample was used for each sample digestion. To initiate the gastric phase of digestion, 10 mL of fresh saline solution (0.9% sodium chloride) was added to each sample and mixed. The pH was then adjusted to 2.0 with 1.0mol/L HCl, and 0.5 mL of the pepsin solution (containing 1 g pepsin per 50 mL; certified >250 U per mg protein; Sigma #P7000, St. Louis, MO, USA) was added to each mixture. The mixtures were under gastric digestion for 1 h at 37 °C on a rocking platform (model RP-50, Laboratory Instrument, Rockville, MD, USA) located in an incubator. After 1 h of gastric digestion, the pH of the sample mixture was raised to 5.5–6.0 with 1.0 mol/L of $NaHCO_3$ solution. Then, 2.5 mL of the pancreatin–bile extract solution was added to each mixture. The pancreatin–bile extract solution contained 0.35 g pancreatin (Sigma #P1750, St. Louis, MO, USA) and 2.1 g bile extract (Sigma #B8631, St. Louis, MO, USA) in a total volume of 245 mL. The pH of the mixture was then adjusted to approximately 7.0, and the final volume of each mixture was adjusted to 15.0 mL by weight using a salt solution of 140 mmol/L of NaCl and 5.0 mmol/L of KCl at pH 6.7. At this point, the mixture was referred to as a "digest". The samples were then incubated for an additional two hours at 37 °C, at which point the digests were centrifuged, and supernatants and pellet fractions collected and transferred to tubes for analysis. Three independent replications of the in vitro digestion procedure were carried out for all of the food samples. For some samples, as noted in the specific results section, Fe bioavailability was assessed in both the presence and absence of ascorbic acid (AA). The AA was added to the digests at the start of the gastric digestion phase at a concentration of 10 µmol/L. This treatment has been shown to expose some additional differences between samples and thus provides further information on the matrix of the digest.

2.5. Statistical Analysis

Data were analyzed using the software package GraphPad Prism 8 (GraphPad Software, San Diego, CA, USA). Data were analyzed using analysis of variance incorporating normalization of variance, if needed, and Tukey's post test to determine significant differences ($p < 0.05$) between groups. Unless noted otherwise, values are expressed as mean ± standard deviation (SD); $n = 3$ independent replications.

3. Results

3.1. Maize Fe Concentration and Fe Bioavailability

Iron concentration in the maize samples ranged from 12.5 to 30.8 µg/g in the whole kernels (Table 1). The germ fractions contained the highest density of Fe, ranging from 51.0 to 141.3 µg/g. Iron concentration in the non-germ component ranged from 7.4 to 18.9 µg/g. It is notable that the three varieties, M37W, Ki3, and CML333, demonstrating the highest Fe bioavailability also had the highest non-germ Fe concentrations: 15.9–18.9 µg/g (Figure 3). The other three varieties exhibited non-germ Fe concentrations of 7.4–10.4 µg/g and thus exhibited lower Fe bioavailability.

Table 1. Iron and phosphorous [1] concentration in the germ and non-germ (endosperm + pericarp) fractions of maize varieties. Percent values represent percent of total in whole kernel sample.

Maize Variety	Whole Seed Fe (µg/g)	Germ Fe (µg/g)	Germ Fe %	Non Germ Fe (µg/g)	Non Germ Fe %	Whole Seed P (mg/g)	Germ P (mg/g)	Germ P %	Non Germ P (mg/g)	Non Germ P %
B73	20.6	126.4	54.1	10.4	45.9	2.96	20.8	61.8	1.24	38.2
M37W	20.2	71.0	27.5	15.9	72.5	3.06	22.2	56.7	1.44	43.3
Ki3	21.8	51.0	27.4	17.9	72.6	3.43	16.2	55.4	1.73	44.6
CML333	30.8	141.3	44.7	18.9	55.3	3.38	22.5	64.8	1.32	35.2
Tx303	12.5	61.4	46.3	7.4	53.7	3.16	20.8	62.1	1.33	37.9
Pioneer 3245	13.4	75.8	49.2	7.5	50.8	2.04	14.4	61.4	0.87	38.6

[1] Phosphorous was used as an indirect estimate of phytic acid content as insufficient material was available to directly measure phytic acid.

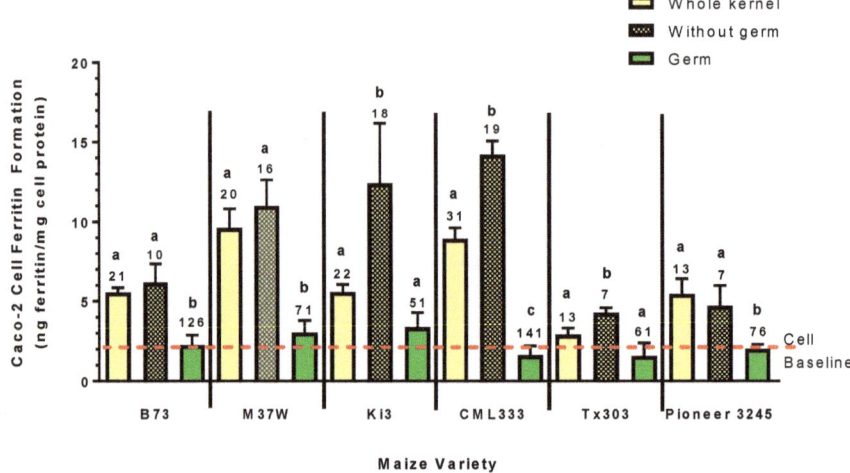

Figure 3. Iron bioavailability from manually dissected maize samples as measured via Caco-2 cell bioassay (cell ferritin formation equals Fe uptake). Numbers on top of the bar values represent Fe concentrations (µg/g) of samples. Bar values within variety with no letter in common are significantly different ($p < 0.05$). Bar values are mean ± SD, $n = 3$. Dashed red line indicates Caco-2 cell baseline ferritin level when exposed only to the in vitro digest solutions without food samples.

The manual dissection of the germ fraction from the maize demonstrated that the germ has the highest density of Fe in the seed, ranging from 51 to 141 µg/g, and accounting for 27–54% of the total Fe (Table 1). The non-germ portion of the kernels from each variety was of lesser Fe density, ranging from 7 to 19 µg/g, and accounting for 46–73% of the total Fe in the seed.

Iron bioavailability from the germ fractions was low for all varieties despite having high Fe concentrations (Figure 3). Despite being significantly lower in Fe content, the non-germ fractions exhibited similar or greater Fe bioavailability than the whole kernel samples; and except for two varieties, M37W and Tx303, the non-germ fractions were higher than the germ fractions.

3.2. Kernel Size

Kernel size was substantially different among the varieties but was not measured in this study; however, the average germ fraction by weight was 9.4%, ranging from 7.8 to 11.7% across the six samples. The commercial line, Pioneer 3245, was clearly the largest in terms of kernel size, with a substantial portion of the kernel comprised of floury endosperm. In contrast, the CML333 and Ki3 samples were smaller kernels, with lesser amounts of floury endosperm (Figure 2).

3.3. Maize Phosphorous Concentration

Due to limited amounts of material, kernel phosphorous levels were used as an indirect estimate of phytic acid levels. The results clearly show that P was more concentrated in the germ fraction of all varieties. Phosphorous density was highest in the germ fraction ranging from 14 to 23 mg/g, and accounting for 55–65% of the total seed P (Table 1). The non-germ fraction of the kernel was less dense in P, ranging from 0.9 to 1.7 mg/g, and accounting for 35–45% of the total seed P.

3.4. Wet-Milled Fractions of Maize

Commercial milling of the Pioneer 3245 variety resulted in the gluten fraction containing the highest Fe bioavailability (Figure 4). The germ fraction was the highest in Fe concentration but significantly lower in bioavailable Fe relative to the gluten fraction. Compared to the hand dissected germ fraction of the Pioneer 3245 variety, it appears that the milled germ fraction was less pure relative to the dissected germ fraction. The Fe in the fiber fractions and the pericarp were poorly available as indicated by ferritin values similar to the cell baseline, which indicates no net increase in Fe uptake as a result of exposure to the in vitro digest. The starch fraction contained only trace levels of Fe (2 µg/g). The steep liquor contained only 4 µg/g and yet exhibited a noticeable increase in ferritin above the cell baseline, indicating that this small amount of Fe could be highly available.

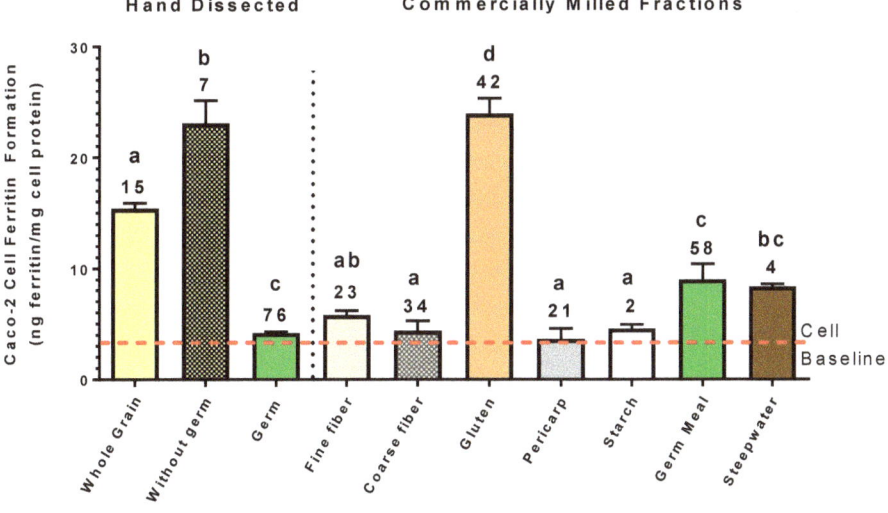

Figure 4. Iron bioavailability from the Pioneer 3245 maize samples that were manually dissected versus wet-milled fractions from a 500 g sample. Caco-2 cell ferritin values represent relative Fe bioavailability as cell ferritin formation is proportional to Fe uptake. Numbers on top of bar values represent Fe concentrations (µg/g) of samples. Bar values within manually dissected or commercial fractions with no letter in common are significantly different ($p < 0.05$). Bar values are mean ± SD, $n = 3$. Dashed red line indicates Caco-2 cell baseline ferritin level when exposed only to the in vitro digest solutions without food samples.

Iron and P analysis of the wet-milled Pioneer 3245 fractions showed that 29.3% of the total Fe was in the gluten fraction, followed by the germ fraction with 16.8% (Table 2). The concentration of

Fe in the germ fraction (58.2 µg/g) was higher than that of the gluten fraction (42 µg/g); however, the P concentration in the gluten fraction was substantially less than that of the germ fraction, which contained seven times more P. This suggests that the phytate:Fe molar ratio was significantly less in the gluten fraction and thus may explain the relatively high Fe bioavailability of the gluten fraction.

Table 2. Iron and phosphorous concentration and amounts in the various fractions from the wet-milling process of the Pioneer 3245 variety [1].

Fraction	Dry Weight (g)	Percent of Total Solids Recovered	Fe Concentration (µg/g)	Percent of Total Fe	P Concentration (µg/g)	Percent of Total P
Fine Fiber	42.8	9.3	22.6	12.6	686	2.7
Coarse Fiber	27.5	6.0	33.7	12.1	698	1.8
Gluten	53.6	11.6	42.0	29.3	2060	10.2
Pericarp	15.9	3.4	20.9	4.3	234	0.3
Starch	255.2	55.4	2.3	7.6	271	6.4
Germ	22.1	4.8	58.2	16.8	14401	29.5
Steep Liquor	—	—	4.2 *	—	938 **	—

[1] A 500 g sample of maize was milled. Recovered total solids (dry weight) were 461 g. Fe concentration of whole kernel sample was 15.4 µg/g. P concentration in whole grain sample was 2159 µg/g. * µg/mL. ** µg/g.

3.5. Comparison of Supermarket Samples vs. Degerminated Maize

Of the cornmeal products purchased in the local supermarket, two were fortified with Fe (Figure 5). Comparison of these samples indicated that the absence of the germ fraction improved Fe bioavailability from the fortified cornmeal. The unfortified whole wheat sample was lower in bioavailable Fe relative to the maize samples, and also lower relative to the 80% extracted wheat flour.

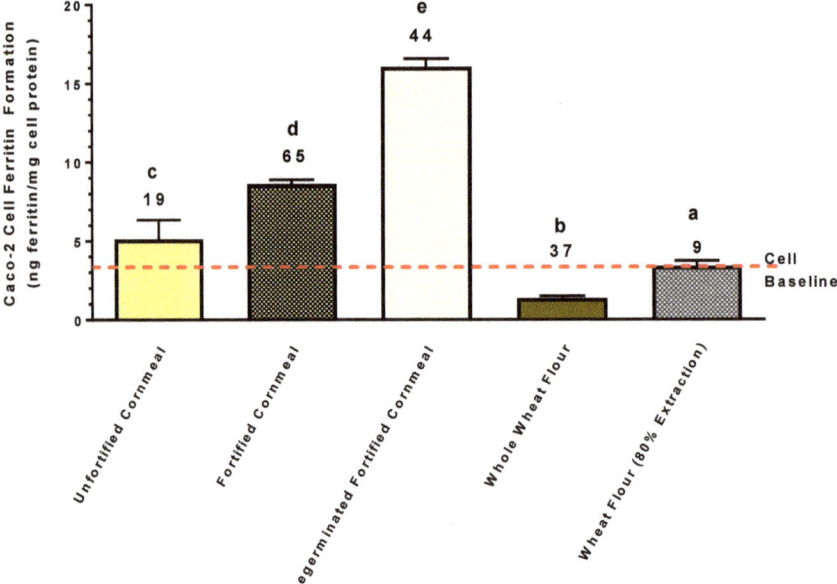

Figure 5. Iron bioavailability from the cornmeal and wheat flours purchased at a local supermarket. Caco-2 cell ferritin values represent relative Fe bioavailability as cell ferritin formation is proportional to Fe uptake. Numbers on top of bar values represent Fe concentrations (µg/g) of samples. Bar values with no letter in common are significantly different ($p < 0.05$). Bar values are mean ± SD, $n = 3$. Dashed red line indicates Caco-2 cell baseline ferritin level when exposed only to the in vitro digest solutions without food samples. A bar value below the baseline indicates strong inhibitory factors that negate the bioavailability of ultra-low background Fe present in the digest solutions.

A direct comparison of Fe bioavailability of white beans, red-mottled beans, and degerminated maize samples is shown in Figure 6. These samples were compared on an equal dry weight basis (0.5 g sample per replicate) in the same run of the bioassay. Relative to the beans, more Fe was taken up by the Caco-2 cells from the degerminated maize samples versus the beans. This occurred despite the fact that the bean samples contained approximately 80% more Fe than the maize. This observation indicated greater fractional bioavailability of the Fe in the maize samples relative to the beans.

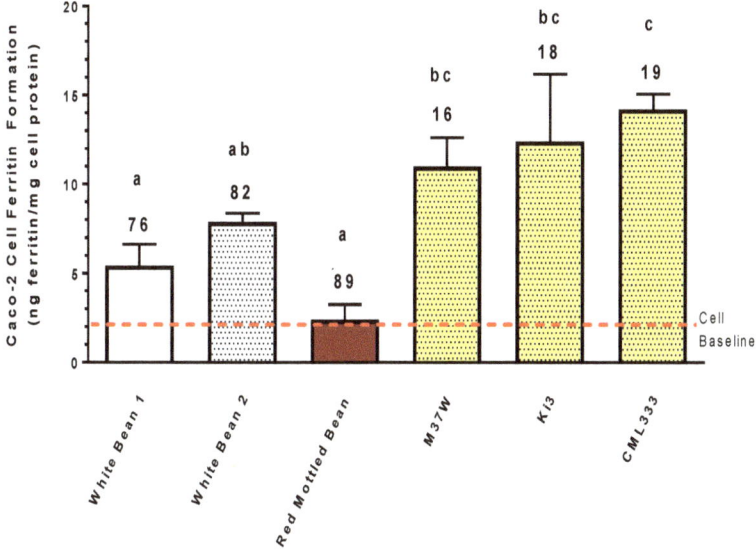

Bean and Degerminated Maize Samples

Figure 6. Iron bioavailability from white bean, red bean, and degerminated maize samples. Caco-2 cell ferritin values represent relative Fe bioavailability as cell ferritin formation is proportional to Fe uptake. Numbers on top of bar values represent Fe concentrations (µg/g) of samples. Bar values with no letter in common are significantly different ($p < 0.05$). Bar values are mean ± SD, $n = 3$. Dashed red line indicates Caco-2 cell baseline ferritin level when exposed only to the in vitro digest solutions without food samples. A bar value below the baseline indicates strong inhibitory factors that negate the bioavailability of ultra-low background Fe present in the digest solutions.

4. Discussion

The present study clearly shows that the Fe in the germ fraction of maize is very low in bioavailability (Figure 3). This was evident by the observation that the Caco-2 cell ferritin formation (i.e., the measure of Fe uptake) from the germ fraction of all six varieties was essentially equal to the baseline ferritin of the cells, despite having Fe concentration of 51–126 µg/g. In addition, the germ fraction appears to inhibit Fe bioavailability from the rest of the kernel. This effect was also evident in all six of the maize varieties analyzed, as Caco-2 cell ferritin formation from the degerminated kernel was either equal to or greater than that of the whole kernel, despite a decrease in Fe content by approximately 20–50% (Figure 3).

Iron bioavailability and Fe content analyses of the commercially wet-milled fractions of the Pioneer 3245 variety also demonstrated that the Fe of the germ fraction was poorly available (Figure 4; Table 2). However, in this experiment, the ferritin formation value for the "germ meal" fraction indicated that more bioavailable Fe was present. Given that the germ meal fraction was lower in Fe concentration relative to the hand-dissected fraction (58 vs. 76 µg/g, respectively), it would reasonably suggest that the wet-milled germ fraction was not as pure in germ composition as the manually excised germ tissue. Alternatively, the wet-milling process may alter the Fe bioavailability, perhaps through dilution in the wet-milling or loss of phytate via endogenous phytase activity during processing. Interestingly, the "gluten" fraction demonstrated the highest Fe bioavailability with an Fe concentration of 42 µg/g. The gluten fraction was also significantly lower in P concentration relative to the germ meal fraction, suggesting the phytate:Fe molar ratio was significantly less in the gluten fraction and thus contributing to the higher Fe bioavailability. Not surprisingly, the fiber fractions and the pericarp were of low Fe bioavailability despite Fe concentrations of 23–34 µg/g. In contrast, the "steepwater" fraction with an Fe concentration of only 4 µg/g yielded a ferritin formation value equal to or greater than that of the pericarp and fiber fractions. Polyphenol analysis of the steepwater was inconclusive as no polyphenols known to promote or inhibit Fe uptake were detected.

Until the present study, very little information was available on the distribution of Fe in maize, and there appears to be no reports of the relative Fe bioavailability between maize fractions. The present study clearly shows in this small set of samples that the germ tissue Fe content can vary substantially, ranging in this study from 27 to 54% of the total kernel Fe; thus, the non-germ fraction can have between 46 to 73% of the total kernel Fe. This relative Fe content suggests that breeding for higher non-germ Fe content may be possible; however, the question remains as to whether or not such an increase could overcome the inhibitory effect of the germ fraction. Such concern is particularly relevant to populations that consume maize as a major dietary staple, where Fe deficiency is prevalent. A broader set of diverse maize samples should clearly be evaluated to address the feasibility of these potential breeding objectives.

The present study clearly indicates that degermed maize and degermed maize products found in the marketplace can provide more absorbable Fe than crops such as beans or wheat, even though these crops have substantially more Fe (Figures 5 and 6). It is important to keep in mind that this Caco-2 bioassay gives a relative measure of the amount of Fe absorbed from the amount of sample provided. Therefore, the results indicate that relative to the bean and wheat samples used in the present study, the degermed maize was a better source of Fe, exhibiting a higher fractional Fe bioavailability and delivering more Fe to the enterocytes. Such observations suggest that Fe biofortification of maize could have a more profound impact relative to beans and wheat on improving Fe status of populations prone to Fe deficiency.

Milling of maize to remove the germ fraction and thus potentially promote Fe absorption in at risk populations may not be a viable or affordable option on a large scale. Indeed, many regions of Africa and Latin America are challenged by having enough maize that is uncontaminated by mycotoxins [13]. However, it is likely that in some regions or for some food applications such as infant complementary foods, a degerminated maize product could be produced, or is already being produced, that would be acceptable to consumers. For that reason alone, further research on the application of degermed maize to improve Fe nutrition is warranted. Animal and or human studies should be conducted to confirm this in vitro observation. If this effect is demonstrated in vivo, then it is clearly an intervention that could be deployed immediately to improve Fe nutrition of maize-based foods.

Iron biofortification research has primarily focused on crops that have been shown to be relatively high in iron and demonstrate a genetic diversity for Fe content [14]. For example, common beans have been shown to have diversity in Fe content, ranging from 50 to 100 µg/g [15,16], and pearl millet has shown a range of 30–80 µg/g [17]. Improvement in Fe status following prolonged consumption has been demonstrated in humans and in an animal model when the Fe concentration in the common bean or pearl millet has been compared at these extreme levels [18–20]. There is also evidence in a poultry model, where a lesser difference in the Fe concentration in beans, 50 vs. 71 µg/g, can have significant benefit [21]. It should be noted that the key assumptions of this approach is that increased Fe concentration and content can deliver additional absorbable Fe within the overall diet, and that such increases in Fe are primarily genetic and can be stable traits.

In contrast to beans, maize has not been extensively pursued for Fe biofortification, possibly because the Fe concentration is approximately 60% lower, and because there is a general perception that Fe bioavailability in maize is very low [14,22]. The low Fe bioavailability is believed to be primarily due to phytic acid, as polyphenols known to influence Fe bioavailability have not been identified as a factor in yellow or white maize varieties (R.P. Glahn, unpublished observations) [23]. Colored varieties of maize certainly have substantial amounts of polyphenols, but these have not been evaluated for Fe bioavailability or polyphenol profiles. Mutant varieties of maize with low phytic acid levels have been developed, but appear to have limited application, primarily due to reduced seedling viability [24]. A transgenic strategy to enhance the nutritional quality of Fe in low phytate maize, the overexpression of soybean ferritin in the endosperm, has been explored and appears to enhance the amount of absorbable Fe [25]. However, a search of the literature finds no additional research on this approach, nor on any large-scale production of low-phytate maize, suggesting that for maize, this approach has been abandoned.

To date, Fe biofortification of staple food crops has focused primarily on crops such as beans and pearl millet, as these crops demonstrate a diversity in range with relatively high Fe content. The assumption in focusing on these crops is that more Fe content should result in delivering more Fe for absorption, and that the Fe content is a genetically tractable trait. In addition, such assumptions require that sufficient bioavailability accompanies the added Fe. The results of the present study clearly suggest an alternative approach to Fe biofortification. More precisely, this study suggests that focusing on identifying the foods and food matrices that result in more Fe may be a more effective and efficient approach. Even though this study presents only in vitro data, it should be noted that the Caco-2 bioassay correctly predicted the beneficial effects of high Fe carioca beans and high Fe pearl millet in human efficacy trials [12]. The Caco-2 cell ferritin values for those crops were much lower on a relative scale than those of the degermed maize samples analyzed in this study. Granted, there are additional nutritional reasons for consuming crops such as beans; however, for many populations, food choices are limited, and to alleviate iron deficiency anemia, all strategies should be considered to improve the nutritional quality of Fe in the food system.

The present study is also evidence that this model is capable of identifying new factors and obstacles to improving Fe quality in staple foods. For example, this model has shown that the cotyledon cell wall of beans represents a significant barrier to the bioaccessibility of Fe in the bean cotyledon [26]. Moreover, it has shown that such obstacles can be overcome by processing or possibly by breeding for faster cooking, a tractable trait that is likely related to cell wall structure and linked to improved Fe bioavailability [27]. This model has also identified seed coat polyphenols, and thus color classes of beans that may be better sources of Fe nutrition [28,29]. In vitro observations should always be viewed with a healthy dose of skepticism; however, as stated previously, this model has correctly predicted numerous in vivo results of Fe biofortified crops. Most recently, this model predicted key interactions between carioca beans and the "food basket" of a common Brazilian diet [30]. Therefore, the in vitro observations from the application of this in vitro approach are now highly accepted as a tool to assess specific foods and diets and to guide plant breeding for enhanced Fe quality.

In summary, by identifying the germ fraction of maize as a significant inhibitor of Fe bioavailability from this crop, and proposing the strategy of increasing the non-germ, mostly endosperm Fe content, an additional breeding strategy is thus exposed to enhance the nutritional quality of maize. It should also be noted that the present study focused only on removing the germ fraction and noted the enhancing effects of removal of the germ fraction. It may be possible to use this approach to identify a germ fraction trait that may be less inhibitory, and thus complement the strategy of increasing Fe content in the non-germ fraction. It is also highly likely that such varieties may already be available in commercial production, and simply need to be identified. Given the broad consumption of maize and the high incidence of Fe deficiency anemia in resource-poor populations, a successful application of the above could have profound effect on human health.

Author Contributions: R.G. was responsible for the conceptualization, experimental design, methodology, technical work, data analysis, and writing—review and editing. M.A.G. provided maize samples and contributed to the review and editing. E.T. contributed to the review and editing.

Funding: This research was funded entirely by the U.S. Department of Agriculture, Agricultural Research Service.

Acknowledgments: The authors gratefully acknowledge Mr. Steven Fox of the Center for Crops Utilization Research, Iowa State University, Ames Iowa for providing the wet-milled maize samples. We also thank Mary Bodis and Yongpei Change of Cornell University for their excellent technical assistance.

Conflicts of Interest: The authors declare no conflict of interest.

References

1. Food and Agriculture Organization of the United Nations. *Crop Prospects and Food Situation: Quarterly Global Report*; Food and Agriculture Organization of the United Nations: Rome, Italy, 2019.
2. Tanumihardjo, S.A.; Ball, A.M.; Kaliwile, C.; Pixley, K.V. The research and implementation continuum of biofortified sweet potato and maize in Africa. *Ann. N. Y. Acad. Sci.* **2017**, *1390*, 88–103. [CrossRef] [PubMed]
3. Hoekenga, O.A.; Lung'aho, M.G.; Tako, E.; Kochian, L.V.; Glahn, R.P. Iron biofortification of maize grain. *Plant Gen. Res.* **2011**, *9*, 327–329. [CrossRef]
4. Oikeh, S.O.; Menkir, A.; Maziya-Dixon, B.; Welch, R.M.; Glahn, R.P. Assessment of concentrations of iron and zinc and bioavailable iron in grains of early-maturing tropical maize varieties. *J. Agric. Food Chem.* **2003**, *51*, 3688–3694. [CrossRef]
5. Oikeh, S.O.; Menkir, A.; Maziya-Dixon, B.; Welch, R.M.; Glahn, R.P. Genotypic differences in concentration and bioavailability of kernel-iron in tropical maize varieties grown under field conditions. *J. Plant Nutr.* **2003**, *26*, 2307–2319. [CrossRef]
6. Oikeh, S.O.; Menkir, A.; Maziya-Dixon, B.; Welch, R.M.; Glahn, R.P. Assessment of iron bioavailability from 20 elite late-maturing tropical maize varieties using an in vitro digestion/Caco-2 cell model. *J. Sci. Food Agric.* **2004**, *84*, 1202–1206. [CrossRef]
7. Pixley, K.V.; Palacios-Rojas, N.; Glahn, R.P. The usefulness of iron bioavailability as a target trait for breeding maize (*Zea mays* L.) with enhanced nutritional value. *Field Crops Res.* **2011**, *123*, 153–160. [CrossRef]
8. Lung'aho, M.G.; Mwaniki, A.M.; Szalma, S.J.; Hart, J.J.; Rutzke, M.A.; Kochian, L.V.; Glahn, R.P.; Hoekenga, O.A. Genetic and physiological analysis of iron biofortification in maize kernels. *PLoS ONE* **2011**, *6*, e20429. [CrossRef]
9. Tako, E.; Hoekenga, O.A.; Kochian, L.V.; Glahn, R.P. Retracted Article: High bioavailability iron maize (Zea mays L.) developed through molecular breeding provides more absorbable iron in vitro (Caco-2 model) and in vivo (Gallus gallus). *Nutr. J.* **2013**, *12*, 3. [CrossRef]
10. Tako, E.; Hoekenga, O.A.; Kochian, L.V.; Glahn, R.P. Retraction Note: High bioavailablilty iron maize (Zea mays L.) developed through molecular breeding provides more absorbable iron in vitro (Caco-2 model) and in vivo (Gallus gallus). *Nutr. J.* **2015**, *14*, 126. [CrossRef] [PubMed]
11. Glahn, R.P.; Lee, O.A.; Yeung, A.; Goldman, M.I.; Miller, D.D. Caco-2 cell ferritin formation predicts nonradiolabeled food iron availability in an in vitro digestion/Caco-2 cell culture model. *J. Nutr.* **1998**, *128*, 1555–1561. [CrossRef] [PubMed]
12. Tako, E.; Bar, H.; Glahn, R.P. The combined application of the Caco-2 cell bioassay coupled with in vivo (Gallus gallus) feeding trial represents an effective approach to predicting Fe bioavailability in humans. *Nutrients* **2016**, *8*, 732. [CrossRef]
13. Ingenbleek, L.; Sulyok, M.; Adegboye, A.; Hossou, S.E.; Koné, A.Z.; Oyedele, A.D.; Kisito, C.S.K.J.; Dembélé, Y.K.; Eyangoh, S.; Verger, P.; et al. Regional sub-saharan africa total diet study in benin, cameroon, mali and nigeria reveals the presence of 164 mycotoxins and other secondary metabolites in foods. *Toxins* **2019**, *11*, 57. [CrossRef]
14. Vasconcelos, M.L.; Gruissem, W.; Bhullar, N.K. Iron biofortification in the 21st century: Setting realistic targets, overcoming obstacles, and new strategies for healthy nutrition. *Curr. Opin. Biotech.* **2017**, *44*, 8–15. [CrossRef]
15. Izquierdo, P.; Astudillo, C.; Blair, M.W.; IqbalBodo Raatz, A.M.; Cichy, K.A. Meta-QTL analysis of seed iron and zinc concentration and content in common bean (Phaseolus vulgaris L.). *Theor. Appl. Gen.* **2018**, *131*, 1645–1658. [CrossRef]

16. Cichy, K.A.; Porch, T.G.; Beaver, J.S.; Cregan, P.B.; Fourie, D.; Glahn, R.P.; Grusak, M.A.; Kamfwa, K.; Katuuramu, D.; McClean, P.; et al. A Phaseolus vulgaris diversity panel for Andean bean improvement. *Crop Sci.* **2015**, *55*, 2149–2160. [CrossRef]
17. Kumar, S.; Hash, C.T.; Nepolean, T.; Mahendrakar, M.D.; Satyavathi, C.T.; Singh, G.; Rathore, A.; Yadav, R.S.; Gupta, R.; Srivastava, R.K. Mapping grain iron and zinc content quantitative trait loci in an iniadi-derived immortal population of pearl millet. *Genes* **2018**, *9*, 248. [CrossRef]
18. Finkelstein, J.L.; Haas, J.D.; Mehta, S. Iron-biofortified staple food crops for improving iron status: A review of the current evidence. *Curr. Opin. Biotechnol.* **2017**, *44*, 138–145. [CrossRef]
19. Tako, E.; Reed, S.M.; Budiman, J.; Hart, J.J.; Glahn, R.P. Higher iron pearl millet (Pennisetum glaucum L.) provides more absorbable iron that is limited by increased polyphenolic content. *Nutr. J.* **2015**, *14*, 11. [CrossRef]
20. Tako, E.; Reed, S.; Anandaraman, A.; Beebe, S.E.; Hart, J.J.; Glahn, R.P. Studies of cream seeded carioca beans (Phaseolus vulgaris L.) from a Rwandan efficacy trial: In vitro and in vivo screening tools reflect human studies and predict beneficial results from iron biofortified beans. *PLoS ONE* **2015**, *10*, e0138479. [CrossRef]
21. Tako, E.; Blair, M.W.; Glahn, R.P. Biofortified red mottled beans (Phaseolus vulgaris L.) in a maize and bean diet provide more bioavailable iron than standard red mottled beans: Studies in poultry (Gallus gallus) and an in vitro digestion/Caco-2 model. *Nutr. J.* **2011**, *14*, 113. [CrossRef]
22. Garcia-Oliveira, A.L.; Chander, S.; Ortiz, R.; Menkir, A.; Gedil1, M. Genetic basis and breeding perspectives of grain iron and zinc enrichment in cereals. *Front. Plant Sci.* **2018**, *9*, 937. [CrossRef]
23. Prasanthi, P.S.; Naveena, N.; Vishnuvardhana Rao, M.; Bhaskarachary, K. Compositional variability of nutrients and phytochemicals in corn after processing. *J. Food Sci. Tech.* **2017**, *54*, 1080–1090. [CrossRef]
24. Raboy, V.; Young, K.A.; Dorsch, J.A.; Cook, A. Genetics and breeding of seed phosphorus and phytic acid. *J. Plant Physiol.* **2001**, *158*, 489–497. [CrossRef]
25. Aluru, M.R.; Rodermel, S.R.; Reddy, M.B. Genetic modification of low phytic acid 1-1 maize to enhance iron content and bioavailability. *J. Agric. Food Chem.* **2011**, *59*, 12954–12962. [CrossRef]
26. Glahn, R.P.; Tako, E.; Cichy, K.A.; Wiesinger, J. The cotyledon cell wall of the common bean (Phaseolus vulgaris) resists digestion in the upper intestine and thus may limit iron bioavailability. *Food Func.* **2016**, *7*, 3193. [CrossRef]
27. Wiesinger, J.A.; Cichy, K.A.; Glahn, R.P.; Grusak, M.A.; Brick, M.A.; Thompson, H.J.; Tako, E. Demonstrating a nutritional advantage to the fast-cooking dry bean (Phaseolus vulgaris L.). *J. Agric. Food Chem.* **2016**, *64*, 8592–8603. [CrossRef]
28. Hart, J.J.; Tako, E.; Glahn, R.P. Characterization of polyphenol effects on inhibition and promotion of iron uptake by Caco-2 cells. *J. Agric. Food Chem.* **2017**, *65*, 3285–3294. [CrossRef]
29. Wiesinger, J.A.; Cichy, K.A.; Tako, E.; Glahn, R.P. The fast cooking and enhanced iron bioavailability properties of the manteca yellow bean (Phaseolus vulgaris L.). *Nutrients* **2018**, *10*, 1609. [CrossRef]
30. Dias, D.M.; Kolba, N.; Binyamin, D.; Ziv, O.; Regini Nutti, M.; Martino, H.S.D.; Glahn, R.P.; Koren, O.; Tako, E. Iron biofortified carioca bean (Phaseolus vulgaris L.)-based brazilian diet delivers more absorbable iron and affects the gut microbiota in vivo (Gallus gallus). *Nutrients* **2018**, *10*, 1970. [CrossRef]

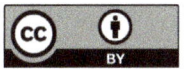

© 2019 by the authors. Licensee MDPI, Basel, Switzerland. This article is an open access article distributed under the terms and conditions of the Creative Commons Attribution (CC BY) license (http://creativecommons.org/licenses/by/4.0/).

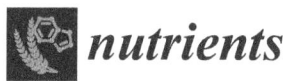

Article

A Randomized Feeding Trial of Iron-Biofortified Beans in School Children in Mexico

Julia L. Finkelstein [1,†], Saurabh Mehta [1,†], Salvador Villalpando [2], Veronica Mundo-Rosas [2], Sarah V. Luna [1], Maike Rahn [1], Teresa Shamah-Levy [2], Stephen E. Beebe [3] and Jere D. Haas [1,*]

1. Division of Nutritional Sciences, Cornell University, Ithaca, NY 14853, USA; jfinkelstein@cornell.edu (J.L.F.); smehta@cornell.edu (S.M.); svl25@cornell.edu (S.V.L.); mr42@cornell.edu (M.R.)
2. Instituto Nacional de Salud Pública, Cuernavaca 62100, Morelos, México; svillalp@insp.mx (S.V.); vmundo@insp.mx (V.M.-R.); tshamah@insp.mx (T.S.-L.)
3. Centro Internacional de Agricultura Tropical, Cali 6713, Colombia; s.beebe@cgiar.org
* Correspondence: jdh12@cornell.edu; Tel.: +607-255-2665; Fax: +607-255-1033
† These authors contributed equally.

Received: 17 December 2018; Accepted: 8 February 2019; Published: 12 February 2019

Abstract: Iron deficiency is a major public health problem worldwide, with the highest burden among children. The objective of this randomized efficacy feeding trial was to determine the effects of consuming iron-biofortified beans (Fe-Beans) on the iron status in children, compared to control beans (Control-Beans). A cluster-randomized trial of biofortified beans (*Phaseolus vulgaris* L.), bred to enhance iron content, was conducted over 6 months. The participants were school-aged children (n = 574; 5–12 years), attending 20 rural public boarding schools in the Mexican state of Oaxaca. Double-blind randomization was conducted at the school level; 20 schools were randomized to receive either Fe-Beans (n = 10 schools, n = 304 students) or Control-Beans (n = 10 schools, n = 366 students). School administrators, children, and research and laboratory staff were blinded to the intervention group. Iron status (hemoglobin (Hb), serum ferritin (SF), soluble transferrin receptor (sTfR), total body iron (TBI), inflammatory biomarkers C-reactive protein (CRP) and α-1-acid glycoprotein (AGP)), and anthropometric indices for individuals were evaluated at the enrollment and at the end of the trial. The hemoglobin concentrations were adjusted for altitude, and anemia was defined in accordance with age-specific World Health Organization (WHO) criteria (i.e., Hb <115 g/L for <12 years and Hb <120 g/L for ≥12 years). Serum ferritin concentrations were adjusted for inflammation using BRINDA methods, and iron deficiency was defined as serum ferritin at less than 15.0 µg/L. Total body iron was calculated using Cook's equation. Mixed models were used to examine the effects of Fe-Beans on hematological outcomes, compared to Control-Beans, adjusting for the baseline indicator, with school as a random effect. An analysis was conducted in 10 schools (n = 269 students) in the Fe-Beans group and in 10 schools (n = 305 students) in the Control-Beans group that completed the follow-up. At baseline, 17.8% of the children were anemic and 11.3% were iron deficient (15.9%, BRINDA-adjusted). A total of 6.3% of children had elevated CRP (>5.0 mg/L), and 11.6% had elevated AGP (>1.0 g/L) concentrations at baseline. During the 104 days when feeding was monitored, the total mean individual iron intake from the study beans (Fe-bean group) was 504 mg (IQR: 352, 616) over 68 mean feeding days, and 295 mg (IQR: 197, 341) over 67 mean feeding days in the control group (p < 0.01). During the cluster-randomized efficacy trial, indicators of iron status, including hemoglobin, serum ferritin, soluble transferrin receptor, and total body iron concentrations improved from the baseline to endline (6 months) in both the intervention and control groups. However, Fe-Beans did not significantly improve the iron status indicators, compared to Control-Beans. Similarly, there were no significant effects of Fe-Beans on dichotomous outcomes, including anemia and iron deficiency, compared to Control-Beans. In this 6-month cluster-randomized efficacy trial of iron-biofortified beans in school children in Mexico, indicators of iron status improved in both the intervention and control groups. However, there were no significant effects of Fe-Beans on iron biomarkers, compared to Control-Beans. This trial was registered at clinicaltrials.gov as NCT03835377.

Keywords: iron; anemia; biofortification; beans; children; Mexico; international nutrition

---

1. Introduction

Global estimates regarding the prevalence of anemia in school-aged children, defined by the World Health Organization as hemoglobin (Hb) <115 g/L for children younger than 12 years and <120 g/L for children 12 years and older [1], range between 25% and 46% [2,3]. Iron deficiency, the most common global micronutrient deficiency [4,5], is the leading cause of anemia, accounting for approximately 25–37% [6] to 50% [7] of anemia cases.

The estimated average requirement for iron in school-aged children is 4.1 for ≤12 y and 5.9 mg for >12 years per day [8,9]. In addition to an inadequate intake of iron and low bioavailability of iron, other nutritional factors, such as vitamin B_{12} and folate, and non-nutritional factors such as inflammation also contribute to the etiology of anemia and impact human health [10,11]. In Mexico, the national nutrition and health survey (2006) reported a prevalence of anemia of 16.6% [12] and iron deficiency of 17.6% (serum ferritin <12.0 µg/L), demonstrating a considerable health risk for children [13]. Other causes of anemia in children identified in this population in Mexico included folate deficiency and vitamin A deficiency [12].

Interventions, including micronutrient supplementation and food fortification, have improved the iron status and reduced the prevalence of anemia in some settings. However, iron deficiency remains an urgent public health problem and threat to child health and development. Young children are at a particularly high risk due to rapid growth, inadequate dietary intake, and a high risk of infection in resource-limited settings [14]. Iron deficiency has been associated with impaired cognitive function in children and long-term impairments in physical work capacity in adulthood [15–17].

One novel approach to reducing micronutrient malnutrition is to enhance the nutrient quality of the diet through the biofortification of staple crops that are already locally accepted and consumed [18]. Consequently, biofortification has been recognized by the Copenhagen Consensus of 2008 as one of the top five solutions to current global health and nutrition challenges [19]. The success and challenges of biofortification have been previously documented [20,21]. We recently reviewed the published evidence from the three randomized efficacy trials of different iron-biofortified crops, including rice in adult Filipino women [22], pearl millet in school-aged children in India [23], and beans in women of reproductive age in Rwanda [24]. The findings demonstrated improvements in serum ferritin concentrations and total body iron concentrations, with an additional potential to benefit individuals who were iron deficient at the baseline [25]. Given this limited evidence and with no studies from Latin America, more studies with diverse populations and locally relevant crops are warranted before the implementation of a potentially important public health intervention.

In order to target at-risk populations in Latin America, the Centro Internacional de Agricultura Tropical (CIAT) in Colombia bred and biofortified a common black bean variety (*Phaseolus vulgaris* L.), the standard black bean currently consumed widely in Central America and Mexico. In Mexico, in 2006, beans were ranked highly among the most consumed foods by school-aged children nationwide, according to Encuesta Nacional de Salud y Nutrición, a nationally representative nutrition survey [26]. Biofortification has nearly doubled the iron concentration (~100 versus ~50 mg/kg) of the standard bean variety. We hypothesized that the daily consumption of iron-biofortified beans (Fe-Beans) would improve hemoglobin, serum ferritin, and total body iron in 6 months, compared to control beans (Control-Beans). In order to examine this hypothesis, we conducted the first randomized efficacy trial of iron-biofortified beans and iron status in primary school-aged children from a low-income setting in

Mexico. Special consideration was applied to assess indicators of iron status with and without anemia and consider the potential impact of inflammatory markers on iron status.

2. Materials and Methods

2.1. Study Population

This study was conducted in boarding schools for children aged 5–12 years between January and June 2010, in the state of Oaxaca, Mexico. In this rural setting, many low-resource children between 5 and 12 years of age (predominantly indigenous *Mixe* speakers) reside at boarding schools (*albergues escolares*) for 5 days per week; they receive 3 meals per day, prepared in common kitchens with fixed daily menus, and the meals are consumed in communal dining rooms. The schools in this setting were selected based on their students' high risk of iron deficiency, willingness to participate, and regular consumption of black beans typical to rural Mexico. Specifically, the inclusion criteria were: boarding schools for children (5–12 years), located in a rural area approximately 60 km east of the city of Oaxaca, a high prevalence of anemia ($\geq 15.0\%$) on the baseline survey, and an adequate infrastructure to sustain a 6-month feeding trial. The exclusion criteria were a prevalence of anemia of less than 15% on the baseline survey and an inadequate infrastructure to sustain a 6-month feeding trial.

2.2. Study Design

Sample selection. Boarding school administrators were contacted to explain the study design and obtain permission for prescreening. An initial prescreening survey was conducted in 30 (of 48 previously surveyed) randomly selected boarding schools, which included information on the school size, past menus, infrastructure, and capacity to support this research project (Figure 1). In all boarding schools, students provided a capillary blood sample analyzed for hemoglobin concentrations (HemoCue AB, Ängelholm, Sweden). A total of 30 schools were assessed for eligibility; 10 boarding schools were excluded based on a low prevalence of anemia in the screening survey (<15.0%) and an inadequate management and infrastructure to sustain a 6-month controlled feeding trial. The 20 boarding schools with the highest prevalence ($\geq 15.0\%$) of anemia were selected; out of a total of 20 schools ($n = 670$ children), 10 were randomized to receive iron-biofortified beans (Fe-Beans; $n = 304$ children) and 10 were randomized to receive control beans (Control-Beans; $n = 366$ children) for 6 months between January and June 2010.

Randomization and masking. The study was a double-blind, cluster-randomized controlled trial (with randomization at the school level) of: (1) iron-biofortified black beans, compared to (2) a commercial variety of beans, with the intervention randomized at the school level. The school administrators, children, research staff (for managing the intervention, food weighing, assessment of outcomes), and laboratory staff were blinded to the intervention group.

Ethics approval. Informed written assent was obtained from each participant, as well as their guardians and institution heads, at the screening and again at baseline. The Commission for Ethics, Biosafety, and Research of the Instituto Nacional de Salud Pública (INSP), Cuernavaca, Mexico, approved the research protocol.

2.3. Intervention

Beans: The iron-biofortified beans (*Phaseolus vulgaris* L. MIB465) were grown at the Centro Internacional de Agricultura Tropical (CIAT) in Cali, Colombia, in 2009. The beans were then shipped to Oaxaca, Mexico, for repackaging and storage. The control beans (*Phaseolus vulgaris* L. Jamapa variety) that were identical in color and size were purchased from local sources in Mexico. The two bean varieties were repackaged into knitted 50-kg plastic sacks with color-coded identifiers to distinguish the Fe-Beans and Control-Beans. The code was not known to any of the field staff, participants, or those involved in the data collection and analysis. The Fe-Beans and Control-Beans were similar in color, taste, and phytochemical content. An analysis of the iron content by inductively coupled plasma mass spectrometry (ICP-MS) before the start of the study indicated a difference of 40 µg iron per g of uncooked beans between the iron-biofortified beans (95 µg/g) and control beans (55 µg/g). All of the beans were stored in a properly ventilated and secure facility. Sacks of beans were distributed monthly to participating boarding schools from January to June 2010.

Baseline and follow-up procedures. Individual children within boarding schools were assessed for their dietary iron intake, blood parameters, and anthropometry. The anthropometric measurements were obtained by trained research assistants using standardized procedures and calibrated instruments at the baseline and endline. Body weight was measured using a digital weighing scale (Tanita, Arlington Heights, Illinois, USA) with a precision of 100 g, calibrated daily. Height was assessed using a stadiometer (Dyna-Top, Mexico City, Mexico) with a precision of 1 mm. Individual z-scores were calculated as per World Health Organization (WHO) guidelines [27]. Mothers or housemothers of the boarding schools were asked about morbidity in children by listing symptoms related to diarrhea, upper respiratory illness, and fever. Morbidity was assessed at the baseline for 2 weeks prior to the blood sampling, as well as at endline.

Dietary intake of iron. Children were offered 2 daily portions (100 g each) of cooked beans, one at lunch and another at dinner. The mean dietary intake for participants in this study was estimated by calculating the nutrient composition of the menus for the three meals per day offered at the boarding schools and the bean intake measured during the trial. Portion sizes were derived from the dietary test weighing performed on a monthly basis in all the boarding schools. For food weighing measurements, 1 out of 10 children were randomly selected at each boarding school in a rotation fashion. For that purpose, the portions of beans and animal-source foods (e.g., meat, eggs, cheese, or milk) were weighed before serving, and the remains were weighed again by trained personnel with OHAUS Compact Scales (Model CS, 5000), at a precision of 2 g.

Blood collection. The venous blood samples (7 mL) were collected from participants for an analysis of iron status by a trained phlebotomist at the baseline and endline. Whole blood was analyzed for hemoglobin using HemoCue (HemoCue AB, Ängelholm, Sweden). Plasma was separated by centrifugation and stored below $-20\ °C$ (for < 4 days) until it was transported to the central laboratory at INSP and stored below $-80\ °C$ until analysis. Serum concentrations of ferritin and the soluble transferrin receptors (sTfR) were measured by an immunoassay method using commercial kits (Dade Behring Inc., Deerfield, IL, USA). C-reactive protein (CRP) and α-1-acid glycoprotein (AGP) were analyzed via the particle-enhanced immunoturbidimetric assay in a Roche Hitachi 902 analyzer (Roche, Basel, Switzerland) at the laboratory at INSP.

Definitions of outcomes. The primary outcomes were: hemoglobin (Hb), serum ferritin (SF), and soluble transferrin receptor (sTfR) concentrations at the individual level. We also assessed total body iron (TBI), anemia, and iron deficiency. Total body iron was estimated using the approach originally proposed by Cook [28]:

$$\text{TBI (mg/kg)} = -[\log_{10}(\text{sTfR(mg/L)} \times 1000/\text{SF}(\mu g/L)) - 2.8229]/\ 0.1207 \qquad (1)$$

Anemia was defined as Hb <11.5 g/dL for children younger than 12 years, and <12.0 g/dL for children 12 years and older [1]. Iron deficiency was defined as SF <15.0 µg/L for the primary analyses, and as TBI <0.0 mg/kg or sTfR >8.3 mg/L in additional analyses.

2.4. Power and Sample Size Calculations

The initial power and sample size calculations were based on the following criteria: alpha (0.05), differential in iron content between the Fe-Bean and Control-Bean varieties (40 ppm), daily dry bean consumption (90 grams per day), duration of feeding (120 days of feeding), between school variance in serum ferritin (0.014 µg/L) and within school variance in serum ferritin (0.15 µg/L) concentrations. We would have an 80% power to detect a 2.7 µg/L difference in serum ferritin concentrations over the course of the study, with a sample size of 17 schools with approximately 664 children.

Statistical analysis. The descriptive statistics were expressed as the median, interquartile range (IQR) and percentages. Hemoglobin concentrations were adjusted for altitude: the hemoglobin values in the samples from children living in communities located more than 1000 m above sea level were corrected using the equation published by Cohen and Haas [29].

The laboratory analyses for serum ferritin concentrations for the baseline and endline were not analyzed in batch. In order to correct for significant analytical differences observed between the baseline and endline ferritin samples, a subset of samples at both time points were analyzed together. Based on these results, we developed the following equation to correct the endline ferritin values:

$$\text{Corrected endline ferritin} = \frac{(4.2464 + \text{uncorrected endline ferritin})}{1.179782} \quad (2)$$

The serum ferritin concentrations were adjusted for inflammation and sex, using the BRINDA method [30], and using methods previously described [31–33]. The variables were natural logarithm-transformed in order to achieve normality prior to the analyses. Mixed models were used to examine the effects of Fe-Beans on hematological outcomes, compared to Control-Beans, with school as a random effect. All the models were also adjusted for the baseline value of the respective iron status indicator. p-values of less than 0.05 were considered statistically significant. The statistical analyses were conducted with SAS 9.4 (SAS Institute Inc., Cary, NC, USA). This trial was registered at clinicaltrials.gov as NCT03835377.

3. Results

3.1. Baseline Characteristics

Recruitment began in January 2010, and the feeding trial was conducted from January 2010 to June 2010. The baseline characteristics of children attending the 20 schools included in these analyses are presented in Table 1. After screening, 10 schools were excluded based on a low prevalence of anemia; 20 schools were randomized to receive either Fe-Beans (n = 10 schools; n = 304 children) or Control-Beans (n = 10 schools; n = 366 children) (Figure 1). Iron biomarker data were available at the endline for a total of 574 children attending 20 schools: 269 children from 10 schools received iron-biofortified beans, and 305 children from 10 schools received control beans. The median age of participants was 9.6 years (Inter-Quartile Range (IQR): 8.1, 10.9 years); 53.3% of the sample were female. There were no significant differences at the baseline between schools in treatment groups in terms of sociodemographic or anthropometric indicators, and there were no significant differences between schools or children initially enrolled (n = 20 schools, n = 670 children) and those who completed the intervention (n = 20 schools, n = 574 children). The a priori assumptions for adequate power were not met, as the number of feeding days was lower than initially anticipated (median number of feeding days was 68 vs. 120 days in power and sample size calculations).

At the baseline, 17.8% of children were anemic; the median hemoglobin concentration was 12.8 g/dL (IQR: 11.8, 13.8 g/dL). A total of 11.3% of children were iron deficient (SF <15.0 µg/L, unadjusted), and the median unadjusted ferritin concentration was 28.7 µg/L (20.4, 38.9 µg/L). The prevalence of inflammation was 6.3% based on CRP (>5.0 mg/L) and 11.6% based on AGP (>1.0 g/L) in the overall sample. However, the prevalence of inflammation (CRP >5.0 mg/L: 8.3% vs. 4.1%; AGP >1.0 g/L: 16.1% vs. 6.4%) and morbidity (i.e., fever, diarrhea, productive cough: 38% vs. 22%) was higher in schools in the Control-Bean group at the baseline, compared to the Fe-Bean group.

After adjusting baseline serum ferritin concentrations for inflammation (using the BRINDA method [30]), the median SF concentration was reduced from 28.7 (IQR: 20.4, 38.9 µg/L) to 24.5 (IQR: 18.2, 33.8 µg/L). The prevalence of iron deficiency at the baseline was 15.9%, after adjusting serum ferritin concentrations for inflammation. The median sTfR concentration of 4.3 mg/L was not affected by inflammation. The unadjusted median value of 5.4 mg/kg for baseline TBI was reduced to 4.8 mg/kg after the BRINDA adjustment.

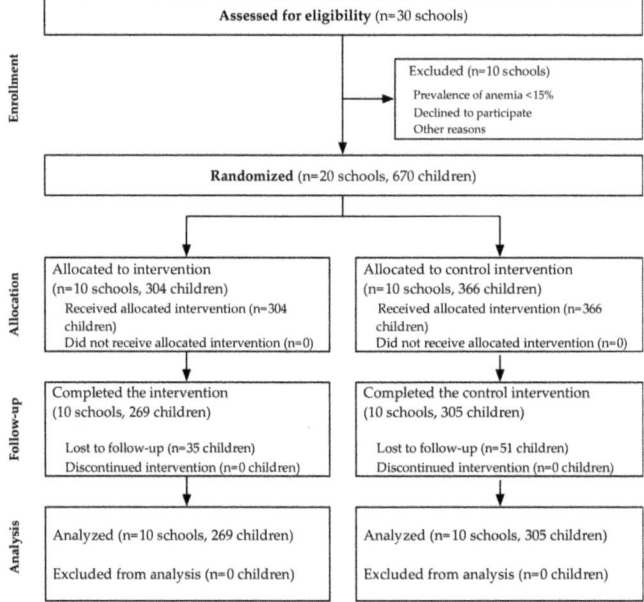

Figure 1. CONSORT Diagram for Cluster-Randomized Trial.

3.2. Effects of the Intervention on Iron Status

The effects of iron-biofortified beans on the iron status in children compared to control beans are presented in Table 2. All the analyses presented show the effects of the intervention on the iron status indicator at the endline, adjusted for the baseline indicator, with school as a random effect. The iron status indicators, including Hb, SF, sTfR, and TBI, improved in both the intervention and control groups during the 6-month trial. However, the Fe-Beans did not significantly improve the iron biomarkers (Hb, SF, TBI), compared to the Control-Beans. The soluble transferrin receptor (sTfR) values were lower in the Fe-Bean group compared to Control-Beans at the endline ($p = 0.054$). At endline, the median hemoglobin level was 13.0 (IQR: 12.2, 13.8 g/dL) in the Control-Bean group, compared to 12.9 (IQR: 11.9, 13.6 g/dL) in the Fe-Bean group. There was a significant difference in serum ferritin ($p = 0.04$) and CRP ($p = 0.03$) concentrations between the groups at the endline. However, after adjusting for inflammation using BRINDA methods, there were no statistically significant differences between the groups with regard to the serum ferritin concentrations. Similarly, compared to Control-Beans, there were no significant Fe-Bean effects on dichotomous outcomes, including anemia (<12 years: Hb <11.5 g/dL; ≥12 years: Hb <12.0 g/dL)), iron deficiency (SF <15.0 µg/L; TBI <0.0 mg/kg; sTfR >8.3 mg/L), or inflammation (CRP >5.0 mg/L; AGP >1.0 g/L).

3.3. Plausability Analyses

The findings from the secondary plausibility analyses of the effects of the total consumed iron from beans on the iron status are presented in Table S1 (Online Supplementary Materials). There were no significant effects of the iron consumed from beans on the iron status biomarkers.

Table 1. Baseline characteristics of the study population and intervention.

Study Population [1]		Total (n = 574) Median ± IQR/n (%)	Fe-Beans (n = 269) Median ± IQR/n (%)	Control-Beans (n = 305) Median ± IQR/n (%)
Age, years		9.57 (8.08, 10.89)	9.46 (8.06, 10.67)	9.67 (8.09, 11.04)
Girls, n (%)		306 (53.31)	134 (49.81)	172 (56.39)
Weight, kg		25.90 (22.10, 30.70)	25.50 (21.80, 30.50)	26.35 (22.50, 31.00)
Height, cm		124.90 (118.00, 132.55)	124.70 (117.60, 132.35)	125.30 (118.40, 132.85)
Body Mass Index (BMI), kg/m²		16.63 (15.73, 17.66)	16.36 (15.49, 17.53)	16.77 (15.96, 17.78)
BMI z-score (BMIZ)		0.16 (−0.30, 0.65)	0.11 (−0.38, 0.65)	0.20 (−0.20, 0.65)
	BMIZ < −2	2 (0.35)	1 (0.37)	1 (0.33)
Biomarkers				
Hemoglobin [2] g/dL		12.82 (11.84, 13.83)	12.89 (11.89, 14.09)	12.74 (11.74, 13.64)
	Anemic	102 (17.77)	47 (17.47)	55 (18.03)
Serum ferritin [4] μg/L		28.70 (20.40, 38.90)	28.00 (19.00, 38.10)	29.20 (21.80, 39.50)
	<15.0 μg/L	65 (11.32)	40 (14.87) [3]	25 (8.20) [3]
	<20.0 μg/L	138 (24.04)	77 (28.62)	61 (20.00)
	<30.0 μg/L	309 (53.83)	147 (54.65)	162 (53.11)
Serum ferritin [4] (BRINDA adjusted), μg/L		24.51 (18.18, 33.80)	24.20 (15.92, 32.12)	25.10 (18.58, 35.61)
	<15.0 μg/L	90 (15.90)	58 (22.05) [3]	32 (10.56) [3]
	<20.0 μg/L	182 (32.16)	97 (36.88)	85 (28.05)
	<30.0 μg/L	383 (67.67)	184 (69.96)	199 (65.68)
sTfR [4] (Ramco corrected), mg/L		4.31 (3.99, 4.68)	4.33 (4.04, 4.69)	4.31 (3.97, 4.65)
	>8.3 mg/L	0 (0.00)	0 (0.00)	0 (0.00)
Total body iron, mg/kg		5.37 (4.14, 6.51)	5.25 (3.80, 6.42)	5.54 (4.40, 6.61)
	<0 mg/kg	4 (0.70)	4 (1.49)	0 (0.00)
Total body iron (BRINDA adjusted), mg/kg		4.79 (3.63, 5.97)	4.63 (3.20, 5.77)	4.94 (3.86, 6.11)
	<0 mg/kg	5 (0.88)	5 (1.90)	0 (0.00)
CRP [4] mg/L		0.37 (0.17, 0.99)	0.38 (0.18, 1.04)	0.35 (0.15, 0.80)
	>5 mg/L	36 (6.32)	11 (4.12) [3]	25 (8.25) [3]
AGP [4] g/L		0.70 (0.56, 0.84)	0.69 (0.56, 0.80)	0.71 (0.57, 0.89)
	>1 g/L	66 (11.58)	17 (6.42) [3]	49 (16.07) [3]
Intervention				
Iron concentration in experimental beans, μg/g		-	94	54
Maximum potential number of feeding days		104.00 (100.00, 108.00)	104.00 (100.00, 104.00)	104.00 (100.00, 109.00)
Actual number of feeding days		68.00 (52.00, 75.00)	68.00 (51.00, 75.00)	67.00 (54.00, 75.00)
Total beans experimentally consumed, g		11965.00 (8042.00, 14090.00)	11786.00 (8227.00, 14405.00)	12022.50 (8006.50, 13876.00)
Total iron intake from dry experimental beans, mg		337.42 (256.28, 493.20)	503.58 (351.52, 615.49)	295.10 (196.52, 340.59)
Total iron absorbed from dry beans (5.0%), mg		16.87 (12.81, 24.66)	25.18 (17.58, 30.77)	14.75 (9.83, 17.03)

[1] Median (IQR) for continuous data or n (%) for categorical data; [2] Hemoglobin was adjusted for altitude; anemia was defined as Hb <11.5 g/dL for <12 y and Hb <12.0 g/dL for ≥12 y. [3] Comparison between randomization arms at the baseline, school adjusted as a random effect; $p < 0.05$; [4] Natural logarithm-transformed to improve normality (results presented are not back-transformed); Abbreviations used: AGP, α-1-acid glycoprotein; CRP (C-Reactive Protein); IQR, interquartile range.

Table 2. Effects of consuming iron-biofortified bean on the iron status in children, compared to control beans (n = 574).

Observed Outcomes at the Endline	n	Fe-Beans Median ± IQR/n (%)	N	Control-Beans Median ± IQR/n (%)	Intervention β (SE) or RR (95% CI)	p-value [1]
Hemoglobin [2] g/dL	269	12.89 (11.92, 13.59)	305	13.00 (12.20, 13.84)	−0.18 (0.26)	0.50
Anemic		41 (15.24)		39 (12.79)	1.19 (0.54, 2.60)	0.66
Serum ferritin [3] µg/L	269	30.55 (23.26, 39.62)	305	35.55 (26.23, 48.44)	−0.17 (0.08)	0.04
<15.0 µg/L		16 (5.95)		4 (1.31)	3.42 (1.07, 10.97)	0.04
<20.0 µg/L		43 (15.99)		23 (7.54)	1.88 (0.97, 3.62)	0.06
<30.0 µg/L		129 (47.96)		117 (38.36)	1.24 (0.88, 1.74)	0.21
Serum ferritin (BRINDA) [3] µg/L	267	29.03 (22.12, 37.00)	305	33.13 (24.04, 43.18)	−0.10 (0.07)	0.17
<15.0 µg/L		20 (7.49)		7 (2.30)	2.32 (0.92, 5.83)	0.07
<20.0 µg/L		48 (17.98)		37 (12.13)	1.30 (0.75, 2.26)	0.35
<30.0 µg/L		143 (53.56)		134 (43.93)	1.15 (0.86, 1.53)	0.35
sTfR (Ramco corrected) [3] mg/L	269	4.28 (4.02, 4.57)	305	4.42 (4.06, 4.89)	−0.05 (0.02)	0.05
Total body iron, mg/kg	269	5.62 (4.64, 6.54)	305	6.00 (5.07, 7.08)	−0.43 (0.21)	0.05
Total body iron (BRINDA), mg/kg	267	5.40 (4.48, 6.32)	305	5.61 (4.79, 6.65)	−0.18 (0.18)	0.34
CRP [3] mg/L	268	0.27 (0.10, 0.63)	305	0.36 (0.10, 0.90)	−0.33 (0.13)	0.03
>5.0 mg/L		10 (3.73)		18 (5.90)	0.60 (0.27, 1.32)	0.20
AGP [3] g/L	268	0.70 (0.62, 0.81)	305	0.66 (0.57, 0.84)	0.05 (0.03)	0.12
>1.0 g/L		18 (6.72)		41 (13.44)	0.51 (0.25, 1.03)	0.06

[1] Effects of the intervention on the endline outcome, adjusted for the baseline indicator, with school as a random effect. Generalized linear mixed models were used to examine the effects of Fe-Beans on hematological outcomes, with school as a random effect. [2] Hemoglobin was adjusted for altitude; anemia was defined as Hb <11.5 g/dL for <12 years and Hb <12.0 g/dL for ≥12 years. [3] Natural logarithm-transformation was used in the model to improve normality (results presented are not back-transformed). Abbreviations used: AGP, α-1-acid glycoprotein; CRP (C-Reactive Protein); SE, standard error; IQR, interquartile range; RR, risk ratio; 95% CI, 95 percent confidence interval.

4. Discussion

Iron-biofortified beans did not significantly improve iron status in school-aged children, compared to control beans in this cluster-randomized trial in Mexico. After BRINDA adjustments for inflammation, there were no significant differences between the intervention and control groups at the endline in hemoglobin, serum ferritin, or total body iron concentrations. The intervention lowered the sTfR concentrations, a marker typically not expected to be affected by inflammation, although this did not achieve any statistical significance ($p = 0.054$). Our initial power calculations were based on 120 total feeding days; however, the median number of actual feeding days achieved was only 68.

To our knowledge, this is the first randomized controlled trial of biofortified black beans that examined their efficacy in improving iron status in children. In this biofortified efficacy trial, it was not possible to include a true placebo, which constitutes a study limitation. Iron-biofortified beans with 95 μg/g of iron were compared to control beans containing 55 μg/g of iron, rendering a difference in iron intake of 40 μg iron per g of uncooked beans. Children received a median total of 503.6 mg iron in the Fe-Bean group, compared to a total of 295.1 mg iron in the Control-Bean group, over the course of a 6-month intervention (i.e., 180 days between the baseline and endline blood collection vs. 104 total feeding days vs. a median of 68 days of bean consumption)–which would be equivalent to 2.80 and 1.64 mg/d, respectively, over 6 months. Since the estimated average requirement for iron in school-aged children ≤ 12 y is between 4.1 and 5.9 mg/day [8], the Fe-Bean group received approximately 47% to 68% of their daily physiological iron requirement from experimental beans while the control group received 28% to 40% of these requirements. It is expected that during the days when experimental beans were not consumed there was still some bean consumption through the children's usual diets at home. This usual dietary consumption was not measured but assumed to be similar between randomized intervention groups. The difference in iron ingested from experimental beans between the intervention groups (i.e., 208.5 mg or approximately 1.16 mg/day) is substantial. This comparison, however, assumes that the school-aged children regularly consume the allotted two-per-day portions of beans over the entire follow-up period. Considering the anticipated low iron absorption of approximately 5% from beans [34], the net effect of the transfer of absorbed iron from the two types of beans to the iron stores and functional pools may have been inadequate to result in any significant differences between the intervention groups in the measured biomarkers. It is important to note that the improvement of the iron status in both groups indicates the baseline potential for benefits to this population, even from consumption of standard black beans.

Other studies with biofortified crops on school-age children include one from India using biofortified pearl millet [23]. In that study, iron-biofortified pearl millet significantly improved the iron status in secondary school children after 4 months compared with control pearl millet. Although the amount of iron in biofortified pearl millet is similar to that in biofortified black beans, there are a few differences that may explain the discrepant findings. First, the amount of pearl millet consumed was far greater than the amount of beans consumed in this study; second, the bioavailability of iron in pearl millet is estimated to be higher (7.3%) [35] compared to that of black beans (5%); third, the prevalence of inflammation was considerably lower in the location in India; fourth, phytates and polyphenols may reduce iron absorption; and fifth, there was no assessment of the midline iron status in the trial in Mexico. In the study from India, one of the key findings was that although the serum ferritin concentrations were similar by the end of the trial (6 months) in both groups, there were significant benefits of biofortification at the midpoint assessment; i.e., the intervention group reached those levels significantly faster than the control group.

The results from this trial are also inconsistent with other trials of iron-biofortified crops. With the assessment of multiple iron biomarkers, previous randomized trials have demonstrated the efficacy of the iron biofortification of other staple crops, including beans in women of reproductive age attending university, in improving the iron status in at-risk populations [22–24]. A meta-analysis synthesizing the evidence from these three trials found that iron biofortification interventions significantly increased serum ferritin concentrations and total body iron, compared to conventional crops, with the most substantial benefits among those who were iron deficient at the baseline [25].

In this study, there was a higher prevalence of elevated AGP and CRP in the control group at baseline, compared to the Fe-Bean group. Adjusting for inflammation sufficiently attenuated the high ferritin values in the control group—consistent with the impact of inflammation on the iron status—effectively reversing the apparent negative intervention effect (Table 2). A major strength of this study was the comprehensive assessment of the iron status, including iron biomarkers and indicators of inflammation (i.e., CRP and AGP). This is consistent with WHO recommendations for iron status assessment in populations, namely the examination of Hb, SF, sTfR, and at least 1 acute phase protein (i.e., CRP or AGP) [36]. Soluble transferrin receptor is a carrier protein required for iron endocytosis and regulated in response to intracellular iron levels, and it is less sensitive to inflammation or to the acute phase response in infections. Therefore, measurements of both SF and sTfR can inform the distinction between the effects of inflammation on the host iron status and changes in the iron status. It should be noted that, in this study, Fe-Beans reduced the sTfR concentrations compared to Control-Beans ($p = 0.054$), supporting the predicted effect of iron-biofortified beans improving the iron status, as this indicator is not expected to be influenced by inflammation.

Another strength of this study was the use of black beans in a population with high baseline intake of this staple crop. In southern Mexico, the mean daily consumption of standard beans for school-aged children is, on average, 50 g of dry weight per day, which is a good iron source and can provide approximately 50% of the daily estimated average requirement of iron. This affirms the use of the black bean as an appropriate carrier for an amplified iron delivery [26].

This study has several limitations. Randomization was implemented at the school level rather than at the individual level, limiting the power of the study. The a priori assumptions for adequate power were not met, as the number of feeding days was lower than that initially anticipated (i.e., the median number of feeding days was 68 vs. the 120 days included in the power and sample size calculations). The school-level randomization also resulted in significant differences between the treatments at the baseline in inflammation, which impacts the iron assessment since ferritin is an acute-phase protein. Children in schools in the control group were significantly more likely to exhibit elevated inflammation (CRP >5 mg/L, AGP >1 g/L) at the baseline, compared to children in boarding schools in the intervention group. As part of the immune response, inflammation is associated with a variety of human disorders and is common on both ends of the spectrum of malnutrition, including obesity and undernutrition [37]. Inflammation is also common in settings with high burdens of infectious diseases. There is an established relationship between iron and inflammation [38]: inflammatory cytokines activate the secretion of the hepatic peptide hormone hepcidin to reduce the circulation of iron, thus increasing serum ferritin and decreasing transferrin-bound iron [37,39]. This can cause an anemia of inflammation, which is typically unresponsive to iron interventions.

The indicators most susceptible to inflammation, serum ferritin and hemoglobin, responded predictably by exhibiting greater increases in the control group, which included a significantly greater proportion of children with chronic, low-grade inflammation. Additionally, the low bioavailability of iron from the high phytate diets (mostly from maize) is a limitation for both groups and may be one of several factors that reduced the likelihood of an improvement in the iron status.

Generalizability must also be considered; the boarding school setting, with relatively low prevalence of anemia (<20%) and high bean intake, may constrain the generalizability of the intervention efficacy to other populations. Future studies should consider other subgroups at risk of iron deficiency, including pregnant and lactating women, as well as broader populations at large.

Overall, as a plant-based, locally consumed source of iron and protein, beans offer an environmentally and economically sustainable approach for delivering nutrients in resource-limited settings, and both control and intervention groups demonstrated an improved iron status in this trial. The present study highlighted the importance of examining inflammation as part of a comprehensive iron status assessment, and adjusting for inflammation. In prospective studies, additional methods are needed to integrate changes in inflammation in the assessment of the iron status over time. Future investigations should assess the effects of iron-biofortified beans on the iron status in at-risk populations and elucidate the association of iron status and inflammatory markers in children with multiple measurements during follow-ups (e.g., random serial sampling). Future randomized efficacy trials are also needed to evaluate the effects of iron-biofortified beans on functional outcomes of iron deficiency, including cognitive development, growth, and physical performance.

Supplementary Materials: The following are available online at http://www.mdpi.com/2072-6643/11/2/381/s1, Table S1: Effect of total iron consumed on on iron status in children, adjusted for intervention ($n = 571$).

Author Contributions: Conceptualization, J.D.H. and S.V.; analysis, J.L.F., S.M.; writing—original draft preparation, J.D.H., J.L.F., S.V.L., and M.R.; writing—review and editing, J.L.F. and S.M.; supervision, S.V. and T.S.-L.; project administration, study implementation, and data collection, V.M.-R. and T.S.-L.; technical development, growth, and provision of the biofortified beans, S.E.B.; funding acquisition, J.D.H. and S.V. All authors contributed to the development of this manuscript and read and approved the final version.

Funding: This research was funded by HarvestPlus/IFPRI and AgroSalud/Centro Internacional de Agricultura Tropical.

Acknowledgments: We thank colleagues and school administrators who facilitated all aspects of the data collection. We are grateful to Ray Glahn, USDA/Agricultural Research Service in Ithaca, NY, for his expertise in laboratory analysis of bean and food samples.

Conflicts of Interest: J.D.H. received funding as an expert consultant for HarvestPlus. S.M. is an unpaid board member for a diagnostic start up focused on measurement of nutritional biomarkers at the point-of-care utilizing the results from his research. The other authors have no conflict of interest to disclose. The funders had no role in the design of the study; in the collection, analyses, or interpretation of data; or in the writing of the manuscript.

References

1. WHO. *Iron Deficiency Anaemia Assessment, Prevention, and Control: A Guide for Programme Managers*; WHO: Geneva, Switzerland, 2001.
2. UNSCN. *4th Report—The World Nutrition Situation: Nutrition Throughout the Life Cycle*; UNSCN: Rome, Italy, 2000.
3. McLean, E.; Cogswell, M.; Egli, I.; Wojdyla, D.; de Benoist, B. Worldwide prevalence of anaemia, WHO Vitamin and Mineral Nutrition Information System, 1993–2005. *Pub. Health Nutr.* **2009**, *12*, 444–454. [CrossRef]
4. ACC/SCN. *Fourth Report on the World Nutrition Situation*; ACC/SCN in collaboration with IFPRI: Geneva, Switzerland, 2000.
5. WHO. *Micronutrient Deficiencies: Iron Deficiency Anaemia*; WHO: Geneva, Switzerland, 2017.
6. Petry, N.; Olofin, I.; Hurrell, R.F.; Boy, E.; Wirth, J.P.; Moursi, M.; Moira, D.A.; Rohner, F. The proportion of anemia associated with iron deficiency in low, medium, and high Human Development Index countries: A systematic analysis of national surveys. *Nutrients* **2016**, *8*, 693. [CrossRef] [PubMed]
7. WHO. *The Global Prevalence of Anaemia in 2011*; World Health Organization: Geneva, Switzerland, 2015.
8. Trumbo, P.; Yates, A.A.; Schlicker, S.; Poos, M. Dietary reference intakes: Vitamin A., vitamin K., arsenic, boron, chromium, copper, iodine, iron, manganese, molybdenum, nickel, silicon, vanadium, and zinc. *J. Am. Diet Assoc.* **2001**, *101*, 294–301. [CrossRef]
9. Flores, M.; Macías, N.; Rivera, M.; Barquera, S.; Hernández, L.; García-Guerra, A.; Rivera, J.A. Energy and nutrient intake among Mexican school-aged children, Mexican National Health and Survey 2006. *Salud Pub. Mex.* **2009**, *51*, 540–550. [CrossRef]
10. Finkelstein, J.L.; Layden, A.J.; Stover, P.J. Vitamin B-12 and perinatal health. *Adv. Nutr.* **2015**, *6*, 552–563. [CrossRef] [PubMed]
11. Finkelstein, J.L.; Kurpad, A.V.; Thomas, T.; Duggan, C. Vitamin B12 status in pregnant women and their infants in South India. *Eur. J. Clin. Nutr.* **2017**, *71*, 1046–1053. [CrossRef]
12. Villalpando, S.; Perez-Exposito, A.B.; Shamah-Levy, T.; Rivera, J.A. Distribution of anemia associated with micronutrient deficiencies other than iron in a probabilistic sample of Mexican children. *Ann. Nutr. Metab.* **2006**, *50*, 506–511. [CrossRef] [PubMed]

13. Morales-Ruán, M.C.; Villalpando, S.; García-Guerra, A.; Shamah-Levy, T.; Robledo-Pérez, R.; Avila-Arcos, M.A.; Rivera, J. Iron, zinc, copper and magnesium nutritional status in Mexican children aged 1 to 11 years. *Salud Pub. Mex.* **2012**, *54*, 125–134. [CrossRef]
14. WHO. *Guideline: Daily Iron Supplementation in Infants and Children*; World Health Organization: Geneva, Switzerland, 2016.
15. McClung, J.P.; Murray-Kolb, L.E. Iron nutrition and premenopausal women: Effects of poor iron status on physical and neuropsychological performance. *Annu. Rev. Nutr.* **2013**, *33*, 271–288. [CrossRef]
16. Haas, J.D.; Brownlie, T., IV. Iron deficiency and reduced work capacity: A critical review of the research to determine a causal relationship. *J. Nutr.* **2001**, *131*, 676S–688S. [CrossRef]
17. Murray-Kolb, L.E.; Beard, J.L. Iron treatment normalizes cognitive functioning in young women. *Am. J. Clin. Nutr.* **2007**, *85*, 778–787. [CrossRef] [PubMed]
18. Graham, R.S.D.; Beebe, S.; Iglesias, C.; Monasterio, I. Breeding for micronutrient density in edile portions of staple food crops: Conventional approaches. *Field Crops Res.* **1999**, *60*, 57–80. [CrossRef]
19. Meenakshi, J.V. *Cost-Effectiveness of Biofortification*; Best Practice Paper; Copenhagen Consensus Center: Copenhagen, Denmark, 2008.
20. Nestel, P.; Bouis, H.E.; Meenakshi, J.V.; Pfeiffer, W. Biofortification of staple food crops. *J. Nutr.* **2006**, *136*, 1064–1067. [CrossRef] [PubMed]
21. Hotz, C.; McClafferty, B. From harvest to health: Challenges for developing biofortified staple foods and determining their impact on micronutrient status. *Food Nutr. Bull.* **2007**, *28*, S271–S279. [CrossRef] [PubMed]
22. Haas, J.D.; Beard, J.L.; Murray-Kolb, L.E.; del Mundo, A.M.; Felix, A.; Gregorio, G.B. Iron-biofortified rice improves the iron stores of nonanemic Filipino women. *J. Nutr.* **2005**, *135*, 2823–2830. [CrossRef] [PubMed]
23. Finkelstein, J.L.; Mehta, S.; Udipi, S.A.; Ghugre, P.S.; Luna, S.V.; Wenger, M.J.; Murray-Kolb, L.E.; Przybyszewski, E.M.; Haas, J.D. A randomized trial of iron-biofortified pearl millet in school children in India. *J. Nutr.* **2015**, *145*, 1576–1581. [CrossRef] [PubMed]
24. Haas, J.D.; Luna, S.V.; Lung'aho, M.G.; Wenger, M.J.; Murray-Kolb, L.E.; Beebe, S.; Gahutu, J.-B.; Egli, I.M. Consuming iron biofortified beans increases iron status in Rwandan women after 128 days in a randomized controlled feeding trial. *J. Nutr.* **2016**, *146*, 1586–1592. [CrossRef] [PubMed]
25. Finkelstein, J.L.; Haas, J.D.; Mehta, S. Iron-biofortified staple food crops for improving iron status: A review of the current evidence. *Curr. Opin. Biotechnol.* **2017**, *44*, 138–145. [CrossRef]
26. Olaiz-Fernández, G.; Rivera-Donmarco, J.; Shamah-Levy, T.; Rojas, R.; Villalpando-Hernández, S.; Hernández-Avila, M.; Sepúlveda-Amor, J. *Encuesta National de Salud y Nutricion 2006*; Instituto Nacional de Salud Pública: Cuernavaca, Mexico, 2006. (In Spanish)
27. De Onis, M.; Blössner, M. The World Health Organization Global Database on Child Growth and Malnutrition: Methodology and applications. *Int. J. Epidemiol.* **2003**, *32*, 518–526. [CrossRef]
28. Cook, J.D.; Flowers, C.H.; Skikne, B.S. The quantitative assessment of body iron. *Blood* **2003**, *101*, 3359–3364. [CrossRef]
29. Cohen, J.H.; Haas, J.D. Hemoglobin correction factors for estimating the prevalence of iron deficiency anemia in pregnant women residing at high altitudes in Bolivia. *Rev. Panam. Salud Publica* **1999**, *6*, 392–399. [CrossRef] [PubMed]
30. Namaste, S.M.; Rohner, F.; Huang, J.; Bhushan, N.L.; Flores-Ayala, R.; Kupka, R.; Mei, Z.; Rawat, R.; Williams, A.M.; Raiten, D.J.; et al. Adjusting ferritin concentrations for inflammation: Biomarkers Reflecting Inflammation and Nutritional Determinants of Anemia (BRINDA) project. *Am. J. Clin. Nutr.* **2017**, *106*, 359S–371S. [PubMed]
31. Thurnham, D.I.; McCabe, L.D.; Haldar, S.; Wieringa, F.T.; Northrop-Clewes, C.A.; McCabe, G.P. Adjusting plasma ferritin concentrations to remove the effects of subclinical inflammation in the assessment of iron deficiency: A meta-analysis. *Am. J. Clin. Nutr.* **2010**, *92*, 546–555. [CrossRef] [PubMed]
32. Thurnham, D.I.; Northrop-Clewes, C.A.; Knowles, J. The use of adjustment factors to address the impact of inflammation on vitamin A and iron status in humans. *J. Nutr.* **2015**, *145*, 1137S–1143S. [CrossRef] [PubMed]
33. Larson, L.M.; Addo, O.; Sandalinas, F.; Faigao, K.; Kupka, R.; Flores-Ayala, R.; Suchdev, P. Accounting for the influence of inflammation on retinol-binding protein in a population survey of Liberian preschool-age children. *Matern. Child Nutr.* **2017**, *13*. [CrossRef] [PubMed]
34. Petry, N.; Egli, I.; Zeder, C.; Walczyk, T.; Hurrell, R. Polyphenols and phytic acid contribute to the low iron bioavailability from common beans in young women. *J. Nutr.* **2010**, *140*, 1977–1982. [CrossRef] [PubMed]

35. Kodkany, B.S.; Bellad, R.M.; Mahantshetti, N.S.; Westcott, J.E.; Krebs, N.F.; Kemp, J.F.; Hambidge, K.M. Biofortification of pearl millet with iron and zinc in a randomized controlled trial increases absorption of these minerals above physiologic requirements in young children. *J. Nutr.* **2013**, *143*, 1489–1493. [CrossRef] [PubMed]
36. World Health Organization; Centers for Disease Control and Prevention. *Assessing the Iron Status of Populations*; WHO: Geneva, Switzerland, 2007.
37. Camaschella, C. New insights into iron deficiency and iron deficiency anemia. *Blood Rev.* **2017**, *31*, 225–233. [CrossRef]
38. Suchdev, P.S.; William, A.M.; Mei, Z.; Flores-Ayala, R.; Pasricha, S.-R.; Rogers, L.M.; Namaste, S.M.L. Assessment of iron status in settings of inflammation: Challenges and potential approaches. *Am. J. Clin. Nutr.* **2017**, *106*, 1626S–1633S. [CrossRef]
39. Ganz, T. Iron and infection. *Int. J. Hematol.* **2017**, *107*, 7–15. [CrossRef]

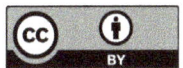

© 2019 by the authors. Licensee MDPI, Basel, Switzerland. This article is an open access article distributed under the terms and conditions of the Creative Commons Attribution (CC BY) license (http://creativecommons.org/licenses/by/4.0/).

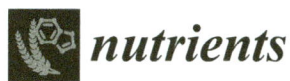

Article

Iron Biofortified Carioca Bean (*Phaseolus vulgaris* L.)—Based Brazilian Diet Delivers More Absorbable Iron and Affects the Gut Microbiota In Vivo (*Gallus gallus*)

Desirrê Morais Dias [1,2], Nikolai Kolba [3], Dana Binyamin [4], Oren Ziv [4], Marilia Regini Nutti [5], Hércia Stampini Duarte Martino [1], Raymond P. Glahn [3], Omry Koren [4] and Elad Tako [3,*]

1. Department of Nutrition and Health, Federal University of Viçosa, 36570000 Viçosa, Minas Gerais, Brazil; desirremorais@hotmail.com (D.M.D.); hercia72@gmail.com (H.S.D.M.)
2. Department of Food Science and Technology, Cornell University, Ithaca, NY 14850, USA
3. USDA-ARS, Robert W. Holley Center for Agriculture and Health, Cornell University, Ithaca, NY 14850, USA; nikolai.kolba@ars.usda.gov (N.K.); raymond.glahn@ars.usda.gov (R.P.G.)
4. Azrieli Faculty of Medicine, Bar-Ilan University, Safed 1311502, Israel; dsimoni925@gmail.com (D.B.); oren.ziv@biu.ac.il (O.Z.); omry.koren@biu.ac.il (O.K.)
5. EMBRAPA Food Technology, 23020-470 Rio de Janeiro, Brazil; m.nuti@cgiar.org
* Correspondence: elad.tako@ars.usda.gov or et79@cornell.edu; Tel.: +1-607-255-5434

Received: 20 November 2018; Accepted: 9 December 2018; Published: 13 December 2018

Abstract: Biofortification aims to improve the micronutrient concentration and bioavailability in staple food crops. Unlike other strategies utilized to alleviate Fe deficiency, studies of the gut microbiota in the context of Fe biofortification are scarce. In this study, we performed a 6-week feeding trial in *Gallus gallus* ($n = 15$), aimed to investigate the Fe status and the alterations in the gut microbiome following the administration of Fe-biofortified carioca bean based diet (BC) versus a Fe-standard carioca bean based diet (SC). The tested diets were designed based on the Brazilian food consumption survey. Two primary outcomes were observed: (1) a significant increase in total body Hb-Fe values in the group receiving the Fe-biofortified carioca bean based diet; and (2) changes in the gut microbiome composition and function were observed, specifically, significant changes in phylogenetic diversity between treatment groups, as there was increased abundance of bacteria linked to phenolic catabolism, and increased abundance of beneficial SCFA-producing bacteria in the BC group. The BC group also presented a higher intestinal villi height compared to the SC group. Our results demonstrate that the Fe-biofortified carioca bean variety was able to moderately improve Fe status and to positively affect the intestinal functionality and bacterial populations.

Keywords: iron deficiency; Biofortification; intestinal morphometry; gut microbiome; metagenome; polyphenols

1. Introduction

Micronutrients deficiency affects approximately two billion people worldwide. Iron (Fe) deficiency is the most prevalent nutrient deficiency, affecting around 40% of the world population, particularly women and children in developing countries [1,2]. It is estimated that around 46% of the population in Africa, 57% in South-East Asia and 19% in America are anemic [3]. Fe deficiency is highly prevalent in low-income countries (~30% in Brazil) due to a lack of meat consumption in addition to a notable dietary reliance on grains containing high amounts of Fe absorption inhibitors (e.g., phytic acid, polyphenolic compounds) [4–7]. Major pathophysiological complications related to insufficient Fe intake may include stunted growth, impaired physical and cognitive development, and increased risk of morbidity and mortality in children [4,8,9]. To alleviate Fe deficiency, an integral step involves the understanding of specific dietary patterns and components that contribute to Fe status in the particular population suffering from a deficiency.

Biofortified staple food crops have become an effective tool by which to address micronutrient deficiencies, especially that of Fe, in many at-risk populations [4,6,10,11]. The common bean (*Phaseolus vulgaris*) is one of the crops target for biofortification program since it exhibits sufficient genetic variability in iron concentration, which is the basic requirement for biofortification [12,13]. This crop is currently estimated to be one of the most important legumes worldwide [13,14], and is an important source of nutrients for more than 300 million people in parts of Eastern Africa and Latin America, representing 65% of total protein consumed, 32% of energy, and a major source of micronutrients (vitamins and minerals) [10,14,15].

Previous studies using Fe biofortified beans in Mexico [16], and Rwanda [17,18] have shown some improvement in Fe status in subjects consuming the biofortified beans versus a standard bean variety. However, a major challenge associated with biofortification of staple food crops, especially common beans, is that they contain factors such as polyphenols and phytic acid that can inhibit Fe bioavailability and absorption, hence limit their nutritional benefit [17,19]. These inhibitory factors may increase with Fe concentration when these crops are biofortified via conventional breeding [17,19,20]. Hence, as was previously suggested, it is necessary to measure the concentration of Fe, the amount of bioavailable Fe, and the concentration of potential inhibitors of Fe bioavailability in these biofortified crops [19,21,22]. It is also important to factor in and assess the other components of the diet in which these crops are consumed as the potential interactions can negate or even enhance the expected benefit of increased Fe content.

Despite containing inhibitory factors, legumes also carry other substances, referred to as promoters, which have the potential to counteract the effects of the inhibitory factors [19,20,23,24]. One of the most notable promoters are prebiotic [19,25,26]. Prebiotics have been characterized as a group of carbohydrates that resist digestion and absorption in the gastrointestinal tract (small intestine), that beneficially affect gut health, by enhancing the growth and activities of probiotics [26–28] and can improve mineral absorption [29]. These compounds can survive the acidic and enzymatic digestion in the small intestine, and thus can be fermented by probiotics that reside in the colon/cecum [30]. The fermentation of prebiotics by probiotics leads to the production of short-chain fatty acids (SCFA), which may improve the intestinal function, increasing the absorption of minerals such as Fe [25,31–33]. At the same time, some polyphenols present in the common beans can stimulate the growth of commensal and beneficial microbiota while pathogenic strains are inhibited or unaffected [34].

Biofortified crops have become an effective tool by which to address micronutrient deficiencies, especially that of Fe, in many at-risk populations [15,35,36]. By using the combination of a Caco-2 cell bioassay and an in vivo (*Gallus gallus*) model that has been used extensively for nutritional research and shown to be an excellent model to assess dietary Fe (and Zinc) bioavailability [4,37–39], the objective of the current study was to evaluate the ability of the Fe biofortified carioca bean line to deliver more Fe for hemoglobin (Hb) synthesis. Also, we aimed to evaluate the effect of the Fe biofortified carioca bean intake on the intestinal microbiota composition and function. If this in vivo assessment indicates that nutritional benefit exists, we suggest to further employ these screening tools to guide future studies aimed to assess biofortified staple food crops, as this approach will allow proceeding to human efficacy studies with greater confidence and success.

2. Materials and Methods

2.1. Sample Preparation

The two carioca bean lines: BRS Perola (Fe Standard) and BRS Cometa (Fe Biofortified) that were used in this study were obtained from Embrapa (Empresa Brasileira de Pesquisa Agropecuaria, Goias, Brazil), and were shipped to Ithaca, New York in sealed containers imported as flours. The beans were cooked in three replicates in a conventional pressure cooker for 40 min using a bean/distilled water ratio of 1:2.7 (w/v) and dried in an air oven for 17 h at 60 °C. The dried beans were ground by stainless steel mill 090 CFT at 3000 rpm and stored at −12 °C [40].

2.2. Polyphenols Analysis

2.2.1. Polyphenol Extraction

1 g of bean flour was added with 5 mL of methanol/water (50:50 v/v). The slurry was vortexed for 1 min, placed in a 24 °C sonication water bath for 20 min, vortexed again for 1 min and centrifuged at 4000× g for 15 min. The supernatant was filtered with a 0.45 μm Teflon syringe, filtered, and stored for later use at −20 °C.

2.2.2. Ultra Performance Liquid Chromatography—Mass Spectrometry (UPLC—MS) Analysis of Polyphenols

Extracts and standards were analyzed with a Waters Acquity UPLC (Waters, Milford, MA, USA). Five microliter samples were injected and passed through an Acquity UPLC BEH Shield RP18, 1.7 μm. 2.1 × 100 mm column (Waters, Milford, MA, USA) at 0.5 mL/min. The column was temperature-controlled at 40 °C. The mobile phase consisted of water with 0.1% formic acid (solvent A) and acetonitrile with 0.1% formic acid (solvent B). Polyphenols were eluted using linear gradients of 86.7–84.4% A in 1.5 min, 84.4–81.5% A in 0.2 min, 81.5–77% A in 2.8 min, 77–55% A in 0.5 min, 55–46% A in 1 min and 46–86.7% A in 0.2 min and a 0.8 min hold at 86.7% A for a total 7 min run time. From the column flow was directed into a Waters Acquity photodiode array detector set at 300–400 nm and a sampling rate of 20/s. Flow was then directed into the source of a Xevo G2 QTOF mass spectrometer (Waters, Milford, MA, USA) and ESI mass spectrometry was performed in negative ionization mode with a scan speed of 5/s in the mass range from 50 to 1200 Da. Capillary and cone gas voltages were set at 2.3 kV and 30 V respectively. Desolvation gas flow was 800 L/h. and desolvation gas temperature was 400 °C. Source temperature was 140 °C. Lock-mass correction was used with leucine encephalin as the lock-mass standard and a scan frequency of 25 s. Instrumentation and data acquisition were controlled by MassLynx software (version 4.2, Waters, Milford, MA, USA). Individual polyphenols in bean samples were tentatively determined by mass using MarkerLynx software (Waters, Milford, MA, USA), and their identities were confirmed by comparison of LC retention times with authentic standards. Polyphenol standard curves for flavonoids were derived from integrated areas under UV absorption peaks from 10 replications. Standard curves for catechin and 3.4-dihydroxybenzoic acid were constructed from MS ion intensities using 10 replications.

2.3. Phytate Analysis

Dietary phytic acid (phytate)/total phosphorus was measured as phosphorus released by phytase and alkaline phosphatase, following the kit manufacturer's instructions ($n = 5$) (K-PHYT 12/12. Megazyme International. Bray, Ireland).

2.4. Iron Content of Bean Flour, Serum and Liver

The bean flour samples and liver samples (0.5 g) and serum (100 μL) were treated with 3.0 mL of 60:40 HNO_3 and $HClO_4$ mixture into a Pyrex glass tube and left for overnight to destroy organic matter. The mixture was then heated to 120 °C for two hours and 0.25 mL of 40 μg/g Yttrium (Sigma-Aldrich, St. Louis, MO, USA) added as an internal standard to compensate for any drift during the subsequent inductively coupled plasma atomic emission spectrometer (ICP-AES) analysis. The temperature of the heating block was then raised to 145 °C for 2 h. Then, the temperature of the heating block raised to 190 °C for ten minutes and turned off. The cooled samples in the tubes were then diluted to 20 mL, vortexed and transferred into auto sample tubes to analyze via ICP-AES. The model of the ICP used was a Thermo iCAP 6500 series (Thermo Jarrell Ash Corp., Franklin, MA, USA).

2.5. Protein and Dietary Fiber Analysis in the Bean Flour

Protein concentration was determined by micro-Kjeldahl method according to the Official Methods of Analysis (AOAC International, Rockville, MD, USA) procedure [41]. The determination of total fiber and soluble and insoluble fractions was performed by the enzymatic-gravimetric method according to AOAC [41], using the enzymatic hydrolysis for a heat-resistant amylase, protease and amyloglucosidase (Total dietary fiber assay Kiyonaga, Sigma®, Kawasaki, Japan).

2.6. In Vitro Iron Bioavailability Assessment

An established in vitro digestion/Caco-2 cell culture model was used to assess Fe-bioavailability [37,42]. The staple food flour samples (biofortified and standard beans, rice, potato) were analyzed by themselves and in a food combination ("food basket"). With this method, the cooked bean samples, additional meal plan components and the formulated diets were subjected to simulated gastric and intestinal digestion. 0.5 g of the freeze dried cooked beans and diet samples were utilized for each replication ($n = 6$) of the in vitro digestion [11,21,43].

2.7. Harvesting of Caco-2 Cells for Ferritin Analysis

The protocols used in the ferritin and the total protein contents analyses of Caco-2 cells were similar to those previously described [19,22,23,37,39,44]. Caco-2 cells synthesize ferritin in response to increases in intracellular Fe concentration. Therefore, we used the ratio of ferritin/total protein (expressed as ng ferritin/mg protein) as an indicator of cellular Fe uptake. All glassware used in the sample preparation and analyses was acid washed.

2.8. Animals, Diets and Study Design

Cornish cross—fertile broiler eggs ($n = 60$) were obtained from a commercial hatchery (Moyer's chicks, Quakertown, PA, USA). The eggs were incubated under optimal conditions at the Cornell University Animal Science poultry farm incubator. Upon hatching (hatchability rate = 50%), chicks were allocated into 2 treatment groups on the basis of body weight and blood hemoglobin concentration (aimed to ensure equal concentration between groups), (1) Fe-standard carioca bean based diet (SC): 42% carioca bean (BRS Perola) based diet ($n = 14$), and (2) Fe-biofortified carioca bean based diet (BC): 42% carioca bean (BRS Cometa) based diet ($n = 14$). Experimental diets (Table 1) had no supplemental Fe. The specific Brazilian dietary formulation used in the study (Table 1) was based on the Brazilian food consumption survey [45]. Chicks were housed in a total confinement building (4 chicks per 1 m^2 metal cage). The birds were under indoor controlled temperatures and were provided 16 h of light. Each cage was equipped with an automatic nipple drinker and a manual self-feeder. All birds were given ad libitum access to water. Feed intakes were measured daily (as from day 1), and Fe intakes were calculated from feed intakes and Fe concentration in the diets. The body weight and the hemoglobin concentration in the blood were measured weekly.

Table 1. Composition of the experimental bean based diets [1–3].

Ingredient	Fe Content (µg Fe/g Sample)	Fe-Standard Carioca Based Diet (SC) (g/kg by Formulation)	Fe-Biofortified Carioca Bean Based Diet (BC) (g/kg by Formulation)
BRS Perola (Fe-standard bean)	64.3 ± 0.54	420	-
BRS Cometa (Fe-biofortified bean)	84.97 ± 2	-	420
Potato	12.89 ± 0.43	320	320
Corn	31.36 ± 4.74	70	70
Pasta (non-enriched)	13.82 ± 1.04	70	70
Rice	4.21 ± 0.8	50	50
Vitamin/mineral premix (no Fe)	0.0	70	70
DL-Methionine	0.0	2.5	2.5
Vegetable oil	0.0	30	30
Choline chloride Total (g) Total (g)	0.0	0.75	0.75
Selected components			
Dietary Fe concentration (µg/g)	-	40.47 ± 1.84	47.04 ± 1.52 *
Phytic acid (µg/g)	-	1.71 ± 0.16 *	1.15 ± 0.053
Phytate:Fe molar ratio	-	35.76	20.84

[1] Vitamin and mineral premix provided/kg diet (330002 Chick vitamin mixture; 235001 Salt mix for chick diet; Dyets Inc. Bethlehem, PA, USA). [2] Iron concentrations in the diets were determined by an inductively-coupled argon-plasma/atomic emission spectrophotometer. [3] Method for determining phytate is described in the materials and method s section.
* Statistical difference by *t*-test at 5% of probability (Comparison between Standard diet and Biofortified diet).

2.9. Blood Analysis, Hemoglobin (Hb) Determination, and Tissue Collection

Blood samples were collected weekly from the wing vein (100 µL) using micro-hematocrit heparinized capillary tubes (Fisher, Pittsburgh, PA, USA). Weekly blood Hb concentrations were determined spectrophotometrically using the Triton/NaOH method following the kit manufacturer's instructions. Fe bioavailability was calculated as hemoglobin maintenance efficiency (HME):

$$\text{HME} = \frac{\text{Hb} - \text{Fe, mg (final)} - \text{Hb} - \text{Fe, mg (initial)}}{\text{Total Fe intake, mg}} \times 100$$

where Hb-Fe (index of Fe absorption) = total body hemoglobin Fe. Hb-Fe was calculated from hemoglobin concentrations and estimates of blood volume based on body weight (a blood volume of 85 mL per kg body weight is assumed):

$$\text{Hb-Fe (mg)} = \text{BW (kg)} \times 0.085 \text{ blood/Kg} \times \text{Hb (g/L)} \times 3.35 \text{ mg Fe/g Hb}$$

At the end of the experiment (day 42), birds were euthanized by CO_2 exposure. The digestive tracts (small intestine and cecum) and livers were quickly removed from the carcass. The samples were immediately frozen in liquid nitrogen, and then stored in a $-80\ ^\circ$C freezer until further analysis.

All animal protocols were approved by the Cornell University Institutional Animal Care and Use Committee (protocol name: Intestinal uptake of Fe and Zn in the duodenum of broiler chicken: extent, frequency, and nutritional implications; approved: 15 December 2016; protocol number: 2007–0129).

2.10. Isolation of Total RNA from Chicken Duodenum and Liver

Total RNA was extracted from 30 mg of the proximal duodenal tissue ($n = 8$) and liver ($n = 8$) using Qiagen RNeasy Mini Kit (RNeasy Mini Kit, Qiagen Inc., Valencia, CA, USA) according to the manufacturer's protocol. Briefly, tissues were disrupted and homogenized with a rotor-stator homogenizer in buffer RLT®, containing β-mercaptoethanol. The tissue lysate was centrifuged for 3 min at 8000× *g* in a micro centrifuge. An aliquot of the supernatant was transferred to another tube, combined with 1 volume of 70% ethanol and mixed immediately. Each sample (700 µL) was applied to an RNeasy mini column, centrifuged for 15 s at 8000× *g*, and the flow through material was discarded. Next, the RN easy columns were transferred to new 2-mL collection tubes, and 500 µL of buffer RPE® was pipetted onto the RNeasy column followed by centrifugation for 15 s at 8000× *g*. An additional 500 µL of buffer RPE were pipetted onto the RNeasy column and centrifuged for 2 min at 8000× *g*. Total RNA was eluted in 50 µL of RNase free water.

All steps were carried out under RNase free conditions. RNA was quantified by absorbance at A 260/280. Integrity of the 28S and 18S ribosomal RNAs was verified by 1.5% agarose gel electrophoresis followed by ethidium bromide staining. DNA contamination was removed using TURBO DNase treatment and removal kit from AMBION (Austin, TX, USA).

2.11. Real Time Polymerase Chain Reaction (RT-PCR)

As was previously described [46], cDNA was used for each 10 µL reaction together with 2× BioRad SSO Advnaced Universal SYBR Green Supermix (BioRad, Hercules, CA, USA) which included buffer, Taq DNA polymerase, dNTPs and SYBR green dye. Specific primers (forward and reverse (Table 2) and cDNA or water (for no template control) were added to each PCR reaction. The specific primers used can be seen in Table 2. For each gene, the optimal $MgCl_2$ concentration produced the amplification plot with the lowest cycle product (Cp), the highest fluorescence intensity and the steepest amplification slope. Master mix (8 µL) was pipetted into the 96-well plate and 2 µL cDNA was added as PCR template. Each run contained seven standard curve points in duplicate. A no template control of nuclease-free water was included to exclude DNA contamination in the PCR mix. The double stranded DNA was amplified in the Bio-Rad CFX96 Touch (Bio-Rad Laboratories, Hercules, CA, USA) using the following PCR conditions: initial denaturing at 95 °C for 30 s, 40 cycles of denaturing at 95 °C for 15 s, various annealing temperatures according to Integrated DNA Technologies (IDT) for 30 s and elongating at 60 °C for 30 s. The data on the expression levels of the genes were obtained as Cp values based on the "second derivative maximum" (automated method) as computed by the software. For each of the 12 genes, the reactions were run in duplicate. All assays were quantified by including a standard curve in the real-time qPCR analysis. The next four points of the standard curve were prepared by a 1:10 dilution. Each point of the standard curve was included in duplicate. A graph of Cp vs. log 10 concentrations was produced by the software and the efficiencies were calculated as 10[1/slope]. The specificity of the amplified real-time RT-PCR products were verified by melting curve analysis (60–95 °C) after 40 cycles, which should result in a number of different specific products, each with a specific melting temperature. In addition, we electrophoresed the resulting PCR products on a 2%-agarose gel, stained the gel with ethidium bromide, and visualized it under UV light. PCR-positive products were purified of primer dimers and other non-specific amplification by-products using QIAquick Gel Kit (Qiagen Inc., Valencia, CA, USA) prior to sequencing. We sequenced the products using BigDye® Terminator v3.1 Cycle Sequencing Kits (Applied Biosystems, Foster City, CA, USA) and ABI Automated 3430xl DNA Analyzer (Applied Biosystems) and analyzed them with Sequencing Analysis ver. 5.2 (Applied Biosystems). We aligned sequences of hepcidin with those from related organisms obtained from Gen Bank using a basic alignment-search tool (BLAST; National Center for Biotechnology Information, Bethesda, MD, USA). Sequence alignments were performed for all samples. We used the ClustalW program for sequence alignment.

Table 2. DNA sequences of the primers used in this study.

Analyte	Forward Primer (5′-3′) (Nucleotide Position)	Reverse Primer (5′-3′)	Base Pairs Length	GI Identifier
Iron metabolism				
DMT1	TTGATTCAGAGCCTCCCATTAG	GCGAGGAGTAGGCTTGTATTT	101	206597489
Ferroportin	CTCAGCAATCACTGGCATCA	ACTGGGCAACTCCAGAAATAAG	98	61098365
DcytB	CATGTGCATTCTCTTCCAAAGTC	CTCCTTGGTGACCGCATTAT	103	20380692
Hepcidin	AGACGACAATGCAGACTAACC	CTGCAGCAATCCCACATTTC	132	
TRCP1	GAGCAAGCCATGTCAAGATTTC	GTCTGGGCCAAGTCTGTTATAG	122	015291382.1
BBM functionality				
SI	CCAGCAATGCCAGCATATTG	CGGTTTCTCCTTACCACTTCTT	95	2246388
SGLT1	GCATCCTTACTCTGTGGTACTG	TATCCGCACATCACACATCC	106	8346783
AP	CGTCAGCCAGTTTGACTATGTA	CTCTCAAAGAAGCTGAGGATGG	138	45382360
18S rRNA	GCAAGACGAACTAAAGCGAAAG	TCGGAACTACGACGGTATCT	100	7262899

DMT-1, Divalent Metal Transporter–1; DcytB, Duodenal cytochrome b; 18S rRNA, 18S Ribosomal subunit; SI, Sucrose isomaltase; SGLT-1: Sodium-Glucose transport protein 1; AP, Amino peptidase; TRCP1: Transferrin Receptor Protein 1; BBM, Brush border membrane.

2.12. 16S rRNA Gene Amplification and Sequencing

Microbial genomic DNA was extracted from cecal samples using the PowerSoil DNA isolation kit, as described by the manufacturer (MoBio Laboratories Ltd., Carlsbad, CA, USA). Bacterial 16S rRNA gene sequences were PCR-amplified from each sample using the 515F-806R primers for the V4 hypervariable region of the 16S rRNA gene, including 12-base barcodes, as previously published [47]. PCR procedure reactions consisted of 25 µL Primestar max PCR mix (Takara Kusatsu, Shiga, Japan), 2 µM of each primer, 17 µL of ultra-pure water, and 4 µL DNA template. Reaction conditions consisted of an initial denaturing step for 3 min at 95 °C followed by 30 cycles of 10 s at 98 °C, 5 s at 55 °C, 20 s at 72 °C, and final elongation at 72 °C for 1 min. PCR products were then purified with Ampure magnetic purification beads (Beckman Coulter, Atlanta, GA, USA) and quantified using a Quant-iT PicoGreen dsDNA quantitation kit (Invitrogen, Carlsbad, CA, USA). Equimolar ratios of total samples were pooled and sequenced at the Faculty of Medicine of the Bar Ilan University (Safed, Israel) using an Illumina MiSeq Sequencer (Illumina, Inc., Madison, WI, USA).

2.13. 16S rRNA Gene Sequence Analysis

Data analysis was performed using QIIME2 [48]. Sequence reads were demultiplexed by per-sample barcodes and Illumina-sequenced amplicon reads errors were corrected by Divisive Amplicon Denoising Algorithm (DADA2) [49]. A phylogenetic tree was generated and sequences were classified taxonomically using the Greengenes [50] reference database at a confidence threshold of 99%. The Greengenes taxonomies were used to generate summaries of the taxonomic distributions of features across different levels (phylum, order, family, and genus). Alpha and beta diversity analysis were calculated based on a feature table with samples containing at least 7026 sequences. Richness and evenness, alpha diversity parameters, were calculated using the Faith's Phylogenetic Diversity and Pielou's Evenness measures [51]. Beta diversity was analyzed using weighted and unweighted UniFrac distances [52]. Linear discriminant analysis Effect Size (LEfSe) [53] was used to determine the features significantly differ between samples according to relative abundances.

Metagenome functional predictive analysis was carried out using phylogenetic investigation of communities by reconstruction of unobserved states (PICRUSt) [54] software (version 1.1.3). Briefly, feature abundance was normalized by 16S rRNA gene copy number, identified and compared to a phylogenetic reference tree using the Greengenes database, and was assigned functional traits and abundance based on known genomes and prediction using the Kyoto Encyclopedia of Genes and Genomes (KEGG). Data representing significant fold-change differences in functional pathways between experimental groups was plotted.

2.14. Morphological Examination

As was previously described [26,46], intestinal samples (duodenal region as the main intestinal Fe absorption site) were collected at the conclusion of the study and from each treatment group. Samples were fixed in fresh 4% (v/v) buffered formaldehyde, dehydrated, cleared, and embedded in paraffin. Serial sections were cut at 5 µm and placed on glass slides. Sections were deparaffinized in xylene, rehydrated in a graded alcohol series, stained with hematoxylin and eosin, and examined by light microscopy. Morphometric measurements of villus height, width and goblet cell diameter were performed with a light microscope using EPIX XCAP software (Standard version, Olympus, Waltham, MA, USA).

2.15. Statistical Analyses

The in vivo and in vitro results were analyzed by ANOVA using the general linear models procedure of SAS software (version 9.4, SAS Institute Inc., Cary, NC, USA), and differences between treatment groups were compared by using the Student's t-test and values were considered statistically different at $p < 0.05$ (values in the text are means ± SEM). For the microbiome results, the Faith's

Phylogenetic Diversity and Pielou's Evenness measures difference between groups were analyzed by Kruskal–Wallis (pairwise) test. Differences between Weighted/Unweighted UniFrac distances were analyzed by Pairwise permanova test. Analysis of composition of microbiomes (ANCOM) is a bioinformatics method to identify features that are differentially abundant (i.e., present in difference abundances) across sample groups. Significant p-values ($p < 0.05$) associated with microbial clades and functions identified by LEfSe were corrected for multiple comparisons using the Benjamini Hochberg false discovery rate (FDR) correction. Statistical analysis was performed using SAS version 9.3 (SAS Institute, Cary, NC, USA). The level of significance was established at $p < 0.05$.

3. Results

3.1. Phytate Concentration and Polyphenol Profile in the Bean Flours

The concentration of the five most prevalent polyphenolic compounds found in the bean seed coats is presented in Table 3. The Fe-standard beans (BRS Perola) presented higher ($p < 0.05$) concentration of epicatechin and quercetin 3-glucoside compared to the Fe-biofortified beans (BRS Cometa). There was no difference ($p > 0.05$) in the phytate ($n = 5$) concentration between the Fe-biofortified and Fe-standard carioca bean flour.

Table 3. Phytate concentration and polyphenol profile (µM) present in common bean flours.

Food Flours	Phytate (g/100 g)	Polyphenol Profile				
		Kaempferol 3-Glucoside	Catechin	Epicatechin	Procyanidin B1	Quercetin 3-Glucoside
BRS Perola (Fe-standard)	1.05 ± 0.03	17.3 ± 1	26.1 ± 1.3	12.8 ± 1.7 *	1.4 ± 0.2	0.2 ± 0.1
BRS Cometa (Fe-biofortified)	1.08 ± 0.005	16.2 ± 1.1	25.9 ± 4.6	11 ± 1.4	1.2 ± 0.2	-

Values are means ± SEM. * Statistical difference by t-test at 5% of probability ($p = 0.0451$).

3.2. Dietary Fiber and Protein Concentration in the Bean Flours

There was no difference ($p > 0.05$) in the insoluble, soluble and total dietary fiber. However, the protein concentration is higher ($p < 0.05$) in the Fe-biofortified bean (BRS Cometa) compared to the Fe-standard bean (BRS Perola) (Table 4).

Table 4. Dietary fiber and protein concentration in the beans (g/100 g).

Beans	Insoluble Fiber	Soluble Fiber	Total Fiber	Total Protein
BRS Perola (Fe-standard)	20.80 ± 0.02	3.77 ± 1.03	24.56 ± 1.05	24.15 ± 0.44
BRS Cometa (Fe-biofortified)	18.71 ± 0.94	4.85 ± 0.33	23.55 ± 1.27	29.01 * ± 0.29

* Statistical difference by t-test ($p = 0.0001$).

3.3. In Vitro Assay (Caco-2 Cell Ferritin Formation)

Ferritin, the cellular Fe storage protein was used as an indicator of Fe bioavailability [42,43]. Ferritin concentrations were significantly higher in cells exposed to the Fe-biofortified (BC) bean based diet versus the Fe-standard (SC) bean based diet ($p < 0.05$, $n = 6$, Table 5). These results indicate greater amounts of bioavailable Fe in the Fe-biofortified bean based diet.

Table 5. Ferritin concentration in Caco-2 cells exposed to samples of bean based diets, and additional meal plan ingredients [1,2].

Tested Sample	Ferritin (ng/mg of Protein)
Tested Diets	
Standard Fe diet (SC) (40.4 ± 1.8 µg/g diet)	5.04 ± 0.37
Biofortified Fe diet (BC) (47.0 ± 1.5 µg/g diet)	6.10 ± 0.29 *

Table 5. *Cont.*

Tested Sample	Ferritin (ng/mg of Protein)
Ingredients	
BRS Perola (Fe-standard bean) (64.3 ± 0.5 µg/g bean)	7.87 ± 1.15 [d]
BRS Cometa (Fe-biofortified bean) (84.9 ± 2 µg/g bean)	5.74 ± 0.34 [d]
Potato flour (12.8 ± 0.4 µg/g flour)	21.74 ± 0.83 [a]
Pasta flour (13.8 ± 1.0 µg/g flour)	12.79 ± 0.60 [b]
Corn flour (31.3 ± 4.7 µg/g flour)	10.38 ± 0.94 [c]
Rice flour (4.2 ± 0.8 µg/g flour)	6.12 ± 1.02 [d]

[1] Caco-2 bioassay procedures and preparation of the digested samples are described in the materials and methods sections. [2] Cells were exposed to only MEM (minimal essential media) without added food digests and Fe ($n = 6$). All samples were run in the same experiment. [a–d] Values are means ± SEM. Different letters indicate statistical differences at 5% by Newman–Keuls test. * Indicates statistical differences at 5% by t-test between the experimental diets.

3.4. In Vivo Assay (Gallus Gallus Model)

3.4.1. Growth Rates, Hb, Hb-Fe, and HME

The feed intake and the Fe intake were higher ($p < 0.0001$) in the BC group (average consumption of 56.49 g diet/day ± 0.8) and cumulative (day 42) Fe intake of 111.3 mg Fe ± 1.5, compared to the SC group (average consumption of 51.06 g diet/day ± 2.1), and cumulative (day 42) Fe intake of 86.9 mg Fe ± 3.3. In addition, as from day 14 of the study, body weights were consistently higher ($p < 0.05$) in the group receiving the Fe-biofortified bean diet versus the group receiving the standard bean diet (Figure 1A). There were no significant differences ($p > 0.05$) in the hemoglobin concentrations between the treatments at any time point (Figure 1B). As from day 21, the total body Hb-Fe was significantly greater in the group receiving the Fe-biofortified carioca bean ($p < 0.05$, Figure 1C). However, no differences in HME values were measured between the groups ($p > 0.05$, Figure 1D)

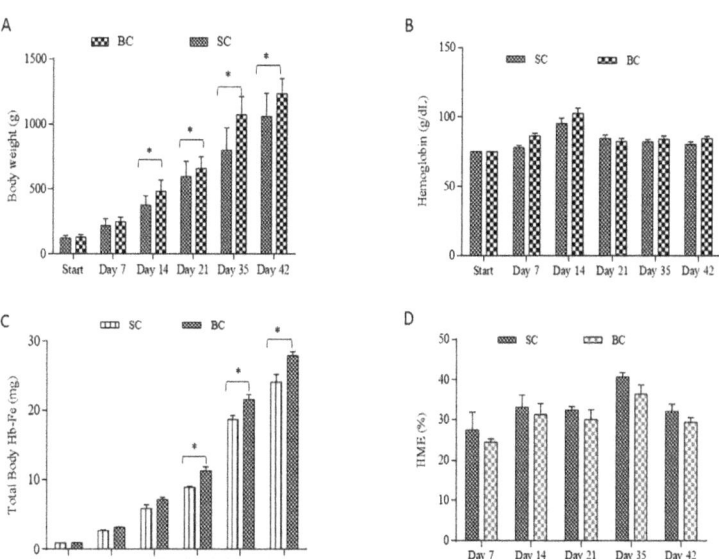

Figure 1. Fe-related parameters assessed during the study. (**A**): Body weight (g); (**B**) Blood hemoglobin concentration (g/L); (**C**): Total body Hb-Fe (mg); (**D**): Hemoglobin maintenance efficiency (%). Values are means ± SEM. * Statistical difference by *t*-test at 5% of probability. SC: Fe-standard carioca bean diet; BC: Fe-biofortified carioca bean diet.

3.4.2. Gene Expression of Fe—Related and BBM Functional Proteins

Relative to 18S rRNA, duodenal gene expression of ferroportin was significantly elevated ($p < 0.05$) in the group receiving the Fe-biofortified carioca bean based diet (BC) (Figure 2). However, no significant differences ($p > 0.05$) in the expression of the other Fe-related proteins were observed between treatment groups (Figure 2).

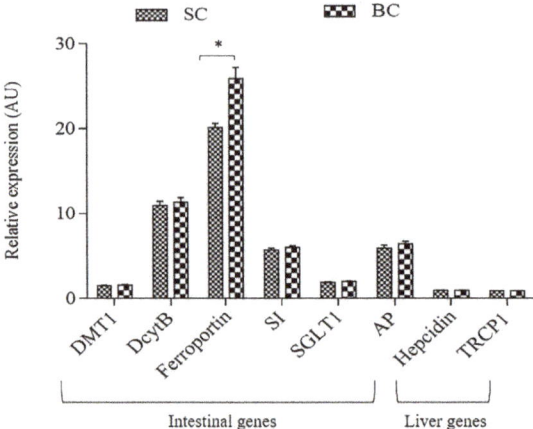

Figure 2. Duodenal and liver mRNA gene expression of Fe-related proteins collected on day 42. Changes in mRNA expression are shown relative to expression of 18S rRNA in arbitrary units (AU, * $p < 0.05$). SC: Fe-standard carioca bean diet; BC: Fe-biofortified carioca bean diet; DMT1: Divalent Metal Transporter 1; DcytB: Duodenal cytochrome b; SI: Sucrose isomaltase; SGLT1: Sucrose isomaltase 1; AP: Amino peptidase; TRCP1: Transferrin Receptor Protein 1.

3.4.3. Morphometric Measurements

The BC group presented higher ($p < 0.0001$) villi height (Figure 3A) and diameter (Figure 3B) compared to the SC group. This serves as a mechanical measurement of brush border membrane absorptive ability and improvement in brush border membrane functionality and overall gut health [46]. It indicates that the consumption of Fe biofortified carioca beans could lead to a proliferation of enterocytes.

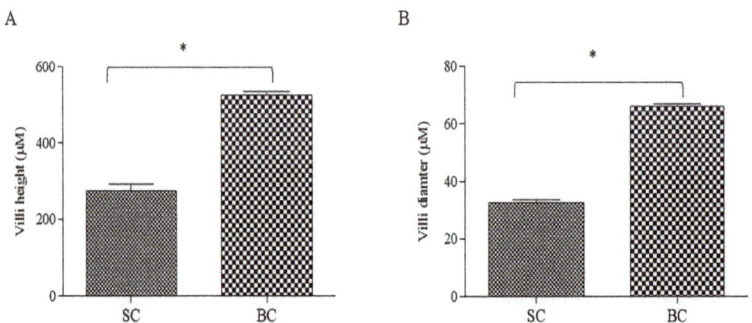

Figure 3. Effect of Standard and Biofortified diets on the duodenal small intestinal parameters: (**A**) Intestinal villi height (μM); (**B**) Intestinal villi diameter. SC: Fe-standard carioca bean diet; BC: Fe-biofortified carioca bean diet. Values are means ± SEM, $n = 5$. * Statistical difference by t-test ($p < 0.0001$).

There were no significant differences ($p > 0.05$) in goblet cells (mucus producing and secreting cells) number per intestinal villi. However, the goblet cell diameter was slightly higher ($p < 0.05$) in the SC group (4.74 µM ± 2.03) compared to the BC group (4.56 µM ± 1.84).

3.4.4. Microbial Analysis

Comparisons were made between Fe-biofortified carioca bean diet (BC) and Fe-standard carioca bean diet (SC) beans groups. Cecal contents samples from the standard and biofortified varieties were collected and used for bacterial DNA extraction and sequencing of the V4 hypervariable region in the 16S rRNA gene. The contents of the cecum highly diverse and abundant microbiota and represent the primary site of bacterial fermentation [55].

The diversity of the cecal microbiota between the standard carioca bean (SC) and biofortified carioca bean (BC) was assessed initially through measures of α and β-diversity. Faith's phylogenetic diversity, used to assess α-diversity (Figure 4A), was not significant between SC and BC groups ($p > 0.05$). We utilized unweighted UniFrac distances as a measure of β-diversity to assess the effect of BC diet on between-individual variation in bacterial community (Figure 4B). Principal coordinate analysis showed statistically significant difference in clustering between the BC and SC groups, suggesting that individual samples were more similar to other samples within the same group, as opposed to samples of the other group ($p > 0.05$). Furthermore, individual samples of the BC group clustered significantly closer to each other than did members of the SC group ($p < 0.05$).

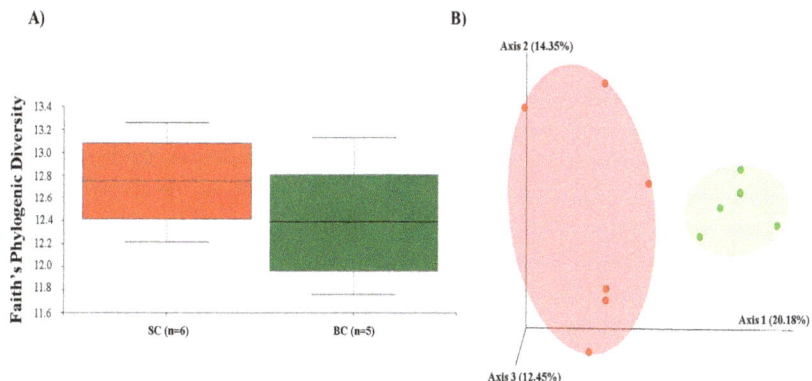

Figure 4. Microbial diversity of the cecal microbiome in Carioca diet. SC: Fe-standard carioca bean diet; BC: Fe-biofortified carioca bean diet. (**A**) Measure of α-diversity using the Faith's Phylogenetic Diversity; and (**B**) Measure of β-diversity using unweighted UniFrac distances separated by the first three principal components (PCoA). Each dot represents one animal, and the colors represent the different treatment groups within Carioca beans (red = SC; green = BC).

Following α and β-diversity, we conducted a taxon-based analysis of the cecal microbiota. 16S rRNA gene sequence revealed that >98% of all bacterial sequences in both treatment groups of the carioca variety. Both of the treatment groups were dominated by two major phyla: Firmicutes and Proteobacteria, whereas sequences of Tenericutes and Verrucomicrobia were also identified, but in much lower abundance. After FDR correction, there were no significant differences between groups at the genus level for the carioca variety (Figure 5A,B). As in the human gut [56], the Firmicutes phyla vastly predominated in the *Gallus gallus* cecum [57].

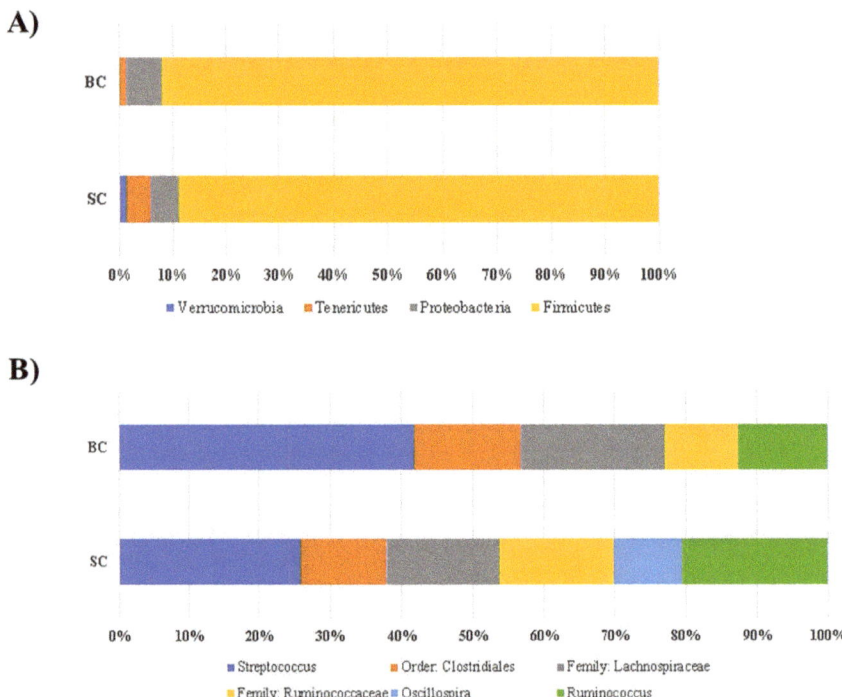

Figure 5. Compositional changes of gut microbiota in response to a Carioca standard versus biofortified diet. SC: Fe-standard carioca bean diet; BC: Fe-biofortified carioca bean diet. (**A**) Phylum level changes in the BC and SC groups as measured at the end of the study (day 42). Only phyla with abundance ≥1% are displayed; (**B**) Genus level changes in the BC and SC groups as measured at the end of the study (day 42). Only genera with abundance ≥5% are displayed.

The final analysis investigation of relative abundances at all taxonomic levels with carioca beans was carried out using the linear discriminant analysis effect size (LEfSe) method to investigate significant bacterial biomarkers that could identify differences in the gut microbiota of SC and BC groups [53]. Figure 6A,B present the differences in abundance between groups at the various taxonomic levels, with their respective LDA (Linear discriminant analysis) scores. We observed a general taxonomic delineation between the SC and BC groups, whereby the SCFA-producing Firmicutes predominated in the BC groups. Specifically, *Eggerthella lenta* (LDA score = 3.65, p = 0.011) and *Clostridium piliforme* (LDA = 3.90, p = 0.006); there were members of the *Coriobacteriaceae* (LDA = 3.65, p = 0.011), *Dehalobacteriaceae* (LDA = 3.52, p = 0.044), *Lachnospiraceae* (LDA = 3.90, p = 0.006) were significantly enriched in the BC group. In the SC group, however, members of the Firmicutes, Tenericutes and Proteobacteria were the predominantly-enriched phyla. Specifically, *Ruminococcus albus* (LDA score = 3.72, p = 0.017), and members of the *Oscillospira* (LDA score = 4.41, p = 0.044) and *Clostridium* (LDA score = 3.75, p = 0.006) genera were significantly enriched in the SC group.

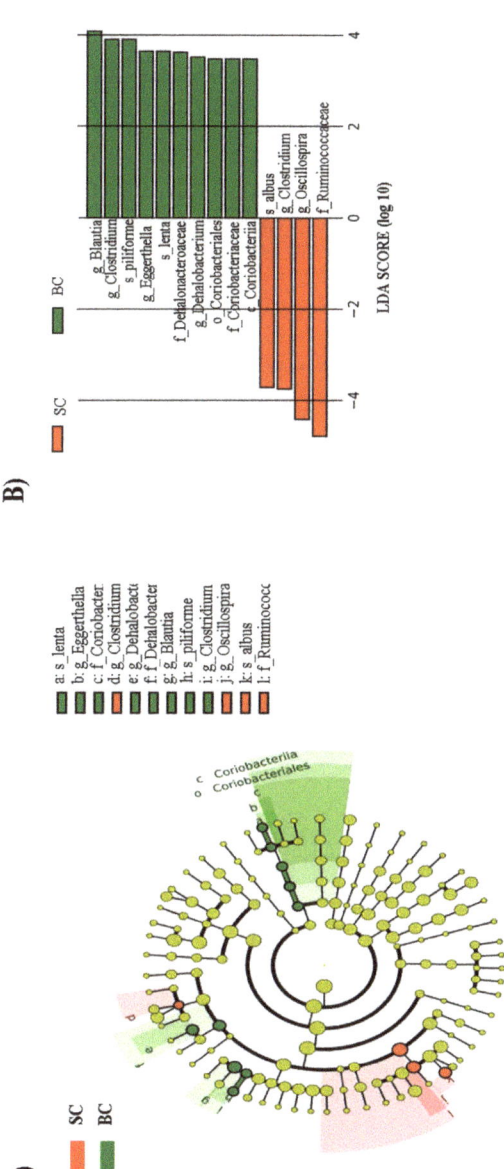

Figure 6. LEfSe method identifying the most differentially enriched taxa in the Standard and Biofortified Carioca diet groups. SC: Fe-standard carioca bean diet; BC: Fe-biofortified carioca bean diet. (**A**) Taxonomic cladogram obtained using LEfSe analysis of the 16S rRNA sequences. Treatment groups are indicated by the different colors, with the brightness of each dot proportional to its effect size; (**B**) Computed LDA (Linear discriminant analysis) scores of the relative abundance difference between the standard Carioca bean diet and the biofortified Carioca bean diet. Negative LDA scores (red) are enriched in standard Carioca bean diet while positive LDA scores (green) are enriched in biofortified Carioca beans.

4. Discussion

In studies of Fe biofortification, there is a clear need and advantage to have in place screening tools capable of evaluating biofortified lines of staple food crops, both individually and in the context of the diet for which they are consumed [4,7,36]. The present study, therefore evolved as an opportunity to demonstrate how the in vitro digestion/Caco-2 cell model and the *Gallus gallus* in vivo model of Fe bioavailability could be applied in the design of an Fe bioavailability study aimed at assessing the Fe bioavailability of Fe biofortified versus standard carioca beans. The diets that were used were specifically formulated according to the Brazilian dietary survey [45] (Table 1). Overall, the data presented in this manuscript are in agreement with previously published research [4,19,22], indicating that this dual in vitro/in vivo screening approach is effective in the assessment of Fe bioavailability of Fe biofortified beans.

The in vivo results showed that although Hb levels were not significantly increased in the Fe biofortified carioca bean group, significant differences in total body Hb-Fe, a sensitive biomarker of dietary Fe bioavailability and status [58], were observed starting on week four of the study (Figure 1), indicating on an improvement in Fe status in the Fe biofortified group. In addition, the animals receiving the standard bean variety had a higher HME at each time point when compared to the group receiving the Fe biofortified carioca beans, indicating an adaptive response (e.g., a relative up-regulation of absorption) to less absorbable dietary Fe [4,22,23,39]. The Fe-biofortified carioca bean diet presented higher Fe content and lower PA: Fe ratio compared to the Fe-standard carioca bean diet (Table 1), which could contribute to the higher dietary Fe bioavailability of this group [59–61].

Additionally, the in vitro assay (Table 5) further supported the in vivo findings. Ferritin values in cells exposed to the Fe-biofortified bean variety only, were low and similar to ferritin values in cells exposed to the standard bean variety only. In contrast, once the Fe biofortified bean variety was included in the experimental bean based diet, an increase in ferritin formation was observed relative to cells exposed to the standard bean based diet. This could be due to the higher Fe content and the lower PA: Fe ratio presented in the Fe-biofortified bean based diet, but can also be attributed to the other dietary ingredients, and their potential effect on dietary Fe bioavailability.

These results are in agreement with previous studies aimed at assessing the Fe promoting effects of Fe-biofortified black beans [19], red mottled beans [37] and pearl millet [22]. Thus, since a number of intrinsic factors, including polyphenol compounds and phytates, may influence the bioavailability of Fe from these beans and other crops [4,17,20,24], and limit their nutritional benefit. This suggests that increased bean Fe concentration alone may not be sufficient to yield significant physiological improvements in Fe status. In this context, it is important to note that in addition to increased Fe content, the Fe-biofortified bean variety had a higher protein content ($p < 0.05$, Table 4), this may further affect the nutritional benefit of this bean variety. Current results are in agreement with recent research indicating that dietary ingredients as potato may enhance the Fe absorption when consumed with beans, whereas other foods consumed with beans, as rice, might negatively affect Fe bioavailability (in vitro) [11].

Previous studies have shown a higher concentration of polyphenolic compounds (PP) and phytate in the Fe-biofortified beans compared to the Fe-standard beans [11,19,62]. However, in the current study the Fe-biofortified carioca bean presented lower concentrations of some PPs and no difference in the phytate concentration compared to the Fe-standard carioca bean (Table 3). This is an interesting finding since the PPs and phytate are known as strong inhibitors of Fe bioavailability [19,23,24,63]. Thus, this Fe-biofortified variety could be a more effective vehicle for the Fe biofortification program. This point was demonstrated, as the totality of the results indicated that the Fe biofortified carioca bean based diet was moderately effective at increasing the bioavailable and therefore absorbable dietary Fe both in vitro and in vivo.

Further, the duodenal gene expression of ferroportin (FPN) was significantly elevated in the group receiving the Fe-biofortified bean diet ($p < 0.05$, Figure 2). However, no significant differences in the expression of the other Fe-related and brush border membrane functional proteins were observed between treatment groups. In contrast, some studies have shown a down-regulation of the gene expression of these proteins (DMT-1, ferroportin and Dcytb) in Fe-biofortified diets compared to the Fe-standard diets [4,22,37,64]. Ferroportin is an Fe exporter protein that transfer the Fe across the basolateral membrane of the enterocyte [34]. Thus, since the BC group presented a higher expression of FPN, more Fe can be released from the enterocyte into the blood circulation, therefore, this mechanism suggests increased amounts of absorbable Fe, hence, the total body Hb-Fe increased in the Fe biofortified group compared to the standard.

As is the case in humans and the vast majority of animals, the *Gallus gallus* model harbor a complex and dynamic gut microbiota [65], heavily influenced by host genetics, environment and diet [66]. There is considerable similarity at the phylum level between the gut microbiota of *Gallus gallus* and humans, with Bacteroidetes, Firmicutes, Proteobacteria, and Actinobacteria representing the four dominant bacterial phyla in both [67]. In the current study, a general taxonomic delineation between the SC and BC group was observed, whereby the SCFA-producing Firmicutes predominated in the BC group. Specifically, *Eggerthella lenta* and *Clostridium piliforme* (Figure 6B). The increase in the SCFA-producing bacteria could lead to an increased SCFA concentration in the intestinal lumen, which in return can promote intestinal cell proliferation [68], as was observed in the BC group that presented an increase in duodenal villi height (Figure 3). This observation is in agreement with previous research indicating that duodenal villi height was significantly increased due to dietary fiber (as xylooligosaccharides) that have led to increased SCFA bacterial production in vivo [69]. Also, the Fe-biofortified bean presented a higher, although not significant, soluble fiber content compared to the Fe-standard bean (Table 4). Soluble fiber can increase the villi height by increasing the intestinal cell proliferation [70] (Figure 3).

In addition, and as was mentioned above, the Fe-biofortified bean presented higher ($p < 0.05$) protein content compared to the Fe-standard bean (Table 4), a higher protein contented in a diet was shown increase villi height and intestinal cell proliferation [71]. Undigested dietary proteins and fibers are fermented in the intestine and this fermentation process produces SCFAs (mainly composed by acetate, propionate, and butyrate). Functionally, SCFAs affect the metabolism and gut health [72]. Acetate and propionate are energy substrates for peripheral tissues and butyrate is preferentially used as an energy source by colonic epithelial cells [73,74].

In this study, the abundance of members of the *Coriobacteriaceae*, specially *Eggerthella lenta* and *Lachnospiracea* were enriched in the BC group (Figure 5B). These results demonstrate a potential beneficial effect of the Fe-biofortified bean diet on the intestinal microbial composition, since these microorganisms can improve the host health [75,76]. *Lachnospiracea* is a butyrate producer family [75]. This short chain fatty acid (SCFA) is an energy source of colonocytes and it stimulates the immunogenicity of cancer cells [76]. *Coriobacteriacea* acts on the conversion of bile salts and steroid hormones, and the *Eggerthella lenta* was recently found to reductively cleave the heterocyclic C-ring of the epicatechin and catechin [77], and the breakdown product (3-(3,4-dihydroxyphenyl) propionic acid) presents anti-inflammatory effects [78]. This result is especially important since in general, carioca beans present these flavonoids (Table 3), thus they can be metabolized by the bacteria from the BC group.

Further, one of the aims of this study was to determine whether ingestion of an Fe biofortified diet would lead to an increased pathogenic bacterial load in the gut microbiota. Dietary Fe supplementation has been associated with an inflammatory-promoting gut microbiota, most likely due to the increased presence of luminal Fe [79], subsequent generation of free radicals, and ensuing epithelial stress and microbial dysbiosis [80]. Many of the nutritional methods used to combat Fe deficiency, such as Fe supplementation and Fe fortification, induce dysbiotic conditions and an expansion of pathogenic bacteria in the gut microbiota of subjects receiving Fe replete diets [79,81]. In contrast to these findings, we did not observe significant increase in pathogenic taxa in the BC group that have been previously associated with dietary Fe intake (e.g., Salmonella and other Enterobacteria) [81]. Therefore, this finding suggests that the use of biofortified beans instead of Fe fortification or Fe supplementation can be an effective and potentially sustainable strategy to reduce the Fe deficiency, with additional improvement in the gut bacterial populations.

Overall, we demonstrate in vitro that the potential consumption of the Fe-biofortified bean in a food basket context may increase the Fe uptake. The in vivo analyses demonstrated a significant remodeling of the gut microbiota in animals receiving a Fe-biofortified diet, which also presented higher amount protein. This microbiota remodeling increased the SCFA-producing bacteria abundance, improving the morphometric parameters (villi height), and increasing the intestinal absorptive surface area, these findings can potentially lead to increased Fe bioavailability and uptake. Therefore, under these experimentalal conditions, the results suggest that the consumption of the Fe biofortified carioca bean with other staple foods (i.e., food basket), increased Fe bioavailability, improved Fe status, and improved the composition and function of the gut microbiota. Understanding the effect of Fe biofortification on the gut microbiota may help to further biofortification efforts by improving the safety and efficacy profile of the food crop, as we understand more about the relationship between biofortified diets and the resident gut microbiota.

5. Conclusions

Nutritional methods aimed to alleviate global Fe deficiency, such as Fe supplementation or Fe fortification, have been moderately efficacious at attaining optimal Fe status. However, any improvement in serum Fe levels comes at the expense of decreased gut health in the form of dysbiosis and infection. This study showed how Fe-biofortification affects the composition and metagenome of the gut microbiota and intestinal function. Animals (*Gallus gallus*) that consumed the Fe biofortified carioca bean-based diet had less abundance of pathogenic bacteria, with concomitant increases in SCFA-producing bacteria that have known phenolic catabolic capacity, which have led to an improvement in intestinal morphology. In addition, and for the first time, the Fe-biofortified carioca bean presented similar concentration of phytate and polyphenols, yet, a higher protein content, in comparison to the Fe-standard bean, which potentially can increase the Fe bioavailability, and intestinal functionality, respectively.

Further and similar to previous data, the current research suggests that increased Fe content may not necessarily result in an increased absorbable Fe, and a key factor is the measurement of dietary Fe bioavailability in Fe biofortified crop varieties based diets, and as part of the breeding process.

Collectively, the findings presented here provide evidence that, unlike other nutritional methods of increasing Fe status, the Fe biofortification appear to improve the gut microbiota, and they raise the possibility that this strategy can further improve the efficacy and safety of the crop Fe biofortification approach. We suggest the utilization of the discussed in vitro and in vivo screening tools to guide studies aimed to develop and evaluate Fe biofortified staple food crops, and their potential nutritional benefit.

Author Contributions: Data curation, D.M.D. and E.T.; Formal analysis, D.M.D. and E.T.; Investigation, D.M.D. and E.T.; Methodology, N.K., D.B., O.Z., O.K. and E.T.; Resources, M.R.N., H.S.D.M. and E.T.; Supervision, E.T.; Writing–original draft, D.M.D. and E.T.; Writing–review & editing, R.P.G. and E.T.

Acknowledgments: The authors would like to thank the Coordination for the Improvement of Higher Education Personnel (CAPES, Brazil) for the Doctor's fellowship.

Conflicts of Interest: The authors declare no conflict of interest.

References

1. Wegmüller, R.; Bah, A.; Kendall, L.; Goheen, M.M.; Mulwa, S.; Cerami, C.; Moretti, D.; Prentice, A.M. Efficacy and safety of hepcidin-based screen-and-treat approaches using two different doses versus a standard universal approach of iron supplementation in young children in rural Gambia: A double-blind randomised controlled trial. *BMC Pediatr.* **2016**, *16*, 149. [CrossRef] [PubMed]
2. World Health Organization. The Global Prevalence of Anaemia in 2011. *WHO Rep.* **2011**, *48*. [CrossRef]

3. Allen, L.; Benoist, B.; Dary, O.; Hurrell, R. *Guidelines on Food Fortification With Micronutrients*; WHO Press: Rome, Italy, 2006; p. 341.
4. Tako, E.; Reed, S.; Anandaraman, A.; Beebe, S.E.; Hart, J.J.; Glahn, R.P. Studies of cream seeded carioca beans (*Phaseolus vulgaris* L.) from a Rwandan efficacy trial: In vitro and in vivo screening tools reflect human studies and predict beneficial results from iron Biofortified beans. *PLoS ONE* **2015**, *10*, 1–15. [CrossRef]
5. WHO. *Guideline: Use of multiple Micronutrient Powders for Home Fortification of Foods Consumed by Infants and Children 6–23 Months of Age*; WHO: Geneva, Switzerland, 2011; pp. 1–30.
6. Bouis, H.E.; Saltzman, A. Improving nutrition through biofortification: A review of evidence from HarvestPlus, 2003 through 2016. *Glob. Food Secur.* **2017**, 49–58. [CrossRef] [PubMed]
7. Nestel, P.; Bouis, H.E.; Meenakshi, J.V.; Pfeiffer, W. Symposium: Food Fortification in Developing Countries Biofortification of Staple Food Crops. *J. Nutr.* **2006**, *136*, 1064–1067. [CrossRef] [PubMed]
8. Bhargava, A.; Bouis, H.E.; Scrimshaw, N.S. Dietary Intakes and Socioeconomic Factors Are Associated with the Hemoglobin Concentration of Bangladeshi Women. *Econ. Stat. Comput. Approaches Food Health Sci.* **2006**, 105–111. [CrossRef]
9. Lozoff, B.; Jimenez, E.; Wolf, A.W. Long-term developmental outcome of infants with iron deficiency. *N. Engl. J. Med.* **1991**, *352*, 687–694. [CrossRef]
10. Broughton, W.J.; Hernandez, G.; Blair, M.; Beebe, S.; Gepts, P.; Vanderleyden, J. Beans (Phaseolus spp.) model food legumes. *Plant Soil.* **2003**, *252*, 55–128. [CrossRef]
11. Glahn, R.; Tako, E.; Hart, J.; Haas, J.; Lung'aho, M.; Beebe, S. Iron Bioavailability Studies of the First Generation of Iron-Biofortified Beans Released in Rwanda. *Nutrients* **2017**, *9*, 787. [CrossRef]
12. White, P.J.; Broadley, M.R. Biofortifying crops with essential mineral elements. *Trends Plant Sci.* **2005**, *10*, 586–593. [CrossRef]
13. HarvestPlus. Biofortification Progress Briefs. 2014, (August): 82. Available online: https://www.harvestplus.org/sites/default/files/Biofortification_Progress_Briefs_August2014_WEB_2.pdf (accessed on 2 September 2016).
14. Petry, N.; Boy, E.; Wirth, J.P.; Hurrell, R.F. Review: The potential of the common bean (*Phaseolus vulgaris*) as a vehicle for iron biofortification. *Nutrients* **2015**, *7*, 1144–1173. [CrossRef]
15. Blair, M.W.; González, L.F.; Kimani, P.M.; Butare, L. Genetic diversity, inter-gene pool introgression and nutritional quality of common beans (*Phaseolus vulgaris* L.) from Central Africa. *Theor. Appl. Genet.* **2010**, *121*, 237–248. [CrossRef] [PubMed]
16. Moura, F.F.; Palmer, A.C.; Finkelstein, J.L.; Haas, J.D.; Murray-Kolb, L.E.; Wenger, M.J.; Birol, E.; Boy, E.; Pena-Rosas, J.P. Are Biofortified Staple Food Crops Improving Vitamin A and Iron Status in Women and Children? New Evidence from Efficacy Trials. *Adv. Nutr.* **2014**, 568–570. [CrossRef]
17. Petry, N.; Egli, I.; Gahutu, J.B.; Tugirimana, P.L.; Boy, E.; Hurrell, R. Phytic Acid Concentration Influences Iron Bioavailability from Biofortified Beans in Rwandese Women with Low Iron Status. *J. Nutr.* **2014**, *144*, 1681–1687. [CrossRef]
18. Haas, J.; Luna, S.; Lung'aho, M.; Ngabo, F.; Wenger, M.; Murray-Kolb, L.; Beebe, S.; Gahutu, J. Iron biofortificatified beans improve bean status in Rwandan university women: Results of a feeding trial. *FASEB J.* **2014**, *28*, 646.1.
19. Tako, E.; Beebe, S.E.; Reed, S.; Hart, J.J.; Glahn, R.P. Polyphenolic compounds appear to limit the nutritional benefit of biofortified higher iron black bean (*Phaseolus vulgaris* L.). *Nutr. J.* **2014**, *13*. [CrossRef] [PubMed]
20. Hart, J.J.; Tako, E.; Glahn, R.P. Characterization of Polyphenol Effects on Inhibition and Promotion of Iron Uptake by Caco-2 Cells. *J. Agric. Food Chem.* **2017**, *65*, 3285–3294. [CrossRef] [PubMed]
21. Hart, J.J.; Tako, E.; Kochian, L.V.; Glahn, R.P. Identification of Black Bean (*Phaseolus vulgaris* L.) Polyphenols That Inhibit and Promote Iron Uptake by Caco-2 Cells. *J. Agric. Food Chem.* **2015**, *63*, 5950–5956. [CrossRef] [PubMed]
22. Tako, E.; Reed, S.M.; Budiman, J.; Hart, J.J.; Glahn, R.P. Higher iron pearl millet (*Pennisetum glaucum* L.) provides more absorbable iron that is limited by increased polyphenolic content. *Nutr. J.* **2015**, *14*, 1–9. [CrossRef]
23. Tako, E.; Glahn, R.P. White beans provide more bioavailable iron than red beans: Studies in poultry (*Gallus gallus*) and an in vitro digestion/Caco-2 model. *Int. J. Vitam. Nutr. Res.* **2010**, *80*, 416–429. [CrossRef]
24. Petry, N.; Egli, I.; Zeder, C.; Walczyk, T.; Hurrell, R. Polyphenols and phytic acid contribute to the low iron bioavailability from common beans in young women. *J. Nutr.* **2010**, *140*, 1977–1982. [CrossRef] [PubMed]

25. Tako, E.; Glahn, R.P.; Knez, M.; Stangoulis, J.C. The effect of wheat prebiotics on the gut bacterial population and iron status of iron deficient broiler chickens. *Nutr. J.* **2014**, *13*, 58. [CrossRef] [PubMed]
26. Pacifici, S.; Song, J.; Zhang, C.; Wang, Q.; Glahn, R.P.; Kolba, N.; Tako, E. Intra amniotic administration of raffinose and stachyose affects the intestinal brush border functionality and alters gut microflora populations. *Nutrients* **2017**, *9*, 304. [CrossRef]
27. Wong, J.M.W.; Souza, R.; Kendall, C.W.C.; Emam, A.; Jenkins, D.J.A. Colonic Health: Fermentation and Short Chain Fatty Acids. *J. Clin. Gastroenterol.* **2006**, *40*, 235–243. [CrossRef] [PubMed]
28. Tuohy, K.M.; Rouzaud, G.C.M.; Brück, W.M.; Gibson, G.R. Modulation of the human gut microflora towards improved health using prebiotics–assessment of efficacy. *Curr. Pharm. Des.* **2005**, *11*, 75–90. [CrossRef]
29. Welch, R.M.; Graham, R.D. Breeding for micronutrients in staple food crops from a human nutrition perspective. *J. Exp. Bot.* **2004**, *55*, 353–364. [CrossRef]
30. Dwivedi, S.; Sahrawat, K.; Puppala, N.; Ortiz, R. Plant prebiotics and human health: Biotechnology to breed prebiotic-rich nutritious food crops. *Electron. J. Biotechnol.* **2014**, *17*, 238–245. [CrossRef]
31. Tako, E.; Glahn, R.P.; Welch, R.M.; Lei, X.; Yasuda, K.; Miller, D.D. Dietary inulin affects the expression of intestinal enterocyte iron transporters, receptors and storage protein and alters the microbiota in the pig intestine. *Br. J. Nutr.* **2008**, *99*, 472–480. [CrossRef] [PubMed]
32. Zimmermann, M.B.; Chassard, C.; Rohner, F.; N'goran, E.K.; Nindjin, C.; Dostal, A.; Utzinger, J.; Ghattas, H.; Lacroix, C.; Hurrell, R.F. The effects of iron fortification on the gut microbiota in African children: A randomized controlled trial in Cote d'Ivoire. *Am. J. Clin. Nutr.* **2010**, *92*, 1406–1415. [CrossRef] [PubMed]
33. Chen, T.; Kim, C.Y.; Kaur, A.; Lamothe, L.; Shaikh, M.; Keshavarzian, A.; Hamaker, B.R. Dietary fibre-based SCFA mixtures promote both protection and repair of intestinal epithelial barrier function in a Caco-2 cell model. *Food Funct.* **2017**, *8*, 1166–1173. [CrossRef] [PubMed]
34. Duda-Chodak, A.; Tarko, T.; Satora, P.; Sroka, P. Interaction of dietary compounds, especially polyphenols, with the intestinal microbiota: A review. *Eur J Nutr.* **2015**, *54*, 325–341. [CrossRef]
35. Blair, M.W. Mineral biofortification strategies for food staples: The example of common bean. *J. Agric. Food Chem.* **2013**, *61*, 8287–8294. [CrossRef] [PubMed]
36. Bouis, H.E.; Hotz, C.; McClafferty, B.; Meenakshi, J.V.; Pfeiffer, W.H. Biofortification: A New Tool to Reduce Micronutrient Malnutrition. *Food Nutr. Bull.* **2014**, *32*, S31–S40. [CrossRef] [PubMed]
37. Tako, E.; Blair, M.W.; Glahn, R.P. Biofortified red mottled beans (*Phaseolus vulgaris* L.) in a maize and bean diet provide more bioavailable iron than standard red mottled beans: Studies in poultry (*Gallus gallus*) and an in vitro digestion/Caco-2 model. *Nutr. J.* **2011**, *10*, 113. [CrossRef] [PubMed]
38. Tako, E.; Hoekenga, O.; Kochian, L.V.; Glahn, R.P. High bioavailablilty iron maize (*Zea mays* L.) developed through molecular breeding provides more absorbable iron in vitro (Caco-2 model) and in vivo (*Gallus gallus*). *Nutr. J.* **2013**, *12*, 3. [CrossRef] [PubMed]
39. Tako, E.; Rutzke, M.A.; Glahn, R.P. Using the domestic chicken (*Gallus gallus*) as an in vivo model for iron bioavailability. *Poult. Sci.* **2010**, *89*, 514–521. [CrossRef] [PubMed]
40. Dias, D.M.; Castro, M.E.M.; Gomes, M.J.C.; Lopes Toledo, R.C.; Nutti, M.R.; Pinheiro Sant'Ana, H.M.; Martino, H.S. Rice and bean targets for biofortification combined with high carotenoid content crops regulate transcriptional mechanisms increasing iron bioavailability. *Nutrients* **2015**, *7*, 9683–9696. [CrossRef] [PubMed]
41. AOAC, *!!! REPLACE !!!*. Appendix J. In *Proceedings of the AOAC INTERNATIONAL Methods Committee Guidelines for Validation of Microbiological Methods for Food and Environmental Surfaces*; AOAC Off. Methods Anal.: Rockville, MD, USA, 2012; pp. 1–21.
42. Glahn, R.P.; Lee, O.A.; Yeung, A.; Goldman, M.I.; Miller, D.D. Caco-2 cell ferritin formation predicts nonradiolabeled food iron availability in an in vitro digestion/Caco-2 cell culture model. *J. Nutr.* **1998**, *128*, 1555–1561. [CrossRef]
43. Tako, E.; Bar, H.; Glahn, R.P. The combined application of the Caco-2 cell bioassay coupled with in vivo (*Gallus gallus*) feeding trial represents an effective approach to predicting fe bioavailability in humans. *Nutrients* **2016**, *8*, 732. [CrossRef]
44. Tako, E.; Glahn, R.P.; Laparra, J.M.; Welch, R.M.; Lei, X.; Kelly, J.D.; Rutzke, M.A.; Miller, D.D. Iron and zinc bioavailabilites to pigs from red and white beans (*Phaseolus vulgaris* L.) are similar. *J. Agric. Food Chem.* **2009**, *57*, 3134–3140. [CrossRef]

45. IBGE. Instituto Brasileiro de Geografia e Estatística, Coordenação de Trabalho e Rendimento. In *Pesquisa de Orçamentos Familiares: 2008–2009. Análise Do Consumo Alimentar Pessoal No Brasil*; IBGE: Rio de Janeiro, Brazil, 2011.
46. Hou, T.; Kolba, N.; Glahn, R.; Tako, E. Intra-Amniotic Administration (*Gallus gallus*) of Cicer arietinum and Lens culinaris Prebiotics Extracts and Duck Egg White Peptides Affects Calcium Status and Intestinal Functionality. *Nutrients* **2017**, *9*, 785. [CrossRef]
47. Caporaso, J.G.; Lauber, C.L.; Walters, W.A.; Berg-Lyons, D.; Huntley, J.; Fierer, N.; Owens, S.M.; Betley, J.; Fraser, L.; Bauer, M.; et al. Ultra-high-throughput microbial community analysis on the Illumina HiSeq and MiSeq platforms. *ISME J.* **2012**, *6*, 1621–1624. [CrossRef] [PubMed]
48. Caporaso, G.J.; Kuczynski, J.; Stombaugh, J.; Bittinger, K.; Bushman, F.D.; Costello, E.K.; Fierer, N.; Peña, A.G.; Goodrich, J.K.; Gordon, J.I.; et al. Correspondence QIIME allows analysis of high-throughput community sequencing data Intensity normalization improves color calling in SOLiD sequencing. *Nat. Publ. Gr.* **2010**, *7*, 335–336. [CrossRef]
49. Callahan, B.J.; McMurdie, P.J.; Rosen, M.J.; Han, A.W.; Johnson, A.J.A.; Holmes, S.P. High-resolution sample inference from Illumina amplicon data. *Nat Methods* **2016**, *13*, 581–583. [CrossRef] [PubMed]
50. DeSantis, T.Z.; Hugenholtz, P.; Larsen, N.; Rojas, M.; Brodie, E.L.; Keller, K.; Huber, T.; Dalevi, D.; Hu, P.; Andersen, G.L. Greengenes, a chimera-checked 16S rRNA gene database and workbench compatible with ARB. *Appl. Environ. Microbiol.* **2006**, *72*, 5069–5072. [CrossRef] [PubMed]
51. Faith, D.P. Conservation evaluation and phylogentic diversity. *Biol. Conserv.* **1992**, *61*, 1–10. [CrossRef]
52. Lozupone, C.; Knight, R. UniFrac: A New Phylogenetic Method for Comparing Microbial Communities. *Appl. Environ. Microbiol.* **2005**, *71*, 8228–8235. [CrossRef] [PubMed]
53. Segata, N.; Izard, J.; Waldron, L.; Gevers, D.; Miropolsky, L.; Garrett, W.S.; Huttenhower, C. LEfSe-Metagenomic biomarker discovery and explanation. *Genome Biol.* **2011**, *12*, R60. [CrossRef]
54. Langille, M.G.I.; Zaneveld, J.; Caporaso, J.G.; McDonald, D.; Knights, D.; Reyes, J.A.; Clemente, J.C.; Burkepile, D.E.; Thurber, R.L.V.; Knight, R.; et al. Predictive functional profiling of microbial communities using 16S rRNA marker gene sequences. *Nat. Biotechnol.* **2013**, *31*, 814–821. [CrossRef]
55. Mead, G. Bacteria in the gastrointestinal tract of birds. *Gastrointest. Microbiol.* **1997**, *2*, 216–240.
56. Eckburg, P.B.; Bik, E.M.; Bernstein, C.N.; Purdom, E.; Dethlefsen, L.; Sargent, M.; Gill, S.R.; Nelson, K.E.; Relman, D.A. Diversity of the Human Intestinal Microbial Flora. *Science* **2011**, *1635*, 1635–1639. [CrossRef]
57. Wei, S.; Morrison, M.; Yu, Z. Bacterial census of poultry intestinal microbiome. *Poult. Sci.* **2013**, *92*, 671–683. [CrossRef] [PubMed]
58. Ma, X.Y.; Liu, S.B.; Lu, L.; Li, S.F.; Xie, J.J.; Zhang, L.Y.; Zhang, J.H.; Luo, X.G. Relative bioavailability of iron proteinate for broilers fed a casein-dextrose diet. *Am. Hist. Rev.* **2014**, *119*, 556–563. [CrossRef]
59. Hurrell, R.F.; Juillerat, M.A.; Reddy, M.B.; Lynch, S.R.; Dassenko, S.A.; Cook, J.D. Soy protein, phytate, and iron absorption in humans. *Am. J. Clin. Nutr.* **1992**, *56*, 573–578. [CrossRef] [PubMed]
60. Anton, A.A.; Ross, K.A.; Beta, T.; Gary, F.R.; Arntfield, S.D. Effect of pre-dehulling treatments on some nutritional and physical properties of navy and pinto beans (*Phaseolus vulgaris* L.). *LWT Food Sci. Technol.* **2008**, *41*, 771–778. [CrossRef]
61. Petry, N.; Egli, I.; Campion, B.; Nielsen, E.; Hurrell, R. Genetic Reduction of Phytate in Common Bean (*Phaseolus vulgaris* L.) Seeds Increases Iron Absorption in Young Women 1–4. *J. Nutr.* **2013**, *143*, 1219–1224. [CrossRef] [PubMed]
62. Reed, S.; Neuman, H.; Glahn, R.P.; Koren, O.; Tako, E. Characterizing the gut (*Gallus gallus*) microbiota following the consumption of an iron biofortified Rwandan cream seeded carioca (*Phaseolus vulgaris* L.) bean-based diet. *PLoS ONE* **2017**, *12*, 1–15. [CrossRef] [PubMed]
63. Lesjak, M.; Hoque, R.; Balesaria, S.; Skinner, V.; Debnam, E.S.; Srai, S.K.S.; Sharp, P.A. Quercetin inhibits intestinal iron absorption and ferroportin transporter expression in vivo and in vitro. *PLoS ONE* **2014**, *9*, 1–10. [CrossRef] [PubMed]
64. Tako, E.; Laparra, J.M.; Glahn, R.P.; Welch, R.M.; Lei, X.G.; Beebe, S.; Miller, D.D. Biofortified black beans in a maize and bean diet provide more bioavailable iron to piglets than standard black beans. *J. Nutr.* **2009**, *139*, 305–309. [CrossRef]
65. Zhu, X.Y.; Zhong, T.; Pandya, Y.; Joerger, R.D. 16S rRNA-based analysis of microbiota from the cecum of broiler chickens. *Appl. Environ. Microbiol.* **2002**, *68*, 124–137. [CrossRef]

66. Yegani, M.; Korver, D.R. Factors Affecting Intestinal Health in Poultry. *Poult. Sci.* **2008**, *87*, 2052–2063. [CrossRef]
67. Qin, J.; Li, R.; Raes, J.; Arumugam, M.; Burgdorf, K.S.; Manichanh, C.; Nielsen, T.; Pons, N.; Levenez, F.; Yamada, T.; et al. A human gut microbial gene catalogue established by metagenomic sequencing. *Nature* **2010**, *464*, 59–65. [CrossRef]
68. Sakata, T. Stimulatory effect of short-chain fatty acids on epithelial cell proliferation in the rat intestine: A possible explanation for trophic effects of fermentable fibre, gut microbes and luminal trophic factors. *Br. J. Nutr.* **1987**, *58*, 95–103. [CrossRef]
69. Ding, X.M.; Li, D.D.; Bai, S.P.; Wang, J.P.; Zeng, Q.F.; Su, Z.W.; Xuan, Y.; Zhang, K.Y. Effect of dietary xylooligosaccharides on intestinal characteristics, gut microbiota, cecal short-chain fatty acids, and plasma immune parameters of laying hens. *Poult. Sci.* **2018**, *97*, 874–881. [CrossRef]
70. Adam, C.L.; Williams, P.A.; Garden, K.E.; Thomson, L.M.; Ross, A.W. Dose-dependent effects of a soluble dietary fibre (pectin) on food intake, adiposity, gut hypertrophy and gut satiety hormone secretion in rats. *PLoS ONE* **2015**, *10*, 1–14. [CrossRef] [PubMed]
71. Chen, X.; Song, P.; Fan, P.; He, T.; Jacobs, D.; Levesque, C.L.; Johnston, L.J.; Ji, L.; Ma, N.; Chen, Y.; et al. Moderate Dietary Protein Restriction Optimized Gut Microbiota and Mucosal Barrier in Growing Pig Model. *Front. Cell. Infect. Microbiol.* **2018**, *8*, 246. [CrossRef] [PubMed]
72. Tan, J.; McKenzie, C.; Potamitis, M.; Thorburn, A.; Mackay, C.; Macia, L. The role of short-chain fatty acids in health and disease. *Adv. Immunol.* **2014**, *121*, 91–119. [CrossRef] [PubMed]
73. Tremaroli, V.; Bäckhed, F. Functional interactions between the gut microbiota and host metabolism. *Nature* **2012**, *489*, 242–249. [CrossRef] [PubMed]
74. Backhed, F.; Ding, H.; Wang, T.; Hooper, L.V.; Koh, G.Y.; Nagy, A.; Semenkovich, C.F.; Gordon, J.I. The gut microbiota as an environmental factor that regulates fat storage. *Proc. Natl. Acad. Sci. USA* **2004**, *101*, 15718–15723. [CrossRef] [PubMed]
75. O'Connor, A.; Quizon, P.M.; Albright, J.E.; Lin, F.T.; Bennett, B.J. Responsiveness of cardiometabolic-related microbiota to diet is influenced by host genetics. *Mamm. Genome* **2014**, *25*, 583–599. [CrossRef]
76. Hijova, E.; Chmelarova, A. Short chain fatty acids and colonic health. *Bratisl. Lek. List.* **2007**, *108*, 354–358. [CrossRef]
77. Kutschera, M.; Engst, W.; Blaut, M.; Braune, A. Isolation of catechin-converting human intestinal bacteria. *J. Appl. Microbiol.* **2011**, *111*, 165–175. [CrossRef] [PubMed]
78. Larrosa, M.; Luceri, C.; Vivoli, E.; Pagliuca, C.; Lodovici, M.; Moneti, G.; Dolara, P. Polyphenol metabolites from colonic microbiota exert anti-inflammatory activity on different inflammation models. *Mol. Nutr. Food Res.* **2009**, *53*, 1044–1054. [CrossRef] [PubMed]
79. Weiss, G. Dietary iron supplementation: A proinflammatory attack on the intestine? *Gut* **2015**, *64*, 696–697. [CrossRef] [PubMed]
80. Kortman, G.A.M.; Raffatellu, M.; Swinkels, D.W.; Tjalsma, H. Nutritional iron turned inside out: Intestinal stress from a gut microbial perspective. *FEMS Microbiol. Rev.* **2014**, *38*, 1202–1234. [CrossRef] [PubMed]
81. Jaeggi, T.; Kortman, G.A.M.; Moretti, D.; Chassard, C.; Holding, P.; Dostal, A.; Boekhorst, J.; Timmerman, H.M.; Swinkels, D.W.; Tjalsma, H.; et al. Iron fortification adversely affects the gut microbiome, increases pathogen abundance and induces intestinal inflammation in Kenyan infants. *Gut* **2015**, *64*, 731–742. [CrossRef] [PubMed]

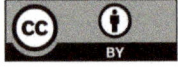

© 2018 by the authors. Licensee MDPI, Basel, Switzerland. This article is an open access article distributed under the terms and conditions of the Creative Commons Attribution (CC BY) license (http://creativecommons.org/licenses/by/4.0/).

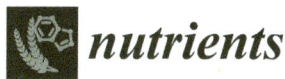

Article

Vitamin D Supplementation Modestly Reduces Serum Iron Indices of Healthy Arab Adolescents

Mohammad S. Masoud, Majed S. Alokail, Sobhy M. Yakout, Malak Nawaz K. Khattak, Marwan M. AlRehaili, Kaiser Wani and Nasser M. Al-Daghri *

Chair for Biomarkers of Chronic Diseases, Biochemistry Department, College of Science, King Saud University, Riyadh 11451, Saudi Arabia; mohammad_masoud@hotmail.com (M.S.M.); msa85@yahoo.co.uk (M.S.A.); sobhy.yakout@gmail.com (S.M.Y.); malaknawaz@yahoo.com (M.N.K.K.); roony607@hotmail.com (M.M.A.); wani.kaiser@gmail.com (K.W.)
* Correspondence: aldaghri2011@gmail.com; Tel.: +966-(11)4675939

Received: 3 October 2018; Accepted: 27 November 2018; Published: 2 December 2018

Abstract: Vitamin D deficiency has been shown to affect iron status via decreased calcitriol production, translating to decreased erythropoiesis. The present study aimed to determine for the first time whether vitamin D supplementation can affect iron levels among Arab adolescents. A total of 125 out of the initial 200 Saudi adolescents with vitamin D deficiency (serum 25(OH)D < 50 nmol/L) were selected from the Vitamin D-School Project of King Saud University in Riyadh, Saudi Arabia. Cluster randomization was done in schools, and students received either vitamin D tablets (1000 IU/day) (N = 53, mean age 14.1 ± 1.0 years) or vitamin D-fortified milk (40IU/200mL) (N = 72, mean age 14.8 ± 1.4 years). Both groups received nutritional counseling. Anthropometrics, glucose, lipids, iron indices, and 25(OH)D were measured at baseline and after six months. Within group analysis showed that post-intervention, serum 25(OH)D significantly increased by as much as 50%, and a parallel decrease of −42% (p-values <0.001 and 0.002, respectively) was observed in serum iron in the tablet group. These changes were not observed in the control group. Between-group analysis showed a clinically significant increase in serum 25(OH)D (p = 0.001) and decrease in iron (p < 0.001) in the tablet group. The present findings suggest a possible inhibitory role of vitamin D supplementation in the iron indices of healthy adolescents whose 25(OH)D levels are sub-optimal but not severely deficient, implying that the causal relationship between both micronutrients may be dependent on the severity of deficiency, type of iron disorder, and other vascular conditions that are known to affect hematologic indices. Well-designed, randomized trials are needed to confirm the present findings.

Keywords: serum iron; vitamin D; adolescents; Arab; vitamin D supplements

1. Introduction

Through the last decade, vitamin D has gained considerable interest in health and biomedical research [1]. Globally, vitamin D deficiency is widespread and is considered a pandemic [2]. The Middle East and North African regions, including the Kingdom of Saudi Arabia (KSA), are not spared from this micronutrient deficiency, and in fact have among the highest rates of vitamin D deficiency in the world [3,4]. Among the most common risk factors for vitamin D deficiency in the Middle-East include female gender and their clothing style, multi-parity, sedentary lifestyle, urban living and socio-economic status for adults, and longer than average breastfeeding as well as low dietary vitamin D and calcium intake in children [5].

Vitamin D is involved in the proliferation and differentiation of bone marrow stem cells and may play a role in red cell production [6]. Vitamin D can also potentially affect circulating iron status by promoting erythropoiesis and by suppressing hepcidin expression [6]. Lower levels of pro-inflammatory cytokines and hepcidin increases iron bioavailability for erythropoiesis and hemoglobin synthesis by preventing iron sequestration in macrophages [7]. On the other hand, iron deficiency damages intestinal absorption of fat soluble vitamins, including vitamin D [8].

Similar to vitamin D deficiency, iron deficiency is also endemic and is, in fact, the most common micronutrient deficiency globally [9]. Adolescent girls are at high risk for iron deficiency because of diet and blood loss during menstruation [10]. Furthermore, according to the World Health Organization, the two main risk target groups for iron deficiency are pre-school children and young women [11,12]. It is also highly prevalent in infants, adolescents, and pregnant women and is believed to account for 75% of all types of anemia in the world, affecting 30% of population [13]. In the Middle East, the prevalence of anemia among women of child-bearing age is 47% in Egypt, 16% in Lebanon, 26.7% in the United Arab Emirates (UAE), and 40% in KSA [14].

Several cross-sectional studies confirm the association of vitamin D status and serum iron. In a large-scale study involving 2526 Korean children and adolescents, they observed that the occurrence of both vitamin D deficiency and anemia were significantly higher in females than males and concluded that the positive correlation between vitamin D and iron may be through the suppressive action of vitamin D in decreasing levels of hepcidin, an iron regulatory hormone [15]. Their results were consistent with the previous observations of Smith and colleagues among African Americans [7].

To date, observational and functional studies suggest a positive relationship between vitamin D status and serum iron, but interventional studies are lacking to prove causality. The recent meta-analysis of Azizi-Soleiman and colleagues indicated that iron supplementation trials conducted so far failed to improve vitamin D status [16], and limited data is available whether the reverse is true. Thus, the present interventional study aims to determine for the first time whether a vitamin D supplementation of six months duration can influence iron status among vitamin D deficient Saudi Arab adolescents.

2. Materials and Methods

2.1. Study Design and Participants

This was a 6-month follow up study involving 200 apparently healthy Saudi adolescents (100 boys and 100 girls) aged 13–17 years (overall mean age 14.1 ± 1.1 years; overall mean body mass index (BMI) 21.2 ± 0.8 kg/m^2) with known vitamin D deficiency (serum 25(OH)D < 50 nmol/L) [17] at baseline and without medical conditions, such as asthma, hypertension, diabetes, liver, and renal diseases. The participants were taken from the Vitamin D School Project database of the Prince Mutaib Chair for Biomarkers of Osteoporosis (PMCO), King Saud University in Riyadh, Saudi Arabia [18,19].

In brief, the Vitamin D School Project is a collaborative project between King Saud University and the Ministry of Education in Riyadh, Saudi Arabia, ascertaining the beneficial effects of 1000 IU/day vitamin D supplementation and other vitamin D correction strategies, including vitamin D-fortified milk consumption and overall public health awareness in raising vitamin D levels. The project database includes information on more than 1000 students and teachers recruited from 34 different schools in the central region of Riyadh during winter-spring season (November–May 2014–2015), when sun exposure for optimum vitamin D$_3$ production in Riyadh was observed to be shorter (10 A.M.–before 2 P.M.) than summer (9 A.M.–3 P.M.) [20]. Government-run school hours were from 6:30 A.M. until 1–2 P.M., Sunday-Thursday. Cluster randomization was done in the 34 schools. This type of randomization was done to prevent 'contamination of allocation', defined as participants in the control group being aware of the interventions given in the test group and adopting it themselves [21]. In the case of the present study, contamination of allocation can occur if both groups are in the same school, since the students in the control group can be influenced by peers/classmates to switch to the tablet group instead. Students from schools assigned to the milk (control) group were allocated to receive daily 200 mL of milk (per 100 mL contains 4.52 g carbohydrates, 3.22 g proteins, 3.0 g fats, 113 mg calcium, 40 IU of vitamin D, 102 IU of vitamin A, and 58 kcal) for 6 months. The milk provided was previously shown to have no effects in serum 25(OH)D levels [18]. Students from schools assigned to the tablet group received 1000 IU/day vitamin D supplementation (VitaD1000®, Synergy Pharma, Dubai, UAE) daily for 6 months. These interventions were monitored by their respective teachers and parents who were assigned to ensure that they were carried out daily in schooldays and weekends, respectively, for the entire duration of the study. Ethical approval was obtained from the Ethics Committee of the College of Science Research Center, King Saud University, Riyadh, Saudi Arabia (Ref No. 15/0502/IRB; Project No. E-15-1667), in accordance with the principles in the Declaration of Helsinki, as well as with the guidelines on good clinical practice. Prior to inclusion in the study, written informed consent was acquired from parents, as well as assent from the students.

The cohort used in the present study were randomly selected from the school database of 2 groups (tablet group (N = 100); milk (control) group (N = 100)). Baseline characteristics of both groups are found in Supplementary Table S1. From the baseline assessment, significant differences were found in the prevalence of severe vitamin D deficiency (25(OH)D < 25 nmol/L) (tablet, 47%, versus control, 28%; p = 0.01) as well as baseline serum iron (p < 0.001), making the groups incomparable for prospective analysis. As extremely low levels of 25(OH)D can alter the overall metabolic profile, participants with severe vitamin D deficiency (25(OH)D <25nmol/L) were excluded in the analysis (N = 28 from the control, and N = 47 from the tablet group). The final overall sample size was N = 125. A flowchart has been provided in Figure 1.

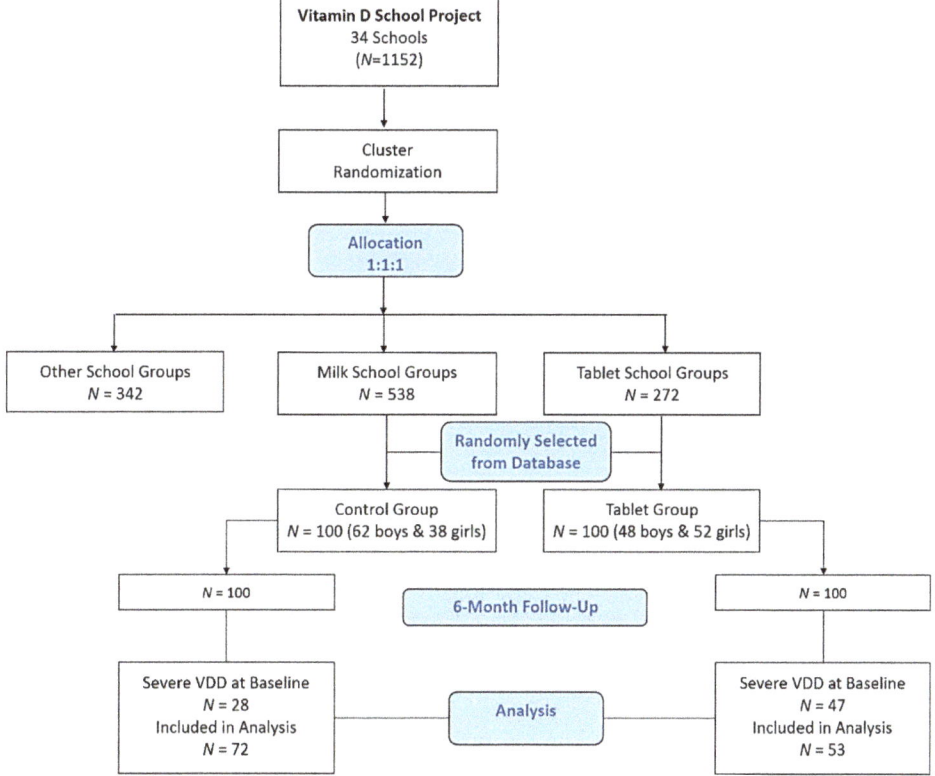

Figure 1. Study flowchart. VDD, vitamin D deficiency.

2.2. Anthropometric and Biochemical Assessment

Information on anthropometrics (height, weight, body mass index, waist and hip circumference, waist-hip ratio, systolic and diastolic blood pressure) were extracted from the database to include values at baseline and after 6 months intervention. Anthropometrics were taken by an assigned research physician using a standard scale (Digital Pearson Scale, ADAM Equipment Inc., Oxford, CT, USA) for the assessment of height (cm) and weight (kg) measured in light clothing and without shoes. Waist and hip circumferences were measured using standard tape measure. Blood pressure (mmHg) was measured twice using a mercurial sphygmomanometer and the appropriate pediatric cuff. The average was noted. Body mass index (kg/m^2) and waist-hip ratio (WHR) were calculated accordingly. Biochemical parameters for baseline and after 6 months, such as glucose, lipid profile (triglycerides, total cholesterol, LDL- and HDL-cholesterol), and calcium, were also retrieved from the database. Morning blood extraction was done twice (at baseline and after 6 months) for each participant after fasting for 8 h. Blood samples were centrifuged and delivered immediately in pre-labeled plain tubes, placed on ice, to King Saud University in Riyadh, Saudi Arabia, for storage and routine analysis using a biochemical analyzer (Konelab, Espoo, Finland).

2.3. Vitamin D and Iron Indices

Serum 25(OH) D was measured using COBAS e-411 automated analyzer (Roche Diagnostics, Indianapolis, IN, USA) in a DEQAS-certified laboratory (PMCO). Colorimetric ferrozine-based assay was used to measure iron and total iron-binding capacity in serum samples using a spectrophotometer. Transferrin saturation (%) was calculated as serum iron ($\mu g/L$)/total iron-binding capacity (TIBC) ($\mu g/L$) × 100.

2.4. Data Analysis

A G*power calculator was used for sample size determination. Using repeated measurement analysis, the observed effect size was 0.40 for a total sample size of 125, and the actual observed power was >0.85. Data were analyzed using SPSS (version 21) (IBM, Armonk, New York, USA). Continuous data were presented as mean ± standard deviation (SD) for variables following Gaussian variables, and non-Gaussian variables were presented in median (minimum-maximum). All continuous variables were checked for normality using Kolmogorov-Smirnov test, and non-normal variables were log-transformed. Categorical variables were presented in percentages (%) and Chi-square tests were performed. Independent *t*-test and paired *t*-test were used to check mean differences between group and time points respectively. Repeated measures analysis of co-variance (ANCOVA) was done to compare control and tablet groups. A *p*-value of <0.05 was considered statistically significant.

3. Results

Table 1 shows the general characteristics of the control and tablet groups after exclusion of participants with severe vitamin D deficiency at baseline. The control group had a higher systolic blood pressure than the tablet group, although this was borderline significant (p = 0.053). The rest of the baseline anthropometrics, biochemical indices, as well as serum 25(OH)D, calcium and iron indices were not significantly different between groups.

Table 1. Baseline characteristics of intervention and control groups.

Parameter	Tablet	Control	p-Value
N	53	72	
Males (%)	30 (56.6)	40 (55.6)	0.68
Anthropometrics			
Age (years)	14.1 ± 1.0	14.8 ± 1.4	0.09
BMI (kg/m^2)	22.8 ± 5.8	22.9 ± 6.2	0.96
Waist circumference (cm)	78.2 ± 15.8	80.1 ± 16.8	0.60
Hip Circumference (cm)	92.3 ± 13.8	94.5 ± 15.9	0.50
Waist-Hip Ratio	0.80 ± 0.1	0.80 ± 0.1	0.98
Systolic Blood Pressure (mmHg)	116.2 ± 12.9	122.5 ± 16.6	0.05
Diastolic Blood Pressure (mmHg)	70.6 ± 11.6	71.1 ± 13.6	0.88
Routine Biochemical Indices			
Glucose (mmol/L)	5.2 ± 0.6	5.4 ± 0.7	0.17
Triglycerides (mmol/L)	1.2 ± 0.6	1.3 ± 0.6	0.43
Total Cholesterol (mmol/L)	4.7 ± 0.8	4.5 ± 1.0	0.22
LDL-Cholesterol (mmol/L)	2.9 ± 0.7	2.5 ± 0.8	0.06
HDL-Cholesterol (mmol/L)	1.1 ± 0.3	1.3 ± 0.3	0.10
Calcium (mmol/L)	2.0 ± 0.1	1.9 ± 0.3	0.11
Vitamin D and Iron Indices			
25(OH)D (nmol/L)	34.6 ± 6.4	37.2 ± 7.5	0.09
Iron (µmol/L) #	18.2 (3–41)	21.5 (8–39)	0.09
Transferrin Iron-Binding Capacity (µmol/L) #	83.4 (19–102)	83.6 (28–99)	0.35
Transferrin Saturation (%) #	23.9 (3–71)	26.3 (2–70)	0.91

Note: # presented as median (interquartile range); p-value significant at <0.05.

Table 2 shows the changes in the anthropometrics and routine biochemical indices over time. Within-group comparisons in the tablet group showed significant increases in waist circumference ($p = 0.01$) and waist-hip ratio ($p < 0.001$). There was also a significant decrease in glucose levels ($p = 0.038$) and triglycerides ($p = 0.015$) over time, parallel to the improvement, although borderline significant, in high density lipoprotein (HDL)-cholesterol levels ($p = 0.06$). Within-group comparison in the control group showed an overall increase in anthropometrics, including weight ($p = 0.006$), BMI ($p = 0.09$), hips ($p = 0.049$), and waist-hip ratio ($p = 0.011$). There was also a significant decrease in HDL-cholesterol levels over time in the control group ($p = 0.008$). Between-group comparisons showed a clinically significant difference in systolic blood pressure ($p = 0.006$), glucose ($p = 0.029$), triglycerides ($p = 0.059$), and HDL-cholesterol ($p = 0.005$) in favor of the tablet group. The rest of the between-group comparisons were not significant (Table 2).

Table 3 shows the effects of vitamin D supplementation in vitamin D status and iron indices over time. Within-group comparison showed a significant increase in 25(OH)D levels in the tablet group by as much as 50% ($p < 0.001$). Also in the tablet group, a significant decrease in iron levels was observed (-42%; $p = 0.002$), as well as in transferrin saturation ($p = 0.01$), parallel to the significant increase in TIBC (8.5%; $p = 0.01$). No significant changes were found in the control group. Between-group comparisons revealed a clinically significant increase in 25(OH)D levels in favor of the tablet group ($p = 0.001$) as well as a clinically significant reduction in iron ($p < 0.001$) and transferrin saturation levels ($p = 0.005$) (Table 3).

Table 2. Changes in anthropometric and clinical parameters at baseline and follow-up.

Parameter	Tablet			Control			Tablet Effects
N	53			72			
	Baseline	Follow-Up	p-Value	Baseline	Follow-Up	p-Value	p-Value
Anthropometrics							
Weight (kg)	55.9 ± 17.3	56.3 ± 18.6	0.65	62.1 ± 19.3	65.0 ± 22.9	0.006	0.07
BMI (kg/m^2)	22.8 ± 5.8	22.9 ± 6.2	0.59	22.9 ± 6.2	23.9 ± 7.5	0.09	0.69
Waist circumference (cm)	78.2 ± 15.8	82.2 ± 17.1	0.01	80.1 ± 16.8	81.4 ± 18.0	0.29	0.87
Hip circumference (cm)	92.3 ± 13.8	91.0 ± 13.4	0.17	94.5 ± 15.9	92.4 ± 14.4	0.049	0.56
Waist-Hip Ratio	0.8 ± 0.1	0.9 ± 0.1	<0.001	0.8 ± 0.1	0.9 ± 0.1	0.011	0.67
SBP (mmHg)	116.2 ± 12.9	113.9 ± 12.3	0.27	122.5 ± 16.6	121.4 ± 13.0	0.61	0.006
DBP (mmHg)	70.6 ± 11.6	69.8 ± 12.6	0.68	71.1 ± 13.6	69.9 ± 15.5	0.6	0.92
Routine Biochemical Indices							
Glucose (mmol/L)	5.2 ± 0.6	5.0 ± 0.5	0.038	5.4 ± 0.7	5.2 ± 0.7	0.15	0.029
Triglycerides (mmol/L) #	1.0 (0.3–3.1)	0.9 (0.3–2.3)	0.015	1.2 (0.3–3.1)	1.3 (0.4–3.0)	0.45	0.059
Total Cholesterol (mmol/L)	4.7 ± 0.8	4.7 ± 0.8	0.84	4.5 ± 1.0	4.6 ± 1.0	0.22	0.33
LDL-Cholesterol (mmol/L)	2.9 ± 0.7	2.8 ± 0.7	0.62	2.4 ± 0.8	2.5 ± 0.7	0.53	0.74
HDL-Cholesterol (mmol/L)	1.1 ± 0.3	1.3 ± 0.3	0.06	1.3 ± 0.3	1.1 ± 0.2	0.008	0.005
Calcium (mmol/L)	2.0 ± 0.2	1.9 ± 0.2	0.07	1.9 ± 0.5	1.8 ± 0.5	0.44	0.062

Note: # presented as median (min-max); significant at $p < 0.05$.

Table 3. Changes in vitamin D and iron indices at baseline and follow-up.

Parameters	Tablet (N = 53)			Control (N = 72)			Intervention Effects
	Baseline	Follow-Up	p-Value	Baseline	Follow-Up	p-Value	
25(OH)D (nmol/L)	34.6 ± 6.4	51.9 ± 13.0	<0.001	37.2 ± 7.5	37.9 ± 10.6	0.69	0.001
Iron (µmol/L) #	18.2 (2.1–40.9)	11.5 (1.3–49.5)	0.002	21.5 (8.1–39.5)	21.7 (8.7–38.0)	0.86	<0.001
TIBC (µmol/L) #	83.4 (18.7–102.8)	90.5 (78.9–102.5)	0.01	83.6 (28.0–99.5)	84.9 (52.7–99.5)	0.90	0.42
Transferrin Saturation (%) #	23.9 (2.1–70.8)	12.3 (1.4–48.7)	0.001	26.3 (1.2–70.7)	25.1 (10.3–80.3)	0.70	0.005

Note: # presented as median (min-max); significant at $p < 0.05$.

4. Discussion

The present interventional study evaluated the changes in circulating serum iron levels and other iron indices in a cohort of Saudi adolescents with suboptimal vitamin D levels before and after six months of daily 1000 IU vitamin D supplementation, as compared to controls. The present study is the first among Arab adolescents in prospectively determining the association between vitamin D and iron status. Among the highlights of the study are the clinically significant decrease in serum iron and transferrin saturation levels post-intervention in the tablet group, parallel to the significant improvements observed in blood pressure, glucose, and selected lipids, also in favor of the tablet group.

The counterintuitive effect of vitamin D supplementation in serum iron levels observed in the present study is in alignment with the observations of Doudin and colleagues conducted among >5000 healthy German adolescents of similar age groups, in that vitamin D levels seems to have an inhibitory role in hematological parameters, including hemoglobin where the bulk of iron is stored [22]. On the other hand, the clinical trial done by Madar and colleagues on healthy adults found that while four months of vitamin D3 (25 µg or 1000 IU) supplementation did not significantly affect any of the iron markers, the observed percentage changes post-intervention in hemoglobin (−0.6%), ferritin (−35%), and iron (−5.9%) were all trending downwards, similar to the present study [23]. Other clinical trials also found no significant changes in iron indices among healthy adults despite mega-doses of vitamin D3 [24,25]. Jastrzebska and colleagues have even taken into consideration the influence of physical activity and intermittent training since it can potentially affect vitamin D and iron metabolism, yet no significant differences were still found in the hematological parameters (Hb, Hct, and ferritin) of athletes given 5000 IU of vitamin D daily for eight weeks over those who did not receive supplementation [26]. All these previous studies, including the present one, suggest that vitamin D correction is unlikely to improve, if not reduce, iron indices, at least in apparently healthy populations.

Given the negative results of previous clinical trials among healthy subjects and the inhibitory effects found in the present study, it appears that the role of vitamin D supplementation in improving iron stores may be limited to those with certain metabolic conditions, such as those with poor vascular and renal function [27,28]. Suboptimal levels of both vitamin D and iron are biomarkers of ill health, and the hypothetical association appears to be reciprocal, as clinical observations demonstrated the role of 1, 25(OH)D in erythropoiesis, and the participation of iron is essential in the second activation of vitamin D in order to be functional [29,30]. The effect of vitamin D in reducing iron levels as observed in the present study, at least in participants who are apparently healthy and with no known vascular diseases, seem to support the mechanistic role of vitamin D as a chemopreventive agent in inhibiting erythropoiesis and angiogenesis, that in turn, suppresses proliferation of certain types of cells, including cancer cells [31].

Other findings include a general improvement in glucose and select lipids in favor of the tablet group. The mean serum vitamin D also significantly increased and almost reached a sufficient level (vitamin D $\geq$ 50 nmol/L) at follow-up. These changes were in alignment with previous vitamin D studies done in the KSA adolescent population [18,19]. Changes in selected anthropometric measures in both groups can be partially explained by dietary intake and physical activity which, unfortunately, were not taken into account in the present study.

The present findings should be interpreted taking into consideration its limitations. The present study is not a randomized controlled trial, and as such, several biases are evident due to non-randomization of participants and the lack of a better placebo group. Differences in baseline characteristics between the tablet and the control groups were minimized by removing all participants with baseline severe vitamin D deficiency. This finally gave a more comparable baseline metabolic profile as the 25(OH)D range was narrowed down (25–50 nmol/L).

Another major limitation is that the control group was given vitamin D-fortified milk, and dairy products have been observed to affect iron absorption due to their calcium content. The effects of dairy products in iron absorption, however, is still debatable since several intervention studies showed no significant change in iron indices from dairy product consumption [32,33]. Current recommendations, however, in milk consumption without affecting vitamin D and iron stores in children are 2 cups (500 mL) per day [34]. The control group in the present study were consuming only 200 mL/day. Serum calcium were also unaffected in both groups. More importantly, the vitamin D and calcium content in the milk products sold in Saudi Arabia are much lower than what the labels claim to be [35].

Other factors, such as dietary intake as a whole, as well as vitamin D intake and sunlight exposure, were also not taken into consideration and can significantly influence vitamin D status independent of the intervention assigned. However, epidemiologic observations done in Arab adolescents of Riyadh show that the majority have darker complexion, are fully clothed during outside activities (especially females), and prefer sunlight exposure before 10 A.M. [36]. These factors significantly reduce any clinically meaningful vitamin D conversion through sunlight exposure in this age group, especially in the present study, which was conducted during winter time when optimum sun light is not only reduced, but the best time to get sun exposure also falls well within their school hours. Other important parameters could not be analyzed, such as hepcidin and ferritin. Hepcidin, in particular, as a master regulator for iron absorption, has been shown to distinguish iron deficiency anemia and anemia of inflammation [37,38], with the latter type of anemia possibly benefiting more from vitamin D correction than the former [39,40].

Despite these limitations, the study remained sufficiently powered and adds value, as it documents the modest but significant effects of vitamin D supplementation in terms of influencing iron status in a relatively understudied ethnic population and age group. To the best of our knowledge, this is also the longest intervention trial done to determine changes in serum iron levels secondary to vitamin D supplementation. As the majority of the limited interventional studies also yielded negative results, given the clear association between vitamin D deficiency and risk of anemia [41,42], identifying which type of anemia will benefit from vitamin D supplementation might give more conclusive evidence.

5. Conclusions

In conclusion, a six-month vitamin D supplementation of 1000 IU/day significantly improved vitamin D status and consequently decreased serum iron levels among Saudi adolescents whose 25(OH)D levels are sub-optimal but not severely deficient. The study adds to the growing literature of the inhibitory and limited effects of vitamin D correction in the iron status of healthy individuals. The identification of the cause of iron deficiency is essential as to which demographics will benefit the most from vitamin D supplementation in terms of improving iron status. Well-designed and adequately powered randomized controlled trials including other iron indices, such as hepcidin, are encouraged to confirm present results.

Supplementary Materials: The following are available online at http://www.mdpi.com/2072-6643/10/12/1870/s1, Table S1: Baseline characteristics of intervention and control groups before exclusion of participants with severe vitamin D deficiency (25(OH)D <25nmol/L).

Author Contributions: Conceptualization, M.S.M., M.S.A., S.M.Y., and N.M.A.; methodology, M.S.M., M.S.A., S.M.Y., and N.M.A.; formal analysis, M.N.K.K., M.M.A., and K.W.; investigation, M.S.M., M.M.A., and S.M.Y.; writing original manuscript, M.S.M.; writing-review and editing, M.S.A., S.M.Y, K.W; funding acquisition, N.M.A.

Funding: This study is supported by the Deanship of Scientific Research Chairs, Chair for Biomarkers of Chronic Diseases, Department of Biochemistry College of Science in King Saud University, Riyadh, Saudi Arabia.

Acknowledgments: The authors are grateful to Syed Danish Hussain for the statistical analysis provided and to Dr. Yousef Al-Saleh for his clinical inputs.

Conflicts of Interest: The authors declare no conflict of interest. The funders, including the company who provided the vitamin D supplements, had no role in the design of the study; in the collection, analyses, or interpretation of data; in the writing of the manuscript; or in the decision to publish the results.

References

1. Holick, M.F.; Binkley, N.C.; Bischoff-Ferrari, H.A.; Gordon, C.M.; Hanley, D.A.; Heaney, R.P.; Murad, M.H.; Weaver, C.M.; Endocrine Society. Evaluation, treatment, and prevention of vitamin D deficiency: An Endocrine Society clinical practice guideline. *J. Clin. Endocrinol. Metab.* **2011**, *96*, 1911–1930. [CrossRef] [PubMed]
2. Holick, M.F.; Chen, T.C. Vitamin D deficiency: A worldwide problem with health consequences. *Am. J. Clin. Nutr.* **2008**, *87*, 1080S–1086S. [CrossRef] [PubMed]
3. Maalouf, G.; Gannage-Yared, M.H.; Ezzedine, J.; Larijani, B.; Badawi, S.; Rached, A.; Zakroui, L.; Masri, B.; Azar, E.; Saba, E.; et al. Middle East and North Africa consensus on osteoporosis. *J. Musculoskelet. Neuronal Interact.* **2007**, *7*, 131–143.
4. Chakhtoura, M.; Rahme, M.; Chamoun, M.; El-Hajj Fuleihan, G. Vitamin D in the Middle East and North Africa. *Bone Rep.* **2018**, *8*, 135–146. [CrossRef] [PubMed]
5. Bassil, D.; Rahme, M.; Hoteit, M.; Fuleihan, G.E. Hypovitaminosis D in the Middle East and North Africa: Prevalence, risk factors and impact on outcomes. *Dermatoendocrinol* **2013**, *5*, 274–298. [CrossRef] [PubMed]
6. Holick, M.F. Vitamin D deficiency. *N. Engl. J. Med.* **2007**, *357*, 266–281. [CrossRef] [PubMed]
7. Smith, E.M.; Tangpricha, V. Vitamin D and anemia: Insights into an emerging association. *Curr. Opin. Endocrinol. Diabetes Obes.* **2015**, *22*, 432–438. [CrossRef] [PubMed]
8. Sim, J.J.; Lac, P.T.; Liu, I.L.; Meguerditchian, S.O.; Kumar, V.A.; Kujubu, D.A.; Rasgon, S.A. Vitamin D deficiency and anemia: A cross-sectional study. *Ann. Hematol.* **2010**, *89*, 447–452. [CrossRef] [PubMed]
9. Bailey, R.L.; West, K.P., Jr.; Black, R.E. The epidemiology of global micronutrient deficiencies. *Ann. Nutr. Metab.* **2015**, *66* (Suppl. 2), 22–33. [CrossRef] [PubMed]
10. Centers for Disease Control and Prevention. Iron and Iron Deficiency. Nutrition for Everyone. 2012. Available online: http://www.cdc.gov/nutrition/everyone/basics/vitamins/iron.html (accessed on 8 November 2018).
11. Assessing the Iron Status of Populations. Available online: http://www.who.int/nutrition/publications/micronutrients/anaemia_iron_deficiency/9789241596107/en (accessed on 8 November 2018).
12. Global Target 2025. Available online: http://www.who.int/nutrition/global-target-2025/en/ (accessed on 8 November 2018).
13. Kassebaum, N.J.; Jasrasaria, R.; Naghavi, M.; Wulf, S.K.; Johns, N.; Lozano, R.; Regan, M.; Weatherall, D.; Chou, D.P.; Eisele, T.P.; et al. systematic analysis of global anemia burden from 1990 to 2010. *Blood* **2014**, *123*, 615–624. [CrossRef]
14. Hwalla, N.; Al Dhaheri, A.S.; Radwan, H.; Alfawaz, H.A.; Fouda, M.A.; Al-Daghri, N.M.; Zaghloul, S.; Blumberg, J.B. The prevalence of micronutrient deficiencies and inadequacies in the Middle-East and approaches to interventions. *Nutrients* **2017**, *9*, 229. [CrossRef] [PubMed]
15. Suh, Y.J.; Lee, J.E.; Lee, D.H.; Yi, H.G.; Lee, M.H.; Kim, C.S.; Nah, J.W.; Kim, S.K. Prevalence and Relationships of Iron Deficiency Anemia with Blood Cadmium and Vitamin D Levels in Korean Women. *J. Korean Med. Sci.* **2016**, *31*, 25–32.
16. Azizi-Soleiman, F.; Vafa, M.; Abiri, M.; Safavi, M. Effects of iron on vitamin D metabolism: A systematic review. *Int. J. Prev. Med.* **2016**, *7*, 126. [CrossRef] [PubMed]
17. Al-Daghri, N.M.; Al-Saleh, Y.; Aljohani, N.; Sulimani, R.; Al-Othman, A.M.; Alfawaz, H.; Fouda, M.; Al-Amri, F.; Shahrani, A.; Alharbi, M.; et al. Vitamin D status correction in Saudi Arabia: An experts' consensus under the auspices of the European Society for Clinical and Economic Aspects of Osteoporosis, Osteoarthritis and Musculoskeletal Diseases (ESCEO). *Arch. Osteoporos.* **2017**, *12*, 1. [CrossRef] [PubMed]
18. Al-Daghri, N.M.; Ansari, M.G.A.; Sabico, S.; Al-Saleh, Y.; Aljohani, N.J.; Alfawaz, H.; Alharbi, M.; Alokail, M.S.; Wimalawansa, S.J. Efficacy of different modes of vitamin D supplementation strategies in Saudi adolescents. *J. Steroid Biochem. Mol. Biol.* **2018**, *180*, 23–28. [CrossRef] [PubMed]
19. Al-Daghri, N.M.; Abd-Alrahman, S.H.; Panigrahy, A.; Al-Saleh, Y.; Aljohani, N.; Al-Attas, O.S.; Khattak, M.N.K.; Alokail, M. Efficacy of vitamin D interventional strategies in Saudi children and adults. *J. Steroid Biochem. Mol. Biol.* **2018**, *180*, 29–34. [CrossRef] [PubMed]
20. Alshahrani, F.M.; Almalki, M.H.; Aljohani, N.; Alzahrani, A.; Alsaleh, Y.; Holick, M.F. Vitamin D: Light side and best time of sunshine in Riyadh, Saudi Arabia. *Dermatoendocrinol* **2013**, *5*, 177–180. [CrossRef]

21. Torgerson, D.J. Contamination in trials: Is cluster randomization the answer? *BMJ* **2001**, *322*, 355–357. [CrossRef]
22. Doudin, A.; Becker, A.; Rothenberge, A.; Meyer, T. Relationship between serum 25-hydroxyvitamin D and red blood cell indices in German adolescents. *Eur. J. Pediatr.* **2018**, *177*, 583–591. [CrossRef]
23. Madar, A.M.; Stene, L.C.; Meyer, H.E.; Brekke, M.; Lagerløv, P.; Knutsen, K.V. Effect of vitamin D3 supplementation on iron status: A randomized, double-blind, placebo-controlled trial among ethnic minorities living in Norway. *Nutr. J.* **2016**, *15*, 74. [CrossRef]
24. Sooragonda, B.; Bhadada, S.K.; Shah, V.N.; Malhotra, P.; Ahluwalia, J.; Sachdeva, N. Effect of vitamin D replacement on hemoglobin concentration in subjects with concurrent iron-deficiency anemia and vitamin D deficiency: A randomized, single-blinded, placebo-controlled trial. *Acta Haematol.* **2015**, *133*, 31–35. [CrossRef] [PubMed]
25. Smith, E.M.; Alvarez, J.A.; Kearns, M.D.; Hao, L.; Sloan, J.H.; Konrad, R.J.; Ziegler, T.R.; Zughaier, S.M.; Tangpricha, V. High-dose vitamin D3 reduces circulating hepcidin concentrations: A pilot, randomized, double-blind, placebo-controlled trial in healthy adults. *Clin. Nutr.* **2017**, *36*, 980–985. [CrossRef] [PubMed]
26. Jastrzebska, M.; Kaczmarczyk, M.; Suarez, A.D.; Sanchez, G.F.L.; Jastrzebska, J.; Radziminski, L.; Jastrzebski, Z. Iron, hematological parameters and blood plasma lipid profile in vitamin D supplemented and non-supplemented young soccer players subjected to a high-intensity interval training. *J. Nutr. Sci. Vitaminol.* **2017**, *63*, 357–364. [CrossRef] [PubMed]
27. Zittermann, A.; Jungvogel, A.; Prokop, A.; Kuhn, J.; Dreier, J.; Fuchs, U.; Schulz, U.; Gummert, J.F.; Borgermann, J. Vitamin D deficiency is an independent predictor of anemia in end-stage heart failure. *Clin. Res. Cardiol.* **2011**, *100*, 781–788. [CrossRef]
28. Ernst, J.B.; Zittermann, A.; Pilz, S.; Kleber, M.E.; Scharnagl, H.; Brandenburg, V.M.; Konig, W.; Grammer, T.B.; Marz, W. Independent associations of vitamin D metabolites with anemia in patients referred to coronary angiography. *Eur. J. Nutr.* **2017**, *56*, 1017–1024. [CrossRef] [PubMed]
29. Autier, P.; Boniol, M.; Pizot, C.; Mullie, P. Vitamin D status and ill-health: A systematic review. *Lancet Diabetes Endocrinol.* **2014**, *2*, 76–89. [CrossRef]
30. Blanco-Rojo, R.; Perez-Granados, A.M.; Toxqui, L.; Zazo, P.; de la Piedra, C.; Vaquero, M.P. Relationship between vitamin D deficiency, bone remodelling and iron status in iron-deficient young women consuming an iron-fortified food. *Eur. J. Nutr.* **2013**, *52*, 695–703. [CrossRef]
31. Ma, Y.; Johnson, C.S.; Trump, D.L. Mechanistic insights of vitamin D anticancer effects. *Vitam. Horm.* **2016**, *100*, 395–491.
32. Lonnerdal, B. Calcium and iron absorption—Mechanisms and public health relevance. *Int. J. Vitam. Nutr. Res.* **2010**, *80*, 293–299. [CrossRef]
33. Grinder-Pedersen, L.; Bukhave, K.; Jensen, M.; Hojgaard, L.; Hansen, M. Calcium and milk or calcium fortified foods does not inhibit nonheme-iron absorption from a whole diet consumed over a 4-d period. *Am. J. Clin. Nutr.* **2004**, *80*, 404–409. [CrossRef]
34. Maguire, J.L.; Lebovic, G.; Kandasamy, S.; Khovratovich, M.; Mamdani, M.; Birken, C.S.; Parkin, P.C. The relationship between cow's milk and stores of vitamin D and iron in early childhood. *Pediatrics* **2013**, *13*, e144–e151. [CrossRef] [PubMed]
35. Sadat-Ali, M.; Al Elq, A.; Al-Farhan, M.; Sadat, N.A. Fortification with vitamin D: Comparative study in the Saudi Arabian and US markets. *J. Family Community Med.* **2013**, *20*, 49–52. [CrossRef]
36. Al-Daghri, N.M.; Al-Saleh, Y.; Khan, N.; Sabico, S.; Aljohani, N.; Alfawaz, H.; Alsulaimani, M.; Al-Othman, A.M.; Alokail, M.S. Sun exposure, skin color and vitamin D status in Arab children and adolescents. *J. Steroid Biochem. Mol. Biol.* **2016**, *164*, 235–238. [CrossRef] [PubMed]
37. Pasricha, S.R.; Atkinson, S.H.; Armitage, A.E.; Khandwala, S.; Veenemans, J.; Cox, S.E.; Eddowes, L.A.; Hayes, T.; Doherty, C.P.; Demir, A.Y.; et al. Expression of the iron hormone hepcidin distinguishes different types of anemia in African children. *Sci. Transl. Med.* **2014**, *6*, 235re3. [CrossRef] [PubMed]
38. Girelli, D.; Nemeth, E.; Swinkels, D.W. Hepcidin in the diagnosis of iron disorders. *Blood* **2016**, *127*, 2809–2813. [CrossRef] [PubMed]
39. Altemose, K.E.; Kumar, J.; Portale, A.A.; Warady, B.A.; Furth, S.L.; Fadrowski, J.J.; Atkinson, M.A. Vitamin D insufficiency, hemoglobin, and anemia in children with chronic kidney disease. *Pediatr. Nephrol.* **2018**. [CrossRef] [PubMed]

40. Icardi, A.; Paoletti, E.; De Nicola, L.; Mazzaferro, S.; Russo, R.; Cozzolino, M. Renal anaemia and EPO hyporesponsiveness is associated with vitamin D deficiency: The potential role of inflammation. *Nephrol. Dial. Transplant.* **2013**, *28*, 1672–1679. [CrossRef]
41. Atkinson, M.A.; Melamed, M.L.; Kumar, J.; Roy, C.N.; Miller, E.R., 3rd; Furth, S.L.; Fadrowski, J.J. Vitamin D, race and risk for anemia in children. *J. Pediatr.* **2014**, *164*, 153–158. [CrossRef]
42. Monlezun, D.J.; Camargo, C.A., Jr.; Mullen, J.T.; Quraishi, S.A. Vitamin D status and the risk of anemia in community-dwelling adults: Results from the national health and nutrition examination survey 2001–2006. *Medicine* **2015**, *94*, 1799. [CrossRef]

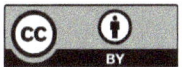

© 2018 by the authors. Licensee MDPI, Basel, Switzerland. This article is an open access article distributed under the terms and conditions of the Creative Commons Attribution (CC BY) license (http://creativecommons.org/licenses/by/4.0/).

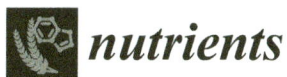

Review

Silver Ions as a Tool for Understanding Different Aspects of Copper Metabolism

Ludmila V. Puchkova [1,2,3,*], Massimo Broggini [1,4], Elena V. Polishchuk [1,5], Ekaterina Y. Ilyechova [1] and Roman S. Polishchuk [5]

1. Laboratory of Trace elements metabolism, ITMO University, Kronverksky av., 49, St.-Petersburg 197101, Russia; massimo.broggini@marionegri.it (M.B.); epolish@tigem.it (E.V.P.); ikaterina2705@yandex.ru (E.Y.I.)
2. Department of Molecular Genetics, Research Institute of Experimental Medicine, Acad. Pavlov str., 12, St.-Petersburg 197376, Russia
3. Department of Biophysics, Peter the Great St. Petersburg Polytechnic University, Politekhnicheskaya str., 29, St.-Petersburg 195251, Russia
4. Laboratory of molecular pharmacology, Istituto di Ricerche Farmacologiche "Mario Negri" IRCCS, Via La Masa, 19, Milan 20156, Italy
5. Telethon Institute of Genetics and Medicine, Via Campi Flegrei 34, Pozzuoli (NA) 80078, Italy; polish@tigem.it
* Correspondence: puchkovalv@yandex.ru; Tel.: +7-921-881-8470

Received: 1 May 2019; Accepted: 12 June 2019; Published: 17 June 2019

Abstract: In humans, copper is an important micronutrient because it is a cofactor of ubiquitous and brain-specific cuproenzymes, as well as a secondary messenger. Failure of the mechanisms supporting copper balance leads to the development of neurodegenerative, oncological, and other severe disorders, whose treatment requires a detailed understanding of copper metabolism. In the body, bioavailable copper exists in two stable oxidation states, Cu(I) and Cu(II), both of which are highly toxic. The toxicity of copper ions is usually overcome by coordinating them with a wide range of ligands. These include the active cuproenzyme centers, copper-binding protein motifs to ensure the safe delivery of copper to its physiological location, and participants in the Cu(I) ↔ Cu(II) redox cycle, in which cellular copper is stored. The use of modern experimental approaches has allowed the overall picture of copper turnover in the cells and the organism to be clarified. However, many aspects of this process remain poorly understood. Some of them can be found out using abiogenic silver ions (Ag(I)), which are isoelectronic to Cu(I). This review covers the physicochemical principles of the ability of Ag(I) to substitute for copper ions in transport proteins and cuproenzyme active sites, the effectiveness of using Ag(I) to study copper routes in the cells and the body, and the limitations associated with Ag(I) remaining stable in only one oxidation state. The use of Ag(I) to restrict copper transport to tumors and the consequences of large-scale use of silver nanoparticles for human health are also discussed.

Keywords: copper metabolic system; copper/silver transport; silver nanoparticles

1. Introduction

Copper is an essential micronutrient that belongs to the group of ubiquitous trace elements [1]. In biosphere, copper has been documented as the third most abundant trace element after iron and zinc. A normal human body (~70 kg) contains about 100 mg of copper, 10 times less than the amounts of iron (4–5 g) and zinc (1.4–2.3 g) [2]. However, the biological role of copper in aerobic organisms cannot be underestimated. The ground state electron configuration of the copper atom is [Ar]$3d^{10}4s^1$. Similarly, to other group 11 elements (Ag, Au), only one electron is left in the 4s shell, allowing the 3d shell to close ($3d^{10}$) and producing a more stable configuration. This explains, to a large extent, the transient properties of copper. Copper has two stable oxidation states, Cu(I) ↔ Cu(II), which are reversible under physiological conditions. The redox potential of this couple is widely used for the catalysis of redox reactions, which involves molecular oxygen [3–6] and one electron transfer [7]. Consequently, in the biosphere, global energy production (respiration and photosynthesis) is not feasible without copper. In mammals, copper operates as a structural and catalytic cofactor of enzymes (cuproenzymes) involved in vitally important processes, including protection from active oxygen metabolites, oxidative phosphorylation, connective tissue biogenesis, post-translational neuropeptide activation, neurotransmitter synthesis, and transmembrane iron transport [8,9]. In addition, copper regulates angiogenesis [10], the number of intracellular signaling pathways [11–14], mitochondria-mediated apoptosis [15], and communication between neurons and astrocytes [13,16,17] as well as participating in the regulation of transcription [18]. Therefore, some functions of copper resemble secondary messenger functions. It has been shown that mammalian odorant receptors in olfactory sensory neurons responsible for recognizing strong-smelling sex attractants [19] and thiol compounds [20] have sites that chelate Cu(I), the loss of which leads to a loss of receptor activity. This phenomenon can be attributed to copper's role as a co-receptor or biosensor.

Since copper carries out its essential functions during changes in oxidation state, it is a potential source of electrons for the catalysis of Fenton reactions. The products of such reactions induce oxidative stress, in turn, damaging the cells, for example, in ionizing irradiation [21]. In the active centers of enzymes, copper is coordinated by many various ligands (as many as six) and is strongly held in both oxidation states [22]. Copper mobilization mechanisms evolved in parallel with a safe intracellular copper transport system (CTS). The CTS is highly conserved among different species and comprises transmembrane and soluble Cu-transporting and Cu-reserving proteins and peptides. CTS members contain Cu-binding motifs that coordinate Cu(I) with the help of a few sulfur atoms in cysteine and methionine. Usually, the number of Cu/S coordinating in the Cu-binding protein domains is two, but this can vary from one to four. The transfer of copper between such domains happens in the direction of increased affinity and without valence change, which requires the activity of the metallothionein/glutathione redox cycle [23]. Components of the CTS not only deliver copper to the cuproenzymes but also facilitate its integration into the active sites [24], exchange copper between themselves [25], generate local copper concentration gradients [26], control copper functions via its redistribution between organelles/compartments, and regulate its recycling and excretion [27,28]. According to this, the dynamic behavior of the copper in the CTS can be considered as an additional function that might be tightly related to intracellular signaling [29].

Currently, aberrations in the system supporting the homeostasis of copper are considered among the reasons for the development of neurodegenerative, oncological, and cardiovascular diseases [30–33]. This quite numerous and heterogeneous group of diseases can be defined as copper-related disorders (CRD). Only some CRDs are caused by mutations in genes that encode proteins with well-established functions in the CTS. These include Menkes [34] and Wilson [35] diseases, occipital horn syndrome, Menkes ATPase-related distal motor neuropathy [36], MEDNIK syndrome [37,38], aceruloplasminemia [39], and amyotrophic lateral sclerosis [40]. The contributions of Cu-dependent mechanisms have been documented widespread pathologies, such as Alzheimer's [41] and Parkinson's [42] diseases, diabetes mellitus [43], cancer [44], and cardio-vascular disorders [31]). However, these mechanisms are yet to be fully understood [45].

In this context, the experimental use of silver ions might help to better characterize the Cu-dependent processes behind the pathogenesis of these disorders. The silver atom has a ground state electron configuration of [Kr]$4d^{10}5s^1$. Again, one of the electrons of the top 5s-shell is borrowed into the 4d-shell, producing an energetically favorable closed $4d^{10}$ shell. Thus, the structures of the valence shell of silver atom and its respective silver ion (Ag(I)), which is formed by the loss of the single top s-shell electron, are highly like those of copper and the Cu(I) ion. Given the close values of ionic radii, the coordination properties of Ag(I) are similar to those of Cu(I) [46,47]. In proteins, the redox-inactive Ag(I) may occupy only Cu(I) coordination sites. In contrast to copper, silver does not reach the Ag(II) oxidation state in the aquatic environment, and the known individual Ag(II) complexes in the presence of water are instantly restored to Ag(I) [48]. As an antibacterial agent, silver has long been used in medical practice. In recent years, the production of silver nanoparticles (AgNPs) has increased exponentially, and they are used not only in engineering but also in various fields of biomedicine, including acting as substitutes for antibiotics [49]. This has led to increased silver contents in both the environment and the human body itself, contributing to ecotoxicity, primarily due to the production of reactive oxygen species (ROS) [50,51]. Recent research suggests that silver toxicity may be the result of Cu(I) and Ag(I) forming non-identical coordination spheres in CTS proteins, causing the integration of Ag(I) into the Cu(I) metabolic system to result in copper dyshomeostasis [46,47]. Studying the influence of silver ions on the copper metabolic system should help in assessing the undesirable impact of silver use on the biosphere and human health and will allow yet unknown mechanisms of copper homeostasis to be identified. This review focuses on the prospects of silver as a tool for investigating in new aspects of copper metabolism and on the adverse consequences of silver interference with copper transport, distribution, and turnover in mammals.

2. Expedients Used to Treat Biological Objects with Silver Ions

For more than 50 years, silver ions have been used to study the systems that control the copper turnover and the mechanisms supporting its homeostasis [52]. For this purpose, silver nitrate is used in the form of a low-toxicity, highly soluble silver salt (K_{sp} = 1.44 at 25 °C). Silver nitrate solutions have been added to cell culture medium, injected into the tail vein of rat [53], intraperitoneally [54], subcutaneously [55], directly into the stomach, or into a 7.0 cm segment of intestine immediately distal to the pylorus [52], and added to fodder [56]. However, in many studies it has not been considered that Ag(I) from AgNO$_3$ in the cell culture medium, food or the body extracellular spaces, is immediately converted to poorly soluble AgCl (K_{sp} = 1.78 × 10^{-10} at 25 °C) while not compensating the possible toxic effect of the nitrate ion. To avoid undesirable effects, the silver chloride grains are added to powdered moistened fodder [57] or the cell growth medium is saturated by AgCl and then diluted with medium [58]. The concentrations and total doses of silver used in studies vary over a wide range (0.2–50 mg/kg body weight daily, from a single dose to a chronic keep on Ag-diet). In addition to inorganic silver compounds, silver acetate and coordinated silver in N-heterocyclic carbene complexes [59] are used. Silver ions from all the listed compounds are picked up by the CTS.

3. Silver Transport through Extracellular Pathways

The results of the pioneering in vivo studies showed that even though in the gastrointestinal tract (GIT) silver ions should form poorly soluble silver chloride, Ag(I) enters the body. It is likely that Ag(I) is successfully absorbed by enterocytes through coordination by amino acids, short peptides, and possibly bacterial chalkophores produced by symbionts in the GIT [60]. Pulse-chase experiments revealed that the silver is first delivered to the liver, then it was found in peripheral blood in the protein fraction, and only later it was detected in other organs [61]. It was noted that silver is selectively distributed among the organs. It mainly accumulates in the liver and poorly penetrates beyond the cell barriers [62]. Free silver ions, or ions associated with low-molecular substances, were not detected in the blood serum. In Ag-treated mouse liver, silver was found to be associated with both metallothionein and high-molecular-weight proteins residing in the membranes of the secretory pathway [63]. Ag treatment leads to a reduction of two parameters related to copper status in the serum—the total copper concentration and oxidase activity associated with ceruloplasmin (Cp)—but it does not affect the Cp protein concentration [55,64,65]. In rats that received Ag fodder over a long period of time, silver appeared in the urine [63,65], as is observed for copper in Wilson disease [66]. This indicates a substantial overlap between the pathways and molecular players that distribute copper throughout the body.

In this context, silver was employed to investigate the Cp properties related to its actions as a copper carrier. Fairly old studies revealed that constant feeding of female rats with Ag-rich food during pregnancy led to the loss of Cp activity and caused developmental abnormalities or prenatal death of embryos or 100% mortality of the pups within the first 24 h of life [57]. On the other hand, injections of human holo-Cp into pregnant rats strongly attenuated Ag-mediated embryotoxicity [57]. These findings indicate that Cp operates as a copper carrier and supplies copper to extrahepatic cells. The issue of whether Cp is indeed an extracellular copper transporter has been discussed for several decades. Several lines of evidence suggest that Cp has a copper-transporting function. First, it has been shown that all copper that is adsorbed in the GIT enters the liver and then returns to the bloodstream within Cp [67]. Second, injected [^{3}H]Cp was detected in different organs of copper-deficient rats that had scarce levels of their own Cp [68]. Third, Cp can transfer copper ions into cultured cells [69]. Finally, molecular dynamics predicts a specific interaction between the high-affinity copper transporter 1 (CTR1) ectodomain and Cp sites that connect liable copper ions [70].

The main objection against the copper-transporting function of Cp comes from the observation that extrahepatic cells do not manifest significant copper deficiency in patients with aceruloplasminemia, an autosomal recessive hereditary disease that develops due to mutations in the *Cp* gene [39]. However, evidence for this objection is not very strong, because mammals accumulate copper in the liver during the embryonic and early postnatal period to distribute it to the organs, and further maintenance of copper might be supported by its recycling. Therefore, it is difficult to create exogenous copper deficiency in adult mammals [71]. This also explains why, during aceruloplasminemia, the main pathologic manifestations are caused by the loss of ferroxidase functions of Cp rather than by the loss of the copper-transporting function of Cp [72]. However, despite this, the copper-transporting function of Cp appears to be critical for newly forming and rapidly growing cellular communities (like embryos or tumors). It may be possible for Ag(I) to be used to study some aspects of aceruloplasminemia related to ferroxidase activity and the copper-transporting function of Cp during different periods of ontogenesis.

Moreover, it is worth noting that in lactating rats, the silver radioactive isotope [^{110}Ag], enters the mammary gland cells and into the hepatocytes with kinetic characteristics similar to those of [^{64}Cu] [61,73]. Ag(I) included in Cp will disturb its oxidase and ferroxidase activities [65]. Milk Ag-Cp might compromise the copper metabolism of newborn pups, thus helping to highlight yet unknown details of copper transport and turnover in post-natal development [74]. These data suggest that silver could be used as a powerful tool to investigate copper metabolism in newborns.

4. Pathways of Silver Import through the Plasma Membranes

4.1. CTR1

Copper uptake from the extracellular space mainly relies on the plasma membrane protein CTR1 (Figure 1) [75,76]. CTR1 operates as a key component of the safe transport system of copper in all eukaryotes and is ideally adapted for the transport of silver ions.

The physiologically active form of CTR1 is a homotrimer [77–80], and the CTR1 monomer is a type I transmembrane protein. The extracellular N-terminal portion of mammalian CTR1 contains three copper-binding motifs. Motifs 1 and 2 are divided by N-glycosylation sites, while the polyglycine linker is situated between motifs 2 and 3. Motif 1 is formed by Met and His, motif 2 consists of His residues, and motif 3 contains (Met)n-X-Met clusters, where n can vary from 1 to 6. Only motif 3 appears to be both essential and sufficient to complement the loss of free copper ion transport in yeasts [81]. According to the Pearson chemical hardness principle [82], copper-binding motifs 1 and 2 of CTR1 might be involved in Cu(II) binding from extracellular donors. Cu(I) and Ag(I) exhibit high affinity to copper-binding motifs 1 and 3 of CTR1 [83]. The ability of motif 3 to form selective binding sites with Cu(I) and Ag(I), but not with bivalent metals, has been confirmed experimentally [84]. The CTR1 monomer contains three α-helices, which are highly conserved in all eukaryotes and form three transmembrane domains (TM1, TM2, and TM3). In the homotrimer, nine α-helices of identical subunits form a cuprophilic pore, which aligns with the threefold central symmetry axis [77,85]. At the extracellular side of the pore, three pairs of conserved methionine residues in the three TM2s form two thioether rings separated by one turn of the α-helix. These serve as highly selective filters for Cu(I) ions. Each ring creates a coordinate sphere of three sulfur atoms, which can coordinate two Cu(I) or two Ag(I) complexes [48]. The copper/silver ions captured in the thioether trap move inside the pore through an electrostatic gradient in ATP-independent manner [85].

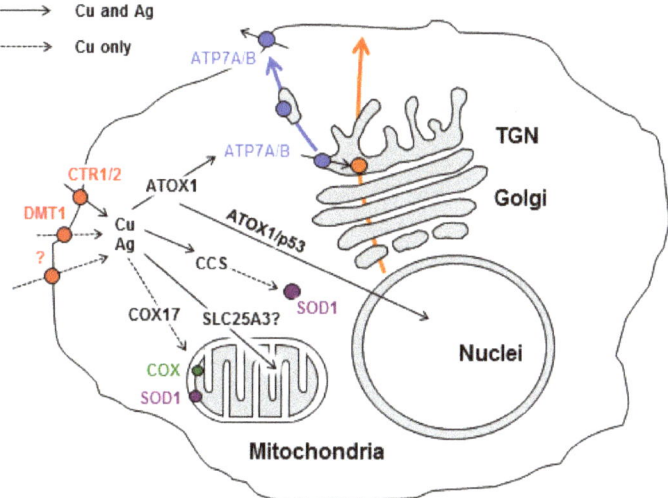

Figure 1. Scheme of copper and silver distribution in a mammalian cell. Copper is taken up via copper transporter 1 (CTR1), divalent metal transporter 1 (DMT1), or the putative transporter (all depicted as red circles). After being imported into the cell, the copper is transferred to chaperone antioxidant protein 1 (ATOX1), copper chaperone (CCS), and cytochrome-c-oxidase (COX17), which ferry it (black arrows) to both copper-transporting ATPase (ATP7A/B, blue) in the Golgi, to Cu, Zn-superoxide dismutase (SOD1, magenta) in the cytosol, and to cytochrome-c-oxidase (COX, green) in the mitochondria. Mitochondrial phosphate carrier protein (SLC25A3) transfers copper into the matrix. In the Golgi, ATP7A/B load Cu on newly synthesized cuproenzymes (orange circle), which transport it along the biosynthetic pathway (orange arrow). A significant increase in intracellular Cu induces the export of ATP7A/B (blue arrow) toward the post-Golgi compartments (TGN) and plasma membrane, where it drives the excretion of excessive Cu from the cell. Silver uses similar copper-transporting routes (solid black arrows). However, several copper-transporting pathways cannot be invaded by silver (dashed black arrows).

The last three amino acids of the short CTR1 cytosolic domain form a His-Cys-His stretch, which contains a sphere of two nitrogen atoms and a sulfur atom for the coordination of Cu(I)/Ag(I) [48]. Thus, the parallel use of Cu(II)/Cu(I) and redox inactive Ag(I) shows that CTR1 only imports Cu(I)/Ag(I), while Cu(II) remains bound to the CTR1 ectodomain and has to be oxidized for import through CTR1.

In mammals, *CTR1* gene is expressed in all cells, and the CTR1 protein serves as the main importer of copper from the bloodstream [86]. However, the pathways of copper absorption in the GIT remain unclear. The first candidate for participation in this process is CTR1, which localizes at the apical membrane of enterocytes. Intestinal epithelial cell-specific CTR1 knockout affects copper accumulation in peripheral tissues and causes hepatic iron overload, cardiac hypertrophy, and severe growth and viability defects [87]. Moreover, a previous study showed that mice fed a copper-deficient diet had elevated levels of apical membrane CTR1 protein [88]. Another study showed that although *CTR1* is expressed in enterocytes, the CTR1 protein resides at the basolateral membrane and [^{64}Cu] is taken up through this surface domain of enterocytes. Thus, basolateral CTR1 has been proposed to participate in the delivery of copper/silver from the blood to the intracellular proteins of enterocytes [89].

4.2. CTR2

CTR2 (low-affinity copper transporter 2) is another potential carrier of copper and silver through the plasma membrane. Its gene was identified by a structural similarity with the *CTR1* gene [75] and presumably, *CTR2* gene arose as a result of duplication and subsequent functional divergence [90]. Further, *CTR1* and *CTR2* are situated in the same chromosome and DNA strand. CTR2 stimulates copper uptake, is expressed in the cells of different internal organs, in the brain, and in the placenta [91] and is localized to late endosomes and lysosomes [92,93] as well as the plasma membrane [91]. The amino acid composition, secondary structure, and topology of CTR2 and CTR1 monomers, as well as their ability to form homotrimers and cuprophilic pores, are highly identical [90]. However, unlike CTR1, CTR2 lacks the ectodomain with copper-binding motifs and hence cannot bind to Cu(II) in the extracellular space. However, the cuprophilic pore of CTR2 still contains two thioether rings composed of two methionine residues, allowing the transport of Cu(I) and Ag(I) across the cell membrane [91]. This might explain why copper and silver absorption decreases in cells lacking *CTR1* and divalent metal transporter 1 (*DMT1*) but is not suppressed completely [94,95].

In addition to the transfer of copper through the plasma membrane, several other functions of CTR2 have been revealed including the regulation of copper influx via the induction of CTR1 ectodomain cleavage [96] and participation in copper mobilization from endolysosomal organelles to the cytosol [93]. CTR2 also plays a role in limiting cisplatin accumulation [97], which is in line with a hypothesis predicting that the transfer of cisplatin through cuprophilic pore of CTR1 requires the binding of copper ions with the ectodomain [98].

4.3. DMT1

The list of copper importers also includes divalent metal transporter 1 (DMT1), a member of the proton-coupled metal ion transporter family, which mediates the transport of ferrous iron from the lumen of the intestine into the enterocytes. DMT1 consists of the only subunit with 12 α-helices, which form transmembrane domains. Both the N- and C-termini of DMT1 are oriented toward the cytosol [99]. The role of DMT1 in importing copper is supported by data showing that knockout of *CTR1* stimulates the expression of *DMT1* and vice versa [94,95]. DMT1 is mainly localized at the apical surface of the enterocytes and the plasma membranes of cells from other organs [100,101]. It plays a relevant role in physiological Cu(I)/Cu(II) entry. However, silver does not inhibit DMT1-mediated copper uptake [102]. Therefore, the participation of DMT1 in the transfer of silver into the cells seems unlikely.

4.4. Other Transporters

In parallel with recognizing the roles of CTR1, CTR2, and DMT1 in transporting copper from the GIT and the blood circulation, a growing body of evidence suggests the existence of an alternative pathway of copper absorption, which appears to be independent from the above-listed transporters. Initially, Lee and coworkers demonstrated that CTR1 knockout cells from mouse embryos remained capable of importing copper [103]. The CTR1-independent copper transport was shown to be saturable, time-, temperature-, and pH-dependent, ATP-independent, and inhibited by biological Cu(II) ligands. Moreover, Ag(I), which is transported to the cells via CTR1 [104], did not inhibit the copper import through the CTR1-independent pathway. Thus, the authors concluded that the CTR1-independent copper transport pathway preferentially transports Cu(II) over Cu(I) [105]. Later, enterocyte- and fibroblast-like cells with CTR1 deletion were incubated with the specific DMT1 inhibitor to show that Cu(II) and Cu(I) uptake still occurred and, importantly, this Cu(I) uptake was not inhibited by Ag(I) [105]. Thus, silver can apparently flow into the cells through CTR1 and CTR2, but not through other copper importers.

5. Interplay between Silver and Pathways Driving Intracellular Copper Distribution

Cu(I), transferred through the CTR1 pore, is bound by the cytosolic His-Cys-His motif [106,107], which is involved in both copper coordination and the transfer mechanism to cytosolic Cu(I) chaperones. The transfer of copper from the cytosolic domain of CTR1 to apo-chaperones occurs on the *cis*-side of the plasma membrane through direct protein–protein contact. Holo-chaperones then transfer the copper to the places where it is loaded into cuproenzymes including the mitochondria, secretory pathway compartments, and cytosolic sites where superoxide dismutase 1 (SOD1), a key enzyme in the antioxidant system of aerobic organisms, resides (Figure 1). The list of Cu(I)-chaperones comprises several well-characterized members. For example, antioxidant protein 1 (in humans, ATOX1 or HAH1) ferries copper to the Cu-transporting ATPases, ATP7A, and ATP7B, which transfer copper to the luminal trans-Golgi spaces for the metalation of secretory cuproenzymes. CCS (copper chaperone for Cu/Zn-SOD1) delivers copper to the active catalytic centers of SOD1. Cox17 transfers copper to the mitochondria, where it is required for the formation of mature cytochrome-*c*-oxidase (COX) and SOD1 localized in the mitochondrial intermembrane space (IMS).

It is worth noting that Cu-chaperones can also obtain Cu(I)/Ag(I) from CTR2, despite it lacking the C-terminal His-Cys-His motif. To do this, the chaperones use lipophilic sites on their surface, which allow them to bind the cell membrane and receive Cu(I)/Ag(I) ions at the exit from the CTR2 pore. Structural, genetic, and biochemical data on Cu-chaperones have been analyzed in several recent reviews [24–26,108–111]. Here, we will discuss the findings related to the role of Cu-chaperones in silver transport through mammalian bodies.

5.1. ATOX1

ATOX1, a small cytosolic protein, contains 68 amino acid residues folded into a $\beta\alpha\beta\beta\alpha\beta$-plait with a single Cu-binding Met-Xaa-Xaa-Cys-Xaa-Xaa-Cys motif coordinated with Cu(I) on a surface-exposed loop. Holo-ATOX1 is more compact than apo-ATOX1, and it has two different conformations through which it can fulfill its dual roles in copper binding and transfer [112–114]. In ATOX1, Ag(I) binds in diagonal coordination to the two cysteine residues of the Cu(I) binding loop and shows high affinity for this protein. X-ray absorption spectroscopy has shown that in the ATOX1 homodimer, the geometric characteristics of the bonds in the coordination sphere differ from those in the [Cu(I)(Atox1)$_2$] complex [115,116]. Several lines of evidence suggest that ATOX1 efficiently participates in the transfer of both Cu(I) and Ag(I) between different chains of CTS. Apo-ATOX1 is capable of binding to Cu(I)/Ag(I) through coordination with histidine and cysteine residues in the cytosolic domain of CTR1 [114]. ATOX1 belongs to the group of so-called moonlighting proteins [117]. The main ATOX1 function consists of delivering copper to ATP7A and ATP7B, which then transport copper ions across the membranes of the biosynthetic pathway (Figure 1). Moreover, ATOX1 has been shown to exchange Cu(I)/Ag(I) ions with CCS and receive Cu(I)/Ag(I) from metallothioneins [25]. Besides the role in delivering copper to the secretory pathway of the cell, holo-ATOX1 seems to be capable of transporting copper to the nucleus with the help of the p53 protein [118]. ATOX1 has also been suggested to act as a copper-dependent transcription activator for the *SOD3* gene. Indeed, Itoh and colleagues demonstrated that ATOX1 is bound to the *SOD3* promoter in a copper-dependent manner in vitro and in vivo [119]. Apo-ATOX1 can extract Cu(I) from the ATP7B metal-binding motif and downregulate its activity [28]. It plays an essential role in the copper export pathway, and it is possible that the ratio of apo- and holo-forms of ATOX1 is involved in the coupling of redox homeostasis to intracellular copper distribution [28]. ATOX1 participates in the differentiation of neurons through local changes in copper concentration [120] and was also recently shown to promote cell migration in breast cancer [121]. Therefore, intracellular transport pathways of Ag(I) can be mediated by the substitution of Cu(I) in ATOX1 and further delivery of ATOX1-bound silver to different intracellular compartments.

5.2. Copper Delivery to the Cellular Secretory Pathway

In mammals, the transfer of copper from the cytosol to the secretory pathway or extracellular space is carried out by two Cu-transporting P1-type ATPases, ATP7A and ATP7B, which normally reside in the TGN (trans-Golgi network) compartment (Figure 1). ATP7A and ATP7B have also been called Menkes ATPase and Wilson ATPase, respectively, due to the inherited diseases that are caused by mutations in the genes encoding these proteins [122–125]. ATP7A and ATP7B proteins are very similar in terms of primary structure and domain topology. Therefore, their functions, catalytic cycles, and mechanisms of copper transfer through the membrane are also highly similar [126]. ATOX1 serves as a cytosolic donor of Cu(I) and Ag(I) for both ATP7A/B. There is a lack of strong specificity between the luminal sites of Cu(I)-ATPases that transmit copper and sites of apo-enzymes that receive copper in the secretory pathway.

ATP7A gene is expressed in all organs, including the newborn liver. The ATP7A protein normally resides in the TGN, where it loads copper onto newly synthesized cuproenzyme that is moving through the secretory pathway. In response to an increase in copper concentration, ATP7A moves toward the plasma membrane to promote the excretion of excess copper from the cell [127]. The Cu-transporting activity of ATP7A is required for the delivery of dietary copper from the enterocytes to the blood [128] and has been shown to participate in copper transfer from astrocytes to neurons [129]. The cuproenzymes, which obtain copper from ATP7A localized in extracellular spaces (blood, extracellular matrix, cerebrospinal fluid, and vesicles derived from the Golgi complex), or are inserted into the membrane. The enzymes to which ATP7A transfers copper belong to several subclasses (Table 1) and have different active center structures. The His/Met-rich segment of the first ATP7A extracytosolic loop, which binds Cu(I) and Ag(I), is likely to play a key role in the metalation of cuproenzymes [130]. Interestingly, a fragment of the second extracellular loop specifically binds to the Cp ($K_d = 1.5 \times 10^{-6}$ M) and, according to protein footprinting, protects a fragment of the Cp domain 6 [131].

Notably, these cuproenzymes are likely to have different affinities for silver (Table 2), which might be employed to selectively inhibit their catalytic activity and hence, to study their functions in the corresponding biological context.

Table 1. Catalyzed reactions by cuproenzyme group (source: ExPASy).

Class Name	Catalyzed Reaction	Electrons Transferred to Dioxygen	Cu Atoms Required
Superoxide dismutase 3, EC 1.15.1.1	2 superoxides + 2 H$^+$ <=> O$_2$ + H$_2$O$_2$	1 + 1	1
Ferroxidase, EC 1.16.3.1	4 Fe^{2+} + 4 H$^+$ + O$_2$ <=> 4 Fe^{3+} + 2 H$_2$O	4	4 (6)
Peptidylglycine monooxygenase, EC 1.14.17.3	[Peptide]-glycine + 2 ascorbates + O$_2$ <=> [peptide]-(2S)-2-hydroxyglycine + 2 monodehydroascorbate + H$_2$O	2 + 2	2
Dopamine beta-monooxygenase, EC 1.14.17.1	3,4-dihydroxyphenethylamine + 2 ascorbates + O$_2$ <=> noradrenaline + 2 monodehydroascorbate + H$_2$O	2 + 2	1
Diamine oxidase, EC 1.4.3.22	Histamine + H$_2$O + O$_2$ <=> (imidazol-4-yl) acetaldehyde + NH$_3$ + H$_2$O$_2$	2	1
Primary-amine oxidase, EC 1.4.3.21	RCH$_2$NH$_2$ + H$_2$O + O$_2$ <=> RCHO + NH$_3$ + H$_2$O$_2$	2	1
Protein-lysine 6-oxidase, EC 1.4.3.13	[Protein]-L-lysine + O$_2$ + H$_2$O <=> [protein]-(S)-2-amino-6-oxohexanoate + NH$_3$ + H$_2$O$_2$	2	1
Tyrosinase, EC 1.14.18.1	L-tyrosine + O$_2$ <=> dopaquinone + H$_2$O 2 L-dopa + O$_2$ <=> 2 dopaquinone + 2 H$_2$O	4	2

Table 2. Theoretical assessment of the ability of Ag(I) to replace copper in the active centers of the major cuproenzymes of mammals.

Enzyme	Class	Reference Structure(s), PDB ID	Copper Coordination Sphere *	Geometry *	Feasibility of Ag(I) Binding ****
COX	Cytochrome-c-oxidase; EC 1.9.3.1,	5IY5 (cow)	*CuA*; Cu pair, subunit 2, C200 (bridge), C196 (bridge), H161, H204, M207, E198 amide	Distorted tetrahedral for each atom; strong Cu–Cu interaction	Low
			CuB; subunit 1, H290, H291, H240, heme	Distorted trigonal pyramidal; Cu–heme interaction	Low
SOD1	Superoxide dismutase, EC 1.15.1.1	1HL5 (human)	H46, H48, H63, H120	Distorted tetrahedral	Low
SOD3	Superoxide dismutase, EC 1.15.1.1	2JLP (human)	H96, H98, H113, H163	Distorted tetrahedral/trigonal	Low
Cp	Ferroxidase, EC 1.16.3.1	1KCW, 2J5W (human)	*Cu21 (blue)*: C319, H276, H324	Distorted trigonal planar	Moderate
			Cu31 **: H163, H980, H1020 (dioxygen)	Trigonal pyramidal (tetrahedral)	Low
			Cu32: H103, H1061, H1022 (dioxygen)	Trigonal (distorted tetrahedral)	Low
			Cu33: H101, H978, (dioxygen, water/OH), η5-bonding from H103 and H980	Linear (square planar, with η-bonds; tetragonal distorted octahedral)	Low
			Cu41 (blue): C680, H637, H685	Distorted trigonal planar	Moderate
			Cu61 (blue): C1021, H975, H1026	Distorted trigonal planar	Moderate
			Cu42 (labile): H692, D684 (water?)	Angular	Very low
			Cu62 (labile): H940, D1025 (water?)	Angular	Very low
Hephaestin (HEPH)	Ferroxidase, EC 1.16.3.1	No data	Putatively similar to Cp, the trinuclear site, Cu21 and Cu41 site are conserved, the presence of blue copper is proven		Moderate for blue sites
Zyklopen (HEPH1)	Ferroxidase, EC 1.16.3.1	No data	Putatively similar to Cp, the trinuclear site and Cu21 site are conserved		Moderate for blue sites
Peptidyl-glycine alpha-amidating monooxygenase	Peptidylglycine monooxygenase, EC 1.14.17.3	1SDW (rat)	*Cu1*, H107, H108, H172	trigonal planar	Low
			Cu2, H242, H244, M314 (dioxygen)	Trigonal pyramidal (tetrahedral)	Low

Table 2. Cont.

Enzyme	Class	Reference Structure(s), PDB ID	Copper Coordination Sphere *	Geometry *	Feasibility of Ag(I) Binding ****
Dopamine beta-monooxygenase	Dopamine beta-monooxygenase, EC 1.14.17.1	4ZEL (human)	H412, H414, M487 (substrate?)	Trigonal pyramidal (tetrahedral?)	Low
Amine oxidase copper-containing 1 (Dopamine oxidase)	Diamine oxidase, EC 1.4.3.22	3HI7	H510, H512; H675, (substrate)	Distorted T-shaped (distorted tetrahedral)	Low
Amine oxidase, copper containing 3 (AOC3)	Primary-amine oxidase, EC 1.4.3.21	2Y73	H520, H522, H684 (substrate, water?)	Distorted T-shaped (seesaw/octahedral?)	Low
Amine oxidase, copper containing 2 (AOC2)	Primary-amine oxidase, 1.4.3.21	No data	Highly similar to AOC3, copper site conserved		Low
LOX	Protein-lysine 6-oxidase, EC 1.4.3.13	1N9E (Pichia pastoris)	H528, H530, H694, modified Y478 (TPQ, O-donor)	Distorted tetrahedral	Low to very low
LOXL2	Protein-lysine 6-oxidase, EC 1.4.3.13; putative	5ZE3	H626, H628, H630, Y689 (putative, Zn instead of Cu)	Distorted tetrahedral	Low to very low
LOXL1,3,4	Protein-lysine 6-oxidase, EC 1.4.3.13; putative	No data	Putatively similar to LOX/LOXL2		Low
TYR	Tyrosinase, EC 1.14.18.1	5Z0D, 5Z0F *** (Streptomyces)	$Cu1$: H38, H54, H63, (η_2-dioxygen)	Distorted trigonal planar (distorted tetrahedral)	Low
			$Cu2$: H190, H194, H216, (η_2-dioxygen)	Distorted trigonal pyramidal (distorted tetrahedral)	Low
Thiol receptor OR2T11		No data	M115, R119, C238, H241	Distorted tetrahedral	High

* The positions of protein-based electron donor groups are given. Substrate(s) and total effective geometry, which accounts for the substrate, are given in brackets. ** Cu31, Cu32, and Cu33 form a dioxygen binding trinuclear site, provided by eight imidazole groups of histidine residues. During dioxygen binding, the donor groups are preserved, but the coordination geometry changes. *** Only the evolutionary conserved active site is discussed. Other copper ions in these structures are not accounted for. **** Feasibility is based on geometry and coordination spheres. N-donor spheres (His-only) are considered inferior for Ag(I) coordination. Coordination of O-donor ligands (tyrosine, water molecules) and intermetallic bonds (different between metal ions) are also considered as unfavorable for Ag(I) binding.

The expression and physiological functions of ATP7B are mainly related to its role in the liver, where it drives the sequestration of excess copper and its excretion through bile [132,133]. Moreover, ATP7B contributes to the maintenance of copper levels in the blood through the synthesis and secretion of Cp [134]. Finally, some reports suggest that ATP7B might be involved in the synthesis of coagulation factors VIII and V [135,136]. Besides the liver, ATP7B expression has been detected in cells of neural origin and vascular endothelial cells [137,138]. It has been assumed that segments of the luminal loops of ATP7B participate in the direct transfer of copper to the active sites of intact Cp [139,140].

Cp is the main protein metalized by ATP7B. However, in cells with ATP7B knockout, ATP7A efficiently substitutes for ATP7B in loading copper onto the newly synthesized Cp [141]. In addition, ATP7A loads copper onto Cp in the liver during early postnatal development when ATP7B is poorly expressed in the hepatocytes [142]. *Cp* gene encodes two mRNA splice variants, which are translated into secretory Cp and membrane-bound Cp with a glycosylphosphatidylinositol anchor

(GPI-Cp) [143]. The expression of *ATP7A* and *GPI-Cp* coincide in different brain regions [137] and in the mammary glands [144], suggesting that GPI-Cp is likely to be mainly metalized by ATP7A rather than ATP7B. In neuronal cells, both *ATP7A* and *ATP7B* can be expressed simultaneously and supply copper to dopamine-beta-hydroxylase in a selective manner, which depends on its localization [145]. Despite structural similarities and co-participation in maintaining the homeostasis of copper, the loss of ATP7B function does not result in an elevation of ATP7A mRNA level [146] and vice versa [147].

N-terminal Cu-binding domains of both ATP7A and ATP7B contain core -Cys-Xaa-Xaa-Cys-stretches, which bind Cu(I) and Ag(I) in a similar manner [148]. These domains receive silver ions from Ag-ATOX1 and participate in their transfer to the lumen of the Golgi compartment or their excretion through the bile (our unpublished results). The silver ions that are transferred to the secretory pathway can be incorporated into the cuproenzymes synthesized de novo.

Indeed, it has been shown that silver ions were included in the Cp molecules synthesized in the liver [56,63,65]. Cp is a blood serum N-glycoprotein, which consists of a single polypeptide chain with a molecular weight of 132 kDa containing 1046 amino acid residues (in human) [134]. About 95% of extracellular copper has been reported to associate with Cp [149]. Cp belongs to the family of multi-copper blue ferroxidases [5,150]. Its active centers contain six copper ions, of which amino acids of domains 3, 4, and 5 form mononuclear centers, and the amino acid residues of domains 1 and 6 form three-nuclear centers [150,151]. Cp belongs to the category of moonlighting proteins [152,153]. Its major function is to facilitate iron redox transitions, which are required for transferrin receptor- and ferroportin-mediated transport of iron through the membranes [154]. In vivo, Cp oxidizes dopamine, serotonin, epinephrine, and norepinephrine, thus inactivating them [134,152]. Cp is an acute-phase protein, as its level increases by several times during processes such as inflammation, ovulation, pregnancy, and lactation [155]. Cp also demonstrates weak antioxidant activity toward ROS and regulates the oxidative status of neutrophils [156].

Cp efficiently binds to silver, which affects its catalytic activity. It was shown that Cp in blood serum from Ag-fed rats exhibits low oxidase and ferroxidase activity. In addition, inactive Cp has been found to contain one to three silver ions per molecule as molten globule [63,65,157]. Presumably, the substitution of copper with silver in the active sites of Cp happens due to the presence of three cysteine residues, each of which creates a coordination area for Cu(I)/Ag(I) with two histidine residues (Table 2). Despite the extensive investigation of active Cp sites using different approaches, including biochemical, chemical, biophysical, and molecular dynamics, some aspects of its enzyme activity and participation in various processes remain unsolved [158]. Thus, further study is required to determine whether the maturation of Cp in the Golgi requires a strict cooperative order of filling of active centers by copper ions. The use of silver may help to solve this issue.

Despite being catalytically inactive, Ag-bound Cp does not undergo rapid degradation like apo-Cp, which is not loaded with copper. In a previous study, Ag-fed rats did not exhibit a significant decrease in overall Cp levels in either blood or isolated Golgi membranes, while blood copper values and Cp oxidase activity remained barely detectable [56,63,65]. These findings differ strikingly from those related to Cp deficiency in Wilson disease, where the loss of ATP7B function does not allow Cp to be loaded with copper in the Golgi. As a result, apo-Cp is rapidly degraded in ATP7B-deficient animals and patients. Indeed, ATP7B-deficient LEC (Long Evans Cinnamon) rats manifest low Cp levels and activity, while Ag treatment does not further affect Cp abundance and function due to a lack of ATP7B-mediated transfer of Ag(I) to Cp. As in the case of copper, previous research found that Ag in LEC rats was bound to metallothionein, excluded from Cp, and not excreted in bile [63]. Interestingly, this suggests that silver allows Cp oxidase activity to be selectively inhibited without significantly impacting the overall protein expression. This finding should aid in the understanding of the pathologic mechanisms associated with the loss or aberrant modulation of Cp function in different diseases.

A recent study revealed that the consumption of a diet including Ag from the first day of life did not dramatically reduce Cp oxidase activity in the blood. In these animals, Cp activity was about half that in the control group [159]. In vivo pulse-chase experiments revealed that de novo synthesis of [^{14}C]Cp in Ag-fed animals occurred even when the liver was isolated from the bloodstream [65]. It turned out that this Cp was synthesized and excreted by the cells of subcutaneous adipose tissue, to which silver was not delivered [160]. Thus, the silver helped to uncover the interorgan control mechanism that supports copper balance in the blood and compensates for the deficit of oxidase Cp.

A growing body of evidence suggests that silver treatment could be of value for various medical purposes. For example, silver might modulate the efficiency of cisplatin chemotherapy, which is widely used to treat solid tumors. As in the case of copper and silver ions, cisplatin uptake into the cells requires CTR1. Thus, modulation of copper status (also with silver) has been considered as an option for the acceleration of cisplatin influx into the cells [161–163]. Indeed, it was recently shown that an Ag diet can be successfully used for this purpose [98]. One of the general signs of tumor development, regardless of its nature, is increased copper consumption, which is manifested in the activation of copper metabolism genes [164]. In this context, Ag(I) might interfere with cuproenzyme synthesis and angiogenesis, which both require copper to promote tumor growth. In line with this notion, a diet including Ag was shown to inhibit the growth of human tumors engrafted into nude mice [164].

Mutations in *ATP7A* cause copper deficiency, which can lead to the development of several disorders such as Menkes disease, occipital horn syndrome, and ATP7A-related distal motor neuropathy [34]. (His)$_2$Cu injections have shown high therapeutic efficiency in patients carrying certain *ATP7A* mutations [165]. The responsiveness of a given patient to such therapy could be predicted using a measurement of the kinetics of copper retention in fibroblasts or in amniotic fluid cell cultures. These in vitro kinetics tests usually require the [^{64}Cu] radioactive isotope, which has a half-life of ~13 h. Radioactive silver [^{110}Ag], which has a half-life of 250 days, is a valuable alternative that has already been used successfully in diagnostic practice [166].

5.3. CCS

CCS operates as a Cu(I) chaperone that ferries Cu(I) to SOD1, one of the main antioxidant enzymes in the cell (Figure 1). Moreover, CCS controls the folding and hence the stability of SOD1. The CCS molecule is composed of three structural-functional domains. Domain 1, which contains the Cys-Xaa-Xaa-Cys motif as ATOX1, acquires Cu(I) from CTR1 during CCS docking to the plasma membrane. Domain 2 appears to be structurally similar to SOD1 and plays a key role in CCS–SOD1 protein recognition. Domain 3 is a short polypeptide segment that lacks a secondary structure but contains a Cys-Xaa-Cys motif that is essential for SOD1 homodimerization via S–S bond formation between SOD1 subunits [167–169]. Thus, CCS participates in all stages of SOD1 post-translational maturation, from metalation of the de novo synthesized polypeptide to the formation of the active enzyme homodimer. In the cells, enzymatically active SOD1 is mainly localized in the cytosol, with a minor fraction (about 5%) in the mitochondrial IMS [170]. Presumably, mitochondrial SOD1 protects the mitochondria from oxidative stress, which might be caused by ROS as a result of electron leakage from the electron transport chain [171,172]. Active cytosolic SOD1 cannot be imported into the mitochondria and vice versa. Both SOD1 and CCS enter the IMS in apo forms through the translocator outer membrane (TOM) and bind to the IMS receptor MIA40 (mitochondrial intermembrane space import and assembly complex), which promotes the formation of disulfide bonds and concomitant protein folding. In the mitochondria, CCS acquires Cu(I) from an unknown Cu(I) transporter.

Although CCS can bind to Ag(I) ions, it does not appear to transfer them to the active site of SOD1. In a previous study, Ag-fed rats and mice did not exhibit a significant loss of SOD1 activity in the cytosol and the mitochondrial IMS [65]. Considering that mRNA, protein levels, and SOD1 activity remain intact in Ag-fed animals, we can conclude that the exchange of Cu(I)/Ag(I) is blocked during SOD1 monomer metalation. This might occur because the active site of the SOD1 is formed only by histidine residues (Table 2), which cannot coordinate the Ag(I) [48], or because Ag(I) fails to be oxidized to Ag(II) and hence to donate the electron, which is needed at the last stage of active SOD1 formation. In any case, silver has no toxic impact on SOD1. Similarly, secretory (extracellular) SOD3 exhibits quite similar resistance to silver incorporation [65]. Ag-fed rats do not manifest changes in the activity of SOD3, which is synthesized in endothelial cells and metalized by ATP7A [173]. Considering the high homology of SOD1 and SOD3, we can assume that silver does not replace copper because the active site of SOD3 also consists of histidine residues (Table 2).

5.4. COX17

The cytosolic Cu(I) chaperone COX17 has been identified as an essential component in the biogenesis of COX, a terminal complex of the mitochondrial electron transport chain [174]. COX consists of 13–14 different subunits (SU), three of which (SU1, SU2, and SU3) form a catalytic center. In mammals, they are encoded by mitochondrial DNA and integrated into the inner membrane using the OXA (oxidase assembly translocase complex). The assembly of mature COX is a complex process requiring high accuracy, which relies on numerous accessory proteins [111,175]. COX activity requires hemes (a + a$_3$) and three copper ions, which are included in the di-copper centers SU1 and SU2 (also known as Cu$_A$ and Cu$_B$). The assembly of both centers depends on copper, which is delivered by the COX17 from the cytosol (Figure 1) [29]. COX17, a small soluble protein with a molecular mass of approximately 8 kDa, contains two Cu-binding motifs, C-X$_9$-C flanked by two neighbor cysteines, which cooperatively bind four Cu(I) ions into a Cu$_4$S$_6$ complex. Ag(I) apparently cannot be embedded into the COX17 molecule at any stage of holo-COX17 formation [176]. It seems that holo-COX17 ferries copper ions from the cytosol toward the mitochondria. Then, COX17 must be unfolded for TOM40-mediated transfer to the IMS, where it subsequently recovers its appropriate 3D structural organization in a MIA40-dependent manner and binds to four Cu(I) complexes [108,177].

Holo-COX17 operates as a copper donor for both COX mitochondrial SUs. Each SU receives copper ions from COX17 through the different systems of mitochondrial Cu-chaperones. In SU1 (Cu$_B$ center), this function is executed by COX11 through three invariant residues of the histidine which form the coordination sphere for the copper ion [109,178]. SU2 (Cu$_A$ center) receives two copper ions from Cu-chaperones SCO1/2, which, in turn, obtain Cu from COX17. SCO1/2 promote the oxidation of Cu(I) to Cu(II), which is required for the integration of copper ions into the COX active site. In mature COX, two copper ions are connected by the –SH of two Cys residues. As a result, a unique electronic structure is formed that allows them to carry out the oxidation of one electron.

This suggests that Ag(I) cannot be transferred to the active sites of COX because COX17 does not bind silver ions, and coordination spheres in SUs do not possess enough affinity for Ag(I). Indeed, COX activity was shown to be unaffected in rats and mice receiving Ag-fodder [58]. In contrast, in proteo- and eubacteria, Ag(I) were found to suppresses COX activity via direct interaction with membranous copper transporting proteins [179]. At the same time in vivo studies suggest that mammalian hepatic mitochondria are capable of accumulating silver, most of which resides in the mitochondrial matrix [58,62]. Therefore, the delivery of silver ions to the mitochondria apparently occurs through COX17-independent pathways, which are probably also used by copper. Mitochondria have been seen to accumulate copper both under physiological conditions (for example, in livers of newborns) [142] and during the development of Wilson disease [66]. The outer membranes of mitochondria can apparently host DMT1, which transports iron, copper, and manganese ions [99,102,180,181]. It might potentially deliver copper (but not silver) ions to the mitochondria. However, DMT1 knockout does not reduce mitochondrial levels of copper [94]. The transfer of copper through the inner membrane is executed by a phosphate transporter, PIC2, in yeast [182] and by its mammalian ortholog encoded by SLC25A3 [183]. The assembly of active COX is associated with the expression of this gene. Since Cu$_A$ and Cu$_B$ are metalized in the IMS while PIC2/SLC25A3 transports copper to the matrix, a copper transporter from the matrix to the IMS is required. Anionic fluorescent molecular complex CuL (copper ligand) has been proposed to play this role, which requires CuL shuttling in the cytosol ↔ IMS ↔ matrix directions [184–186]. It is likely that CuL also participates in Ag(I) transfer. Moreover, the use of silver ions might help to reveal yet unidentified mitochondrial transporters of Cu(I)/Ag(I). This, in turn, would contribute to the understanding of other mechanisms used by mitochondria to support the overall homeostasis of copper in the cell.

6. Interference of Silver Nanoparticles (AgNPs) in Copper Metabolism of Eukaryotes

The properties of silver, high antibacterial activity, excellent thermal and electrical conductivity, make it a widely used metal, and fabrication of AgNPs is economically beneficial. An uncontrolled increase in the application of AgNPs in various areas (technical industry, textile production, agriculture, food industry) has inevitably led to an increased risk of human contact with them in everyday life. AgNP bioactivity indicates chemical instability as a result of the conversion of Ag(0) to Ag(I). In the environment, AgNP corroding is accompanied by sulfidation and chlorination, with the formation of practically insoluble silver salts [187]. If the transformation of AgNPs were to stop at this stage, the AgNPs and their transformation products would not pose threats to humans and the environment. However, silver ions from AgNPs interfere with cellular metabolism, perhaps due to the presence in the biological media of electron carriers, amino acids, and small peptides capable of coordinating Ag(I) by repeatedly increasing the solubility of silver. This raises issues related to the safety of AgNPs for the environment and human health [188]. Therefore, a growing number of studies are aimed at determining the toxic impact of AgNPs on molecular processes in the cells and their mechanisms. The relationships between the bioactivity of AgNPs and their linear size, surface shape, corrosion rate, aggregation state, stability, and biodegradability have been studied [50]. Most investigations have been performed on prokaryotes as targets of AgNP antibacterial action, and cultured cells of higher eukaryotes as models for assessing the toxicity of AgNPs in mammals.

In recent years, more in vivo studies of the effects of AgNPs on cell and molecular processes in higher eukaryotes have been carried out, predominantly on animal models with a short lifespan, well-studied stages of ontogenesis, sequenced genomes, and inexpensive maintenance (such as *Danio rerio, Caenorhabditis elegans*, and *Drosophila melanogaster*). AgNPs with different physicochemical properties has been shown to result in decreased lifespan, fertility, growth, body size, and locomotion [189–192]. It is generally recognized that the toxic effect of particles is based on AgNP-mediated oxidative stress [50,51]. AgNPs overcome intestinal barriers and are absorbed by the cells through clathrin-mediated endocytosis, stimulating lipid peroxidation, DNA and protein damage, and the induction of apoptosis [193–196]. In response to ROS-mediated oxidative stress, genes involved in heat shock, DNA repair, cytosol (glutathione peroxidase), mitochondrial Mn-SOD2, and autophagy are activated, possibly through the p38 MAPK/PMK-1 pathway [195,197,198]. Interestingly, the levels of copper-containing enzymes (tyrosinase and SOD1) are significantly decreased in invertebrate animals following treatment with AgNPs, despite the copper level in tissues remaining unchanged [199]. It was proposed that silver ions dissociated from AgNPs bind with copper transporter proteins and cause copper sequestration, thus creating a condition that resembles copper starvation [199]. In mice treated with AgNPs, Cp oxidase activity in the blood serum was shown to decrease [200]. However, Cp expression and the relative contents of Cp protein in the Golgi complex and in the serum did not change [200]. In addition, treatment with AgNPs did not influence liver SOD1 activity or serum alanine aminotransferase and aspartate aminotransferase content, i.e., AgNPs had no apparent toxic effects in mice. Dark-colored inclusions were observed in the abdominal cavities of the mice, but only in those that received the largest dose of AgNPs [200]. A woman who ingested 1 L of colloidal silver solution (34 mg silver) daily for approximately 16 months as an alternative medical practice showed evidence of argyrosis [201]. The patient had a serum silver concentration of about 381 ng/mL, 25-fold higher than the reference level. In the intercellular space of her sweat glands and hair follicular epithelia, brown-black granules containing silver were deposited, but other signs of toxicity were not observed. In total, the data show that the release of large masses of AgNPs into the environment, e.g., during industrial disasters, will lead to severe consequences. However, moderate concentrations, which can typically be achieved by eating foods containing AgNPs, lead to the interference of silver ions from the AgNPs in copper metabolism, affecting the various processes in the cell (Figure 2).

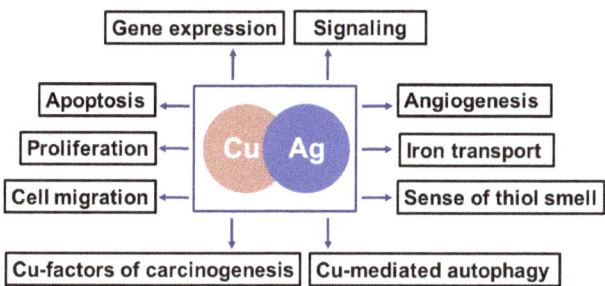

Figure 2. Copper-required cellular processes, in which Cu(I) can be replaced by Ag(I).

Thence, the long-term effects of such interventions have not been assessed, and data obtained from studying the Ag(I) routes in the bodies and cells of mammals are required.

7. Conclusions

In sum, this analysis of the existing studies highlights the usefulness of silver for investigating various metabolic pathways that require copper as an essential participant. Moreover, silver itself has started to gain interest from different research fields due to its emerging role in bioengineering, medicine, nutrition, and environmental pollution. Thus, we expect that biological studies focusing on silver will expand to reveal new mechanisms and pathways that are involved in its transport, turnover, and metabolism.

Author Contributions: Conceptualization, L.V.P., M.B., and R.S.P.; writing—original draft preparation, L.V.P., M.B., E.V.P., E.Y.P., and R.S.P.; funding acquisition, L.V.P., E.Y.I., and R.S.P.; cartoon scheme, L.V.P., E.Y.I., R.S.P., and E.V.P.; writing—review and editing L.V.P., M.B., and R.S.P.; supervision, R.S.P.

Funding: The work was supported by grants: Russian Foundation for Basic Research N18-015-00481, N18-515-7811 and MK 2718.2018.4, 6.7509.2017/8.9; Telethon, Italy, TIGEM-CBDM9; AIRC, Italy, IG 17118.

Acknowledgments: The authors thank Alexey Skvortsov and Tatiyana Sankova for constructive discussion and Ivan Grishchuk for technical help.

Conflicts of Interest: The authors declare no conflict of interest.

Abbreviations

AgNPs	silver nanoparticles
ATOX1	antioxidant protein 1 (copper chaperon for ATP7A/B)
ATP7A and ATP7B	copper transporting ATPases (Menkes ATPase and Wilson ATPase, respectively)
CCS	copper chaperone for SOD1
COX	cytochrome-c-oxidase
COX17	copper chaperon for cytochrome-c-oxidase
Cp	ceruloplasmin
CRD	copper related diseases
CTR1	high affinity copper transporter 1
CTR2	low affinity copper transporter 2
CTS	copper transporting system
CuL	copper ligand (complex anionic fluorescent substance with copper)
DMT1	divalent metal transporter 1
GIT	gastrointestinal tract
IMS	mitochondrial intermembrane space
LEC rats	Long Evans Cinnamon rats
MIA40	mitochondrial intermembrane space import and assembly complex
OXA	oxidase assembly translocase complex
PIC2	yeast phosphate carrier protein of mitochondria

ROS	reactive oxygen species
SLC25A3	mammalian phosphate carrier protein of mitochondria
SOD1	Cu,Zn-superoxide dismutase
SU	subunit
TOM	translocator outer membrane
TGN	trans-Golgi network

References

1. Uauy, R.; Olivares, M.; Gonzalez, M. Essentiality of copper in humans. *Am. J. Clin. Nutr.* **1998**, *67* (Suppl. 5), 952S–959S. [CrossRef] [PubMed]
2. Mason, K.E. A conspectus of research on copper metabolism and requirements of man. *J. Nutr.* **1979**, *109*, 1979–2066. [CrossRef] [PubMed]
3. Wikström, M. Active site intermediates in the reduction of O(2) by cytochrome oxidase, and their derivatives. *Biochim. Biophys. Acta* **2012**, *1817*, 468–475. [CrossRef] [PubMed]
4. Mot, A.C.; Silaghi-Dumitrescu, R. Laccases: Complex architectures for one-electron oxidations. *Biochemistry* **2012**, *77*, 1395–1407. [CrossRef] [PubMed]
5. Vasin, A.; Klotchenko, S.; Puchkova, L. Phylogenetic analysis of six-domain multi-copper blue proteins. *PLoS Curr.* **2013**, *5*. [CrossRef]
6. Ramsden, C.A.; Riley, P.A. Tyrosinase: The four oxidation states of the active site and their relevance to enzymatic activation, oxidation and inactivation. *Bioorg. Med. Chem.* **2014**, *22*, 2388–2395. [CrossRef]
7. Redinbo, M.R.; Yeates, T.O.; Merchant, S. Plastocyanin: Structural and functional analysis. *J. Bioenerg. Biomembr.* **1994**, *26*, 49–66. [CrossRef]
8. Palm-Espling, M.E.; Niemiec, M.S.; Wittung-Stafshede, P. Role of metal in folding and stability of copper proteins in vitro. *Biochim. Biophys. Acta* **2012**, *1823*, 1594–1603. [CrossRef]
9. Hordyjewska, A.; Popiołek, Ł.; Kocot, J. The many "faces" of copper in medicine and treatment. *Biometals* **2014**, *27*, 611–621. [CrossRef]
10. Bharathi Devi, S.R.; Dhivya, M.A.; Sulochana, K.N. Copper transporters and chaperones: Their function on angiogenesis and cellular signalling. *J. Biosci.* **2016**, *41*, 487–496. [CrossRef]
11. Zheng, L.; You, N.; Huang, X.; Gu, H.; Wu, K.; Mi, N.; Li, J. COMMD7 regulates NF-κB signaling pathway in hepatocellular carcinoma stem-like cells. *Mol. Ther. Oncolytics* **2018**, *12*, 112–123. [CrossRef] [PubMed]
12. Tanaka, K.I.; Shimoda, M.; Kasai, M.; Ikeda, M.; Ishima, Y.; Kawahara, M. Involvement of SAPK/JNK signaling pathway in copper enhanced zinc-induced neuronal cell death. *Toxicol. Sci.* **2019**, *169*, 293–302. [CrossRef] [PubMed]
13. Ackerman, C.M.; Chang, C.J. Copper signaling in the brain and beyond. *J. Biol. Chem.* **2018**, *293*, 4628–4635. [CrossRef] [PubMed]
14. Maine, G.N.; Mao, X.; Muller, P.A.; Komarck, C.M.; Klomp, L.W.; Burstein, E. COMMD1 expression is controlled by critical residues that determine XIAP binding. *Biochem. J.* **2009**, *417*, 601–609. [CrossRef] [PubMed]
15. Zhang, H.; Chang, Z.; Mehmood, K.; Abbas, R.Z.; Nabi, F.; Rehman, M.U.; Wu, X.; Tian, X.; Yuan, X.; Li, Z.; et al. Nano Copper Induces Apoptosis in PK-15 Cells via a Mitochondria-Mediated Pathway. *Biol. Trace Elem. Res.* **2018**, *181*, 62–70. [CrossRef]
16. Grubman, A.; White, A.R. Copper as a key regulator of cell signalling pathways. *Expert Rev. Mol. Med.* **2014**, *16*, e11. [CrossRef] [PubMed]
17. Kardos, J.; Héja, L.; Simon, Á.; Jablonkai, I.; Kovács, R.; Jemnitz, K. Copper signalling: Causes and consequences. *Cell Commun. Signal.* **2018**, *16*, 71. [CrossRef] [PubMed]
18. Yuan, S.; Chen, S.; Xi, Z.; Liu, Y. Copper-finger protein of Sp1: The molecular basis of copper sensing. *Metallomics* **2017**, *9*, 1169–1175. [CrossRef]
19. Duan, X.; Block, E.; Li, Z.; Connelly, T.; Zhang, J.; Huang, Z.; Su, X.; Pan, Y.; Wu, L.; Chi, Q.; et al. Crucial role of copper in detection of metal-coordinating odorants. *Proc. Natl. Acad. Sci. USA* **2012**, *109*, 3492–3497. [CrossRef]

20. Li, S.; Ahmed, L.; Zhang, R.; Pan, Y.; Matsunami, H.; Burger, J.L.; Block, E.; Batista, V.S.; Zhuang, H. Smelling sulfur: Copper and silver regulate the response of human odorant receptor OR2T11 to low-molecular-weight thiols. *J. Am. Chem. Soc.* **2016**, *138*, 13281–13288. [CrossRef]
21. Linder, M.C. The relationship of copper to DNA damage and damage prevention in humans. *Mutat. Res.* **2012**, *733*, 83–91. [CrossRef] [PubMed]
22. Rubino, J.T.; Franz, K.J. Coordination chemistry of copper proteins: How nature handles a toxic cargo for essential function. *J. Inorg. Biochem.* **2012**, *107*, 129–143. [CrossRef] [PubMed]
23. Bhattacharjee, A.; Chakraborty, K.; Shukla, A. Cellular copper homeostasis: Current concepts on its interplay with glutathione homeostasis and its implication in physiology and human diseases. *Metallomics* **2017**, *9*, 1376–1388. [CrossRef] [PubMed]
24. Robinson, N.J.; Winge, D.R. Copper metallochaperones. *Annu. Rev. Biochem.* **2010**, *79*, 537–562. [CrossRef] [PubMed]
25. Petzoldt, S.; Kahra, D.; Kovermann, M.; Dingeldein, A.P.; Niemiec, M.S.; Ådén, J.; Wittung-Stafshede, P. Human cytoplasmic copper chaperones Atox1 and CCS exchange copper ions in vitro. *Biometals* **2015**, *28*, 577–585. [CrossRef] [PubMed]
26. Hatori, Y.; Inouye, S.; Akagi, R. Thiol-based copper handling by the copper chaperone Atox1. *IUBMB Life* **2017**, *69*, 246–254. [CrossRef] [PubMed]
27. Hatori, Y.; Lutsenko, S. An expanding range of functions for the copper chaperone/antioxidant protein Atox1. *Antioxid. Redox Signal.* **2013**, *19*, 945–957. [CrossRef]
28. Hatori, Y.; Lutsenko, S. The role of copper chaperone Atox1 in coupling redox homeostasis to intracellular copper distribution. *Antioxidants* **2016**, *5*, 25. [CrossRef]
29. Matson Dzebo, M.; Ariöz, C.; Wittung-Stafshede, P. Extended functional repertoire for human copper chaperones. *Biomol. Concepts* **2016**, *7*, 29–39. [CrossRef]
30. Gaggelli, E.; Kozlowski, H.; Valensin, D.; Valensin, G. Copper homeostasis and neurodegenerative disorders (Alzheimer's, prion, and Parkinson's diseases and amyotrophic lateral sclerosis). *Chem. Rev.* **2006**, *106*, 1995–2044. [CrossRef]
31. Weber, K.T.; Weglicki, W.B.; Simpson, R.U. Macro- and micronutrient dyshomeostasis in the adverse structural remodelling of myocardium. *Cardiovasc. Res.* **2009**, *81*, 500–508. [CrossRef] [PubMed]
32. Kozlowski, H.; Kolkowska, P.; Watly, J.; Krzywoszynska, K.; Potocki, S. General aspects of metal toxicity. *Curr. Med. Chem.* **2014**, *21*, 3721–3740. [CrossRef] [PubMed]
33. Giampietro, R.; Spinelli, F.; Contino, M.; Colabufo, N.A. The pivotal role of copper in neurodegeneration: A new strategy for the therapy of neurodegenerative disorders. *Mol. Pharm.* **2018**, *15*, 808–820. [CrossRef] [PubMed]
34. Ojha, R.; Prasad, A.N. Menkes disease: What a multidisciplinary approach can do. *J. Multidiscip. Healthc.* **2016**, *9*, 371–385. [CrossRef]
35. Członkowska, A.; Litwin, T.; Dusek, P.; Ferenci, P.; Lutsenko, S.; Medici, V.; Rybakowski, J.K.; Weiss, K.H.; Schilsky, M.L. Wilson disease. *Nat. Rev. Dis. Primers* **2018**, *4*, 21. [CrossRef] [PubMed]
36. Montpetit, A.; Côté, S.; Brustein, E.; Drouin, C.A.; Lapointe, L.; Boudreau, M.; Meloche, C.; Drouin, R.; Hudson, T.J.; Drapeau, P.; et al. Disruption of AP1S1, causing a novel neurocutaneous syndrome, perturbs development of the skin and spinal cord. *PLoS Genet.* **2008**, *4*, e1000296. [CrossRef] [PubMed]
37. Kaler, S.G. Inborn errors of copper metabolism. *Handb. Clin. Neurol.* **2013**, *113*, 1745–1754. [CrossRef]
38. Bandmann, O.; Weiss, K.H.; Kaler, S.G. Wilson's disease and other neurological copper disorders. *Lancet Neurol.* **2015**, *14*, 103–113. [CrossRef]
39. Miyajima, H. Aceruloplasminemia. *Neuropathology* **2015**, *35*, 83–90. [CrossRef]
40. Bonafede, R.; Mariotti, R. ALS pathogenesis and therapeutic approaches: The role of mesenchymal stem cells and extracellular vesicles. *Front. Cell. Neurosci.* **2017**, *11*, 80. [CrossRef]
41. Bagheri, S.; Squitti, R.; Haertlé, T.; Siotto, M.; Saboury, A.A. Role of copper in the onset of Alzheimer's disease compared to other metals. *Front. Aging Neurosci.* **2018**, *9*, 446. [CrossRef] [PubMed]
42. Pal, A.; Kumar, A.; Prasad, R. Predictive association of copper metabolism proteins with Alzheimer's disease and Parkinson's disease: A preliminary perspective. *Biometals* **2014**, *27*, 25–31. [CrossRef] [PubMed]
43. Lowe, J.; Taveira-da-Silva, R.; Hilário-Souza, E. Dissecting copper homeostasis in diabetes mellitus. *IUBMB Life* **2017**, *69*, 255–262. [CrossRef] [PubMed]

44. Mendola, D.; Giacomelli, C.; Rizzarelli, E. Intracellular bioinorganic chemistry and cross talk among different -omics. *Curr. Top. Med. Chem.* **2016**, *16*, 3103–3130. [CrossRef] [PubMed]
45. Wittung-Stafshede, P. Unresolved questions in human copper pump mechanisms. *Q. Rev. Biophys.* **2015**, *48*, 471–478. [CrossRef] [PubMed]
46. Palacios, O.; Polec-Pawlak, K.; Lobinski, R.; Capdevila, M.; Gonzalez-Duarte, P. Is Ag(I) an adequate probe for Cu(I) in structural copper–metallothionein studies? The binding features of Ag(I) to mammalian metallothionein 1. *J. Biol. Inorg. Chem.* **2003**, *8*, 831–842. [CrossRef]
47. Veronesi, G.; Gallon, T.; Deniaud, A.; Boff, B.; Gateau, C.; Lebrun, C.; Vidaud, C.; Rollin-Genetet, F.; Carrière, M.; Kieffer, I.; et al. XAS investigation of silver(I) coordination in copper(I) biological binding sites. *Inorg. Chem.* **2015**, *54*, 11688–11696. [CrossRef]
48. Mukherjee, R.; Concepcion Gimeno, M.; Laguna, A. *Comprehensive Coordination Chemistry*; Wilkinson, G., Ed.; Pergamon Press: Oxford, UK, 1987; Volume 5, Chapters 53 and 54; pp. 869–909, 919–991.
49. Khan, K.; Javed, S. Functionalization of inorganic nanoparticles to augment antimicrobial efficiency: A critical analysis. *Curr. Pharm. Biotechnol.* **2018**, *19*, 523–536. [CrossRef]
50. Akter, M.; Sikder, M.T.; Rahman, M.M.; Ullah, A.A.; Hossain, K.F.; Banik, S.; Hosokawa, T.; Saito, T.; Kurasaki, M. A systematic review on silver nanoparticles-induced cytotoxicity: Physicochemical properties and perspectives. *J. Adv. Res.* **2017**, *9*, 1–16. [CrossRef]
51. Mao, B.H.; Tsai, J.C.; Chen, C.W.; Yan, S.J.; Wang, Y.J. Mechanisms of silver nanoparticle-induced toxicity and important role of autophagy. *Nanotoxicology* **2016**, *10*, 1021–1040. [CrossRef]
52. Van Campen, D.R. Effects of zinc, cadmium, silver and mercury on the absorption and distribution of copper-64 in rats. *J. Nutr.* **1966**, *88*, 125–130. [CrossRef] [PubMed]
53. Whanger, P.D.; Weswig, P.H. Effect of some copper antagonists on induction of ceruloplasmin in the rat. *J. Nutr.* **1970**, *100*, 341–348. [CrossRef] [PubMed]
54. Sugawara, N.; Sugawara, C. Comparative study of effect of acute administration of cadmium and silver on ceruloplasmin and metallothionein: Involvement of disposition of copper, iron, and zinc. *Environ. Res.* **1984**, *35*, 507–515. [CrossRef]
55. Pribyl, T.; Jahodová, J.; Schreiber, V. Partial inhibition of oestrogen-induced adenohypophyseal growth by silver nitrate. *Horm. Res.* **1980**, *12*, 296–303. [CrossRef] [PubMed]
56. Pribyl, T.; Monakhov, N.K.; Vasilyev, V.B.; Shavlovsky, M.M.; Gorbunova, V.N.; Aleynikova, T.D. Silver-containing ceruloplasmin without polyphenol oxidase activity in rat serum. *Physiol. Bohemoslov.* **1982**, *31*, 569–571.
57. Shavlovski, M.M.; Chebotar, N.A.; Konopistseva, L.A.; Zakharova, E.T.; Kachourin, A.M.; Vassiliev, V.B.; Gaitskhoki, V.S. Embryotoxicity of silver ions is diminished by ceruloplasmin–further evidence for its role in the transport of copper. *Biometals* **1995**, *8*, 122–128. [CrossRef] [PubMed]
58. Zatulovskiy, E.A.; Skvortsov, A.N.; Rusconi, P.; Ilyechova, E.Y.; Babich, P.S.; Tsymbalenko, N.V.; Broggini, M.; Puchkova, L.V. Serum depletion of holo-ceruloplasmin induced by silver ions in vivo reduces uptake of cisplatin. *J. Inorg. Biochem.* **2012**, *116*, 88–96. [CrossRef] [PubMed]
59. Hindi, K.M.; Siciliano, T.J.; Durmus, S.; Panzner, M.J.; Medvetz, D.A.; Reddy, D.V.; Hogue, L.A.; Hovis, C.E.; Hilliard, J.K.; Mallet, R.J.; et al. Synthesis, stability, and antimicrobial studies of electronically tuned silver acetate N-heterocyclic carbenes. *J. Med. Chem.* **2008**, *51*, 1577–1583. [CrossRef]
60. McCabe, J.W.; Vangala, R.; Angel, L.A. Binding selectivity of methanobactin from methylosinus trichosporium OB3b for copper(I), silver(I), zinc(II), nickel(II), cobalt(II), manganese(II), lead(II), and iron(II). *J. Am. Soc. Mass Spectrom.* **2017**, *28*, 2588–2601. [CrossRef]
61. Hanson, S.R.; Donley, S.A.; Linder, M.C. Transport of silver in virgin and lactating rats and relation to copper. *J. Trace Elem. Med. Biol.* **2001**, *15*, 243–253. [CrossRef]
62. Klotchenko, S.A.; Tsymbalenko, N.V.; Solov'ev, K.V.; Skvortsov, A.N.; Zatulovskii, E.A.; Babich, P.S.; Platonova, N.A.; Shavlovskii, M.M.; Puchkova, L.V.; Broggini, M. The effect of silver ions on copper metabolism and expression of genes encoding copper transport proteins in rat liver. *Dokl. Biochem. Biophys.* **2008**, *418*, 24–27. [CrossRef] [PubMed]
63. Sugawara, N.; Sugawara, C. Competition between copper and silver in Fischer rats with a normal copper metabolism and in Long-Evans Cinnamon rats with an abnormal copper metabolism. *Arch. Toxicol.* **2000**, *74*, 190–195. [CrossRef] [PubMed]

64. Hill, C.H.; Starcher, B.; Matrone, G. Mercury and silver interrelationships with copper. *J. Nutr.* **1964**, *83*, 107–110. [CrossRef] [PubMed]
65. Ilyechova, E.Y.; Saveliev, A.N.; Skvortsov, A.N.; Babich, P.S.; Zatulovskaia, Y.A.; Pliss, M.G.; Korzhevskii, D.E.; Tsymbalenko, N.V.; Puchkova, L.V. The effects of silver ions on copper metabolism in rats. *Metallomics* **2014**, *6*, 1970–1987. [CrossRef] [PubMed]
66. Schilsky, M.L. Wilson Disease: Diagnosis, Treatment, and Follow-up. *Clin. Liver Dis.* **2017**, *21*, 755–767. [CrossRef]
67. Cousin, R.J. Absorption, transport, and hepatic metabolism of copper and zinc: Special reference to metallothionein and ceruloplasmin. *Physiol. Rev.* **1985**, *65*, 238–309. [CrossRef]
68. Linder, M.C.; Moor, J.R. Plasma ceruloplasmin. Evidence for its presence in and uptake by heart and other organs of the rat. *Biochim. Biophys. Acta* **1977**, *499*, 329–336. [CrossRef]
69. Ramos, D.; Mar, D.; Ishida, M.; Vargas, R.; Gaite, M.; Montgomery, A.; Linder, M.C. Mechanism of copper uptake from bood plasma ceruloplasmin by mammalian cells. *PLoS ONE* **2016**, *11*, 0149516. [CrossRef]
70. Zatulovskiy, E.; Samsonov, S.; Skvortsov, A. Docking study on mammalian CTR1 copper importer motifs. *BMC Syst. Biol.* **2007**, *1* (Suppl. 1), 54. [CrossRef]
71. Broderius, M.; Mostad, E.; Wendroth, K.; Prohaska, J.R. Levels of plasma ceruloplasmin protein are markedly lower following dietary copper deficiency in rodents. *Comp. Biochem. Physiol. C Toxicol. Pharmacol.* **2010**, *151*, 473–479. [CrossRef]
72. Gray, L.W.; Kidane, T.Z.; Nguyen, A.; Akagi, S.; Petrasek, K.; Chu, Y.L.; Cabrera, A.; Kantardjieff, K.; Mason, A.Z.; Linder, M.C. Copper proteins and ferroxidases in human plasma and that of wild-type and ceruloplasmin knockout mice. *Biochem. J.* **2009**, *419*, 237–245. [CrossRef] [PubMed]
73. McArdle, H.J.; Danks, D.M. Secretion of copper 64 into breast milk following intravenous injection in a human subject. *J. Trace Elements Exp. Med.* **1991**, *4*, 81–84.
74. Puchkova, L.V.; Babich, P.S.; Zatulovskaia, Y.A.; Ilyechova, E.Y.; Di Sole, F. Copper metabolism of newborns is adapted to milk ceruloplasmin as a nutritive source of copper: Overview of the current data. *Nutrients* **2018**, *10*, 1591. [CrossRef] [PubMed]
75. Zhou, B.; Gitschier, J. hCTR1: A human gene for copper uptake identified by complementation in yeast. *Proc. Natl. Acad. Sci. USA* **1997**, *94*, 7481–7486. [CrossRef] [PubMed]
76. Lee, J.; Pena, M.M.; Nose, Y.; Thiele, D.J. Biochemical characterization of the human copper transporter Ctr1. *J. Biol. Chem.* **2002**, *277*, 4380–4387. [CrossRef] [PubMed]
77. Sharp, P.A. Ctr1 and its role in body copper homeostasis. *Int. J. Biochem. Cell Biol.* **2003**, *35*, 288–291. [CrossRef]
78. De Feo, C.J.; Aller, S.G.; Siluvai, G.S.; Blackburn, N.J.; Unger, V.M. Three-dimensional structure of the human copper transporter hCTR1. *Proc. Natl. Acad. Sci. USA* **2009**, *106*, 4237–4242. [CrossRef] [PubMed]
79. Guo, Y.; Smith, K.; Lee, J.; Thiele, D.J.; Petris, M.J. Identification of methionine-rich clusters that regulate copper-stimulated endocytosis of the human Ctr1 copper transporter. *J. Biol. Chem.* **2004**, *279*, 17428–17433. [CrossRef] [PubMed]
80. Puig, S.; Lee, J.; Lau, M.; Thiele, D.J. Biochemical and genetic analyses of yeast and human high affinity copper transporters suggest a conserved mechanism for copper uptake. *J. Biol. Chem.* **2002**, *277*, 26021–26030. [CrossRef]
81. Jiang, J.; Nadas, I.A.; Kim, A.M.; Franz, K.J. A mets motif peptide found in copper transport proteins selectively binds Cu(I) with methionine only coordination. *Inorg. Chem.* **2005**, *44*, 9787–9794. [CrossRef]
82. Parr, R.G.; Pearson, R.G. Absolute hardness: Companion parameter to absolute electronegativity. *J. Am. Chem. Soc.* **1983**, *105*, 7512–7516. [CrossRef]
83. Skvortsov, A.N.; Zatulovskiĭ, E.A.; Puchkova, L.V. Structure-functional organization of eukaryotic high-affinity copper importerCTR1 determines its ability to transport copper, silver and cisplatin. *Mol. Biol.* **2012**, *46*, 335–347. [CrossRef]
84. Rubino, J.T.; Riggs-Gelasco, P.; Franz, K.J. Methionine motifs of copper transport proteins provide general and flexible thioether-only binding sites for Cu(I) and Ag(I). *J. Biol. Inorg. Chem.* **2010**, *15*, 1033–1049. [CrossRef] [PubMed]
85. Ren, F.; Logeman, B.L.; Zhang, X.; Liu, Y.; Thiele, D.J.; Yuan, P. X-ray structures of the high-affinity copper transporter Ctr1. *Nat. Commun.* **2019**, *10*. [CrossRef] [PubMed]

86. Klomp, A.E.; Tops, B.B.; Van Denberg, I.E.; Berger, R.; Klomp, L.W. Biochemical characterization and subcellular localization of human copper transporter 1 (hCTR1). *Biochem. J.* **2002**, *364*, 497–505. [CrossRef] [PubMed]
87. Nose, Y.; Kim, B.E.; Thiele, D.J. Ctr1 drives intestinal copper absorption and is essential for growth, iron metabolism, and neonatal cardiac function. *Cell Metab.* **2006**, *4*, 235–244. [CrossRef]
88. Nose, Y.; Wood, L.K.; Kim, B.E.; Prohaska, J.R.; Fry, R.S.; Spears, J.W.; Thiele, D.J. Ctr1 is an apical copper transporter in mammalian intestinal epithelial cells in vivo that is controlled at the level of protein stability. *J. Biol. Chem.* **2010**, *285*, 32385–32392. [CrossRef]
89. Zimnicka, A.M.; Maryon, E.B.; Kaplan, J.H. Human copper transporter hCTR1 mediates basolateral uptake of copper into enterocytes: Implications for copper homeostasis. *J. Biol. Chem.* **2007**, *282*, 26471–26480. [CrossRef]
90. Logeman, B.L.; Wood, L.K.; Lee, J.; Thiele, D.J. Gene duplication and neo-functionalization in the evolutionary and functional divergence of the metazoan copper transporters Ctr1 and Ctr2. *J. Biol. Chem.* **2017**, *292*, 11531–11546. [CrossRef]
91. Bertinato, J.; Swist, E.; Plouffe, L.J.; Brooks, S.P.; L'abbé, M.R. Ctr2 is partially localized to the plasma membrane and stimulates copper uptake in COS-7 cells. *Biochem. J.* **2008**, *409*, 731–740. [CrossRef]
92. Van den Berghe, P.V.; Folmer, D.E.; Malingré, H.E.; Van Beurden, E.; Klomp, A.E.; Van de Sluis, B.; Merkx, M.; Berger, R.; Klomp, L.W. Human copper transporter 2 is localized in late endosomes and lysosomes and facilitates cellular copper uptake. *Biochem. J.* **2007**, *407*, 49–59. [CrossRef] [PubMed]
93. Öhrvik, H.; Thiele, D.J. The role of Ctr1 and Ctr2 in mammalian copper homeostasis and platinum-based chemotherapy. *J. Trace Elem. Med. Biol.* **2015**, *31*, 178–182. [CrossRef] [PubMed]
94. Lin, C.; Zhang, Z.; Wang, T.; Chen, C.; Kang, Y.J. Copper uptake by DMT1: A compensatory mechanism for CTR1 deficiency in human umbilical vein endothelial cells. *Metallomics* **2015**, *7*, 1285–1289. [CrossRef] [PubMed]
95. Ilyechova, E.Y.; Bonaldi, E.; Orlov, I.A.; Skomorokhova, E.; Puchkova, L.V.; Broggini, M. CRISP-R/Cas9 mediated deletion of copper transport genes cTR1 and DMT1 in NSCLC cell line H1299. Biological and pharmacological consequences. *Cells* **2019**, *8*, 322. [CrossRef]
96. Öhrvik, H.; Nose, Y.; Wood, L.K.; Kim, B.E.; Gleber, S.C.; Ralle, M.; Thiele, D.J. Ctr2 regulates biogenesis of a cleaved form of mammalian Ctr1 metal transporter lacking the copper- and cisplatin-binding ecto-domain. *Proc. Natl. Acad. Sci. USA* **2013**, *110*, E4279–E4288. [CrossRef]
97. Blair, B.G.; Larson, C.A.; Safaei, R.; Howell, S.B. Copper transporter 2 regulates the cellular accumulation and cytotoxicity of cisplatin and carboplatin. *Clin. Cancer Res.* **2009**, *15*, 4312–4321. [CrossRef]
98. Puchkova, L.V.; Skvortsov, A.N.; Rusconi, P.; Ilyechova, E.Y.; Broggini, M. In vivo effect of copper status on cisplatin-induced nephrotoxicity. *Biometals* **2016**, *29*, 841–849. [CrossRef]
99. Wang, D.; Song, Y.; Li, J.; Wang, C.; Li, F. Structure and metal ion binding of the first transmembrane domain of DMT1. *Biochim. Biophys. Acta* **2011**, *1808*, 1639–1644. [CrossRef] [PubMed]
100. Arredondo, M.; Munoz, P.; Mura, C.V.; Nunez, M.T. DMT1, a physiologically relevant apical Cu1+ transporter of intestinal cells. *Am. J. Physiol. Cell. Physiol.* **2003**, *284*, C1525–C1530. [CrossRef] [PubMed]
101. Coffey, R.; Knutson, M.D. The plasma membrane metal-ion transporter ZIP14 contributes to nontransferrin-bound iron uptake by human β-cells. *Am. J. Physiol. Cell Physiol.* **2017**, *312*, C169–C175. [CrossRef]
102. Arredondo, M.; Mendiburo, M.J.; Flores, S.; Singleton, S.T.; Garrick, M.D. Mouse divalent metal transporter 1 is a copper transporter in HEK293 cells. *BioMetals* **2013**, *27*, 115–123. [CrossRef]
103. Lee, J.; Petris, M.J.; Thiele, D.J. Characterization of mouse embryonic cells deficient in the ctr1 high affinity copper transporter. Identification of a Ctr1-independent copper transport system. *J. Biol. Chem.* **2002**, *277*, 40253–40259. [CrossRef]
104. Bertinato, J.; Cheung, L.; Hoque, R.; Plouffe, L.J. Ctr1 transports silver into mammalian cells. *J. Trace Elem. Med. Biol.* **2010**, *24*, 178–184. [CrossRef]
105. Zimnicka, A.M.; Ivy, K.; Kaplan, J.H. Acquisition of dietary copper: A role for anion transporters in intestinal apical copper uptake. *Am. J. Physiol. Cell. Physiol.* **2011**, *300*, C588–C599. [CrossRef]
106. Pope, C.R.; De Feo, C.J.; Unger, V.M. Cellular distribution of copper to superoxide dismutase involves scaffolding by membranes. *Proc. Natl. Acad. Sci. USA* **2013**, *110*, 20491–20496. [CrossRef]

107. Kahra, D.; Kovermann, M.; Wittung-Stafshede, P. The C-terminus of human copper importer Ctr1 acts as a binding site and transfers copper to Atox1. *Biophys. J.* **2016**, *110*, 95–102. [CrossRef]
108. Nevitt, T.; Öhrvik, H.; Thiele, D.J. Charting the travels of copper in eukaryotes from yeast to mammals. *Biochim. Biophys. Acta* **2012**, *1823*, 1580–1593. [CrossRef]
109. Palumaa, P. Copper chaperones. The concept of conformational control in the metabolism of copper. *FEBS Lett.* **2013**, *587*, 1902–1910. [CrossRef] [PubMed]
110. Fetherolf, M.; Boyd, S.D.; Winkler, D.D.; Winge, D.R. Oxygen-dependent activation of Cu, Zn-superoxide dismutase-1. *Metallomics* **2017**, *9*, 1047–1059. [CrossRef] [PubMed]
111. Signes, A.; Fernandez-Vizarra, E. Assembly of mammalian oxidative phosphorylation complexes I-V and supercomplexes. *Essays Biochem.* **2018**, *62*, 255–270. [CrossRef] [PubMed]
112. Klomp, L.W.; Lin, S.J.; Yuan, D.S.; Klausner, R.D.; Culotta, V.C.; Gitlin, J.D. Identification and functional expression of HAH1, a novel human gene involved in copper homeostasis. *J. Biol. Chem.* **1997**, *272*, 9221–9226. [CrossRef] [PubMed]
113. Wernimont, A.K.; Yatsunyk, L.A.; Rosenzweig, A.C. Binding of copper(I) by the Wilson disease protein and its copper chaperone. *J. Biol. Chem.* **2004**, *279*, 12269–12276. [CrossRef] [PubMed]
114. Levy, A.R.; Turgeman, M.; Gevorkyan-Aiapetov, L.; Ruthstein, S. The structural flexibility of the human copper chaperone Atox1: Insights from combined pulsed EPR studies and computations. *Protein Sci.* **2017**, *26*, 1609–1618. [CrossRef] [PubMed]
115. Rosenzweig, A.C.; Huffman, D.L.; Hou, M.Y.; Wernimont, A.K.; Pufahl, R.A.; O'Halloran, T.V. Crystal structure of the Atx1 metallochaperone protein at 1.02 A resolution. *Structure* **1999**, *7*, 605–617. [CrossRef]
116. Ralle, M.; Lutsenko, S.; Blackburn, N.J. X-ray absorption spectroscopy of the copper chaperone HAH1 reveals a linear two-coordinate Cu(I) center capable of adduct formation with exogenous thiols and phosphines. *J. Biol. Chem.* **2003**, *278*, 23163–23170. [CrossRef] [PubMed]
117. Jeffery, C.J. Protein moonlighting: What is it, and why is it important? *Philos. Trans. R. Soc. B* **2018**, *373*, 20160479. [CrossRef] [PubMed]
118. Beainoa, W.; Guod, Y.; Change, A.J.; Anderson, C.J. Roles of Atox1 and p53 in the trafficking of copper-64 to tumor cell nuclei: Implications for cancer therapy. *J. Biol. Inorg. Chem.* **2014**, *19*, 427–438. [CrossRef]
119. Itoh, S.; Ozumi, K.; Kim, H.W.; Nakagawa, O.; McKinney, R.D.; Folz, R.J.; Zelko, I.N.; Ushio-Fukai, M.; Fukai, T. Novel mechanism for regulation of extracellular SOD transcription and activity by copper: Role of antioxidant-1. *Free Radic. Biol. Med.* **2009**, *46*, 95–104. [CrossRef]
120. Lutsenko, S.; Tsivkovskii, R.; Walker, J.M. Functional properties of the human copper-transporting ATPase ATP7B (the Wilson's disease protein) and regulation by metallochaperone Atox1. *Ann. N. Y. Acad. Sci.* **2003**, *986*, 204–211. [CrossRef]
121. Blockhuys, S.; Wittung-Stafshede, P. Copper chaperone Atox1 plays role in breast cancer cell migration. *Biochem. Biophys. Res. Commun.* **2017**, *483*, 301–304. [CrossRef]
122. Mercer, J.F.; Livingston, J.; Hall, B.; Paynter, J.A.; Begy, C.; Chandrasekharappa, S.; Lockhart, P.; Grimes, A.; Bhave, M.; Siemieniak, D.; et al. Isolation of a partial candidate gene for Menkes disease by positional cloning. *Nat. Genet.* **1993**, *3*, 20–25. [CrossRef] [PubMed]
123. Petrukhin, K.; Lutsenko, S.; Chernov, I.; Ross, B.M.; Kaplan, J.H.; Gilliam, T.C. Characterization of the Wilson disease gene encoding a P-type copper transporting ATPase: Genomic organization, alternative splicing, and structure/function predictions. *Hum. Mol. Genet.* **1994**, *3*, 1647–1656. [CrossRef] [PubMed]
124. Lorincz, M.T. Wilson disease and related copper disorders. *Handb. Clin. Neurol.* **2018**, 279–292. [CrossRef]
125. Kaler, S.G. ATP7A-related copper transport diseases-emerging concepts and future trends. *Nat. Rev. Neurol.* **2011**, *7*, 15–29. [CrossRef]
126. Lutsenko, S.; Barnes, N.L.; Bartee, M.Y.; Dmitriev, O.Y. Function and regulation of human copper-transporting ATPases. *Physiol. Rev.* **2007**, *87*, 1011–1046. [CrossRef] [PubMed]
127. La Fontaine, S.; Mercer, J.F. Trafficking of the copper-ATPases, ATP7A and ATP7B: Role in copper homeostasis. *Arch. Biochem. Biophys.* **2007**, *463*, 149–167. [CrossRef]
128. Lutsenko, S. Copper trafficking to the secretory pathway. *Metallomics* **2016**, *8*, 840–852. [CrossRef]
129. Choi, B.S.; Zheng, W. Copper transport to the brain by the blood-brain barrier and blood-CSF barrier. *Brain Res.* **2009**, *1248*, 14–21. [CrossRef] [PubMed]

130. Barry, A.N.; Otoikhian, A.; Bhatt, S.; Shinde, U.; Tsivkovskii, R.; Blackburn, N.J.; Lutsenko, S. The luminal loop Met672-Pro707 of copper-transporting ATPase ATP7A binds metals and facilitates copper release from the intramembrane sites. *J. Biol. Chem.* **2011**, *286*, 26585–26594. [CrossRef] [PubMed]

131. Tsymbalenko, N.V.; Platonova, N.A.; Puchkova, L.V.; Mokshina, S.V.; Sasina, L.K.; Skvortsova, N.N. Identification of a fragment of ceruloplasmin, interacting with copper-transporting Menkes ATPase. *Bioorg. Khim.* **2000**, *26*, 579–586. [CrossRef] [PubMed]

132. Polishchuk, E.V.; Concilli, M.; Iacobacci, S.; Chesi, G.; Pastore, N.; Piccolo, P.; Paladino, S.; Baldantoni, D.; van IJzendoorn, S.C.; Chan, J.; et al. Wilson disease protein ATP7B utilizes lysosomal exocytosis to maintain copper homeostasis. *Dev. Cell.* **2014**, *29*, 686–700. [CrossRef] [PubMed]

133. Polishchuk, E.V.; Polishchuk, R.S. The emerging role of lysosomes in copper homeostasis. *Metallomics* **2016**, *8*, 853–862. [CrossRef] [PubMed]

134. Hellman, N.E.; Gitlin, J.D. Ceruloplasmin metabolism and function. *Annu. Rev. Nutr.* **2002**, *22*, 439–458. [CrossRef] [PubMed]

135. Mann, K.G.; Lawler, C.M.; Vehar, G.A.; Church, W.R. Coagulation factor contains copper ion. *J. Biol. Chem.* **1984**, *259*, 12949–12951. [PubMed]

136. Hollestelle, M.J.; Geertzen, H.G.; Straatsburg, I.H.; van Gulik, T.M.; van Mourik, J.A. Factor VIII expression in liver disease. *Thromb. Haemost.* **2004**, *91*, 267–275. [CrossRef] [PubMed]

137. Platonova, N.A.; Barabanova, S.V.; Povalikhin, R.G.; Tsymbalenko, N.V.; Danilovskiĭ, M.A.; Voronina, O.V.; Dorokhova, I.I.; Puchkovq, L.V. In vivo expression of copper transporting proteins in rat brain sections. *Izv. Akad. Nauk Ser. Biol.* **2005**, *32*, 108–120.

138. Li, Y.W.; Li, L.; Zhao, J.Y. An inhibition of ceruloplasmin expression induced by cerebral ischemia in the cortex and hippocampus of rats. *Neurosci. Bull.* **2008**, *24*, 13–20. [CrossRef]

139. Maio, N.; Polticelli, F.; De Francesco, G.; Rizzo, G.; Bonaccorsi di Patti, M.C.; Musci, G. Role of external loops of human ceruloplasmin in copper loading by ATP7B and Ccc2p. *J. Biol. Chem.* **2010**, *285*, 20507–20513. [CrossRef]

140. di Patti, M.C.; Maio, N.; Rizzo, G.; De Francesco, G.; Persichini, T.; Colasanti, M.; Polticelli, F.; Musci, G. Dominant mutants of ceruloplasmin impair the copper loading machinery in aceruloplasminemia. *J. Biol. Chem.* **2009**, *284*, 4545–4554. [CrossRef]

141. Barnes, N.; Tsivkovskii, R.; Tsivkovskaia, N.; Lutsenko, S. The copper-transporting ATPases, Menkes and Wilson disease proteins, have distinct roles in adult and developing cerebellum. *J. Biol. Chem.* **2005**, *280*, 9640–9645. [CrossRef]

142. Zatulovskaia, Y.A.; Ilyechova, E.Y.; Puchkova, L.V. The features of copper metabolism in the rat liver during development. *PLoS ONE* **2015**, *10*, e0140797. [CrossRef] [PubMed]

143. Patel, B.N.; Dunn, R.J.; David, S. Alternative RNA splicing generates a glycosylphosphatidylinositol-anchored form of ceruloplasmin in mammalian brain. *J. Biol. Chem.* **2000**, *275*, 4305–4310. [CrossRef]

144. Platonova, N.A.; Orlov, I.A.; Klotchenko, S.A.; Babich, V.S.; Ilyechova, E.Y.; Babich, P.S.; Garmai, Y.P.; Vasin, A.V.; Tsymbalenko, N.V.; Puchkova, L.V. Ceruloplasmin gene expression profile changes in the rat mammary gland during pregnancy, lactation and involution. *J. Trace Elem. Med. Biol.* **2017**, *43*, 126–134. [CrossRef]

145. Schmidt, K.; Ralle, M.; Schaffer, T.; Jayakanthan, S.; Bari, B.; Muchenditsi, A.; Lutsenko, S. ATP7A and ATP7B copper transporters have distinct functions in the regulation of neuronal dopamine-β-hydroxylase. *J. Biol. Chem.* **2018**, *293*, 20085–20098. [CrossRef] [PubMed]

146. Huster, D.; Finegold, M.J.; Morgan, C.T.; Burkhead, J.L.; Nixon, R.; Vanderwerf, S.M.; Gilliam, C.T.; Lutsenko, S. Consequences of copper accumulation in the livers of the Atp7b-/- (Wilson disease gene) knockout mice. *Am. J. Pathol.* **2006**, *168*, 423–434. [CrossRef]

147. Niciu, M.J.; Ma, X.M.; El Meskini, R.; Pachter, J.S.; Mains, R.E.; Eipper, B.A. Altered ATP7A expression and other compensatory responses in a murine model of Menkes disease. *Neurobiol. Dis.* **2007**, *27*, 278–291. [CrossRef]

148. Gitschier, J.; Moffat, B.; Reilly, D.; Wood, W.I.; Fairbrother, W.J. Solution structure of the fourth metal-binding domain from the Menkes copper-transporting ATPase. *Nat. Struct. Biol.* **1998**, *5*, 47–54. [CrossRef] [PubMed]

149. Bernevic, B.; El-Khatib, A.H.; Jakubowski, N.; Weller, M.G. Online immunocapture ICP-MS for the determination of the metalloprotein ceruloplasmin in human serum. *BMC Res. Notes* **2018**, *11*, 213. [CrossRef] [PubMed]

150. Zaitsev, V.N.; Zaitseva, I.; Papiz, M.; Lindley, P.F. An X-ray crystallographic study of the binding sites of the azide inhibitor and organic substrates to ceruloplasmin, a multi-copper oxidase in the plasma. *J. Biol. Inorg. Chem.* **1999**, *4*, 579–587. [CrossRef] [PubMed]
151. Samygina, V.R.; Sokolov, A.V.; Bourenkov, G.; Schneider, T.R.; Anashkin, V.A.; Kozlov, S.O.; Kolmakov, N.N.; Vasilyev, V.B. Rat ceruloplasmin: A new labile copper binding site and zinc/copper mosaic. *Metallomics* **2017**, *9*, 1828–1838. [CrossRef] [PubMed]
152. Bielli, P.; Calabrese, L. Structure to function relationships in ceruloplasmin: A 'moonlighting' protein. *Cell. Mol. Life Sci.* **2002**, *59*, 1413–1427. [CrossRef] [PubMed]
153. Das, S.; Sahoo, P.K. Ceruloplasmin, a moonlighting protein in fish. *Fish Shellfish Immunol.* **2018**, *82*, 460–468. [CrossRef] [PubMed]
154. Drakesmith, H.; Nemeth, E.; Ganz, T. Ironing out Ferroportin. *Cell. Metab.* **2015**, *22*, 777–787. [CrossRef] [PubMed]
155. Giurgea, N.; Constantinescu, M.I.; Stanciu, R.; Suciu, S.; Muresan, A. Ceruloplasmin—Acute-phase reactant or endogenous antioxidant? The case of cardiovascular disease. *Med. Sci. Monit.* **2005**, *11*, RA48–RA51. [PubMed]
156. Golenkina, E.A.; Viryasova, G.M.; Galkina, S.I.; Gaponova, T.V.; Sud'ina, G.F.; Sokolov, A.V. Fine regulation of neutrophil oxidative status and apoptosis by ceruloplasmin and its derivatives. *Cells* **2018**, *7*, 8. [CrossRef] [PubMed]
157. Kostevich, V.A.; Sokolov, A.V.; Kozlov, S.O.; Vlasenko, A.Y.; Kolmakov, N.N.; Zakharova, E.T.; Vasilyev, V.B. Functional link between ferroxidase activity of ceruloplasmin and protective effect of apo-lactoferrin: Studying rats kept on a silver chloride diet. *Biometals* **2016**, *29*, 691–704. [CrossRef]
158. Mukhopadhyay, B.P. Recognition dynamics of trinuclear copper cluster and associated histidine residues through conserved or semi-conserved water molecules in human ceruloplasmin: The involvement of aspartic and glutamic acid gates. *J. Biomol. Struct. Dyn.* **2018**, *36*, 3829–3842. [CrossRef] [PubMed]
159. Il'icheva, E.Y.; Puchkova, L.V.; Shavlovskii, M.M.; Korzhevskii, D.E.; Petrova, E.S.; Tsymbalenko, N.V. Effect of silver ions on copper metabolism during mammalian ontogenesis. *Russ. J. Dev. Biol.* **2018**, *49*, 166–178. [CrossRef]
160. Ilyechova, E.Y.; Tsymbalenko, N.V.; Puchkova, L.V. The role of subcutaneous adipose tissue in supporting the copper balance in rats with a chronic deficiency in holo-ceruloplasmin. *PLoS ONE* **2017**, *12*, e0175214. [CrossRef]
161. More, S.S.; Akil, O.; Ianculescu, A.G.; Geier, E.G.; Lustig, L.R.; Giacomini, K.M. Role of the copper transporter, CTR1, in platinum-induced ototoxicity. *J. Neurosci.* **2010**, *30*, 9500–9509. [CrossRef]
162. Ishida, S.; McCormick, F.; Smith-McCune, K.; Hanahan, D. Enhancing tumor-specific uptake of the anticancer drug cisplatin with a copper chelator. *Cancer Cell* **2010**, *17*, 574–583. [CrossRef] [PubMed]
163. Akerfeldt, M.C.; Tran, C.M.; Shen, C.; Hambley, T.W.; New, E.J. Interactions of cisplatin and the copper transporter CTR1 in human colon cancer cells. *J. Biol. Inorg. Chem.* **2017**, *22*, 765–774. [CrossRef] [PubMed]
164. Babich, P.S.; Skvortsov, A.N.; Rusconi, P.; Tsymbalenko, N.V.; Mutanen, M.; Puchkova, L.V.; Broggini, M. Non-hepatic tumors change the activity of genes encoding copper trafficking proteins in the liver. *Cancer Biol. Ther.* **2013**, *14*, 614–624. [CrossRef] [PubMed]
165. Vairo, F.P.E.; Chwal, B.C.; Perini, S.; Ferreira, M.A.P.; de Freitas Lopes, A.C.; Saute, J.A.M. A systematic review and evidence-based guideline for diagnosis and treatment of Menkes disease. *Mol. Genet. Metab.* **2019**, *126*, 6–13. [CrossRef] [PubMed]
166. Verheijen, F.V.; Beerens, C.E.M.T.; Havelaar, A.C.; Kleijer, W.J.; Mancini, G.M.S. Fibroblast silver loading for the diagnosis of Menkes disease. *J. Med. Genet.* **1998**, *35*, 849–851. [CrossRef] [PubMed]
167. Lamb, A.L.; Torres, A.S.; O'Halloran, T.V.; Rosenzweig, A.C. Heterodimeric structure of superoxide dismutase in complex with its metallochaperone. *Nat. Struct. Biol.* **2001**, *8*, 751–755. [CrossRef] [PubMed]
168. Boyd, S.D.; Calvo, J.S.; Liu, L.; lrich, M.S.; Skopp, A.; Meloni, G.; Winkler, D.D. The yeast copper chaperone for copper-zinc superoxide dismutase (CCS1) is a multifunctional chaperone promoting all levels of SOD1 maturation. *J. Biol. Chem.* **2019**, *294*, 1956–1966. [CrossRef]
169. Sala, F.A.; Wright, G.S.A.; Antonyuk, S.V.; Garratt, R.C.; Hasnain, S.S. Molecular recognition and maturation of SOD1 by its evolutionarily destabilised cognate chaperone hCCS. *PLoS Biol.* **2019**, *17*, e3000141. [CrossRef]
170. Leitch, J.M.; Yick, P.J.; Culotta, V.C. The right to choose: Multiple pathways for activating copper,zinc superoxide dismutase. *J. Biol. Chem.* **2009**, *284*, 24679–24683. [CrossRef]

171. Kawamata, H.; Manfredi, G. Import, maturation, and function of SOD1 and its copper chaperone CCS in the mitochondrial intermembrane space. *Antioxid. Redox Signal.* **2010**, *13*, 1375–1384. [CrossRef]
172. Backes, S.; Herrmann, J.M. Protein translocation into the intermembrane space and matrix of mitochondria: Mechanisms and driving forces. *Front. Mol. Biosci.* **2017**, *4*, 83. [CrossRef] [PubMed]
173. Zelko, I.N.; Mariani, T.J.; Folz, R.J. Superoxide dismutase multigene family: A comparison of the CuZn-SOD (SOD1), Mn-SOD (SOD2), and EC-SOD (SOD3) gene structures, evolution, and expression. *Free Radic. Biol. Med.* **2002**, *33*, 337–349. [CrossRef]
174. Takahashi, Y.; Kako, K.; Kashiwabara, S.I.; Takehara, A.; Inada, Y.; Arai, H.; Nakada, K.; Kodama, H.; Hayashi, J.I.; Baba, T.; et al. Mammalian copper chaperone Cox17p has an essential role in activation of cytochrome C oxidase and embryonic development. *Mol. Cell. Biol.* **2002**, *22*, 7614–7621. [CrossRef] [PubMed]
175. Timón-Gómez, A.; Nývltová, E.; Abriata, L.A.; Vila, A.J.; Hosler, J.; Barrientos, A. Mitochondrial cytochrome c oxidase biogenesis: Recent developments. *Semin. Cell Dev. Biol.* **2018**, *76*, 163–178. [CrossRef]
176. Leary, S.C. Redox regulation of SCO protein function: Controlling copper at a mitochondrial crossroad. *Antioxid. Redox Signal.* **2010**, *13*, 1403–1416. [CrossRef] [PubMed]
177. Baker, Z.N.; Cobine, P.A.; Leary, S.C. The mitochondrion: A central architect of copper homeostasis. *Metallomics* **2017**, *9*, 1501–1512. [CrossRef]
178. Carr, H.S.; George, G.N.; Winge, D.R. Yeast Cox11, a protein essential for cytochrome c oxidase assembly, is a Cu(I)-binding protein. *J. Biol. Chem.* **2002**, *277*, 31237–31242. [CrossRef]
179. Tambosi, R.; Liotenberg, S.; Bourbon, M.L.; Steunou, A.S.; Babot, M.; Durand, A.; Kebaili, N.; Ouchane, S. Silver and copper acute effects on membrane proteins and impact on photosynthetic and respiratory complexes in bacteria. *MBio* **2018**, *9*, e01535-18. [CrossRef]
180. Wolff, N.A.; Ghio, A.J.; Garrick, L.M.; Garrick, M.D.; Zhao, L.; Fenton, R.A.; Thévenod, F. Evidence for mitochondrial localization of divalent metal transporter 1 (DMT1). *FASEB J.* **2014**, *28*, 2134–2145. [CrossRef]
181. Wolff, N.A.; Garrick, M.D.; Zhao, L.; Garrick, L.M.; Ghio, A.J.; Thévenod, F. A role for divalent metal transporter (DMT1) in mitochondrial uptake of iron and manganese. *Sci. Rep.* **2018**, *8*, 211. [CrossRef]
182. Vest, K.E.; Leary, S.C.; Winge, D.R.; Cobine, P.A. Copper import into the mitochondrial matrix in Saccharomyces cerevisiae is mediated by Pic2, a mitochondrial carrier family protein. *J. Biol. Chem.* **2013**, *288*, 23884–23892. [CrossRef] [PubMed]
183. Boulet, A.; Vest, K.E.; Maynard, M.K.; Gammon, M.G.; Russell, A.C.; Mathews, A.T.; Cole, S.E.; Zhu, X.; Phillips, C.B.; Kwong, J.Q.; et al. The mammalian phosphate carrier SLC25A3 is a mitochondrial copper transporter required for cytochrome *c* oxidase biogenesis. *J. Biol. Chem.* **2018**, *293*, 1887–1896. [CrossRef] [PubMed]
184. Cobine, P.A.; Ojeda, L.D.; Rigby, K.M.; Winge, D.R. Yeast contain a non-proteinaceous pool of copper in the mitochondrial matrix. *J. Biol. Chem.* **2004**, *279*, 14447–14455. [CrossRef] [PubMed]
185. Cobine, P.A.; Pierrel, F.; Bestwick, M.L.; Winge, D.R. Mitochondrial matrix copper complex used in metalation of cytochrome oxidase and superoxide dismutase. *J. Biol. Chem.* **2006**, *281*, 36552–36559. [CrossRef] [PubMed]
186. Lindahl, P.A.; Moore, M.J. Labile low-molecular-mass metal complexes in mitochondria: Trials and tribulations of a burgeoning field. *Biochemistry* **2016**, *55*, 4140–4153. [CrossRef] [PubMed]
187. Zhang, W.; Xiao, B.; Fang, T. Chemical transformation of silver nanoparticles in aquatic environments: Mechanism, morphology and toxicity. *Chemosphere* **2018**, *191*, 324–334. [CrossRef] [PubMed]
188. Du, J.; Tang, J.; Xu, S.; Ge, J.; Dong, Y.; Li, H.; Jin, M. A review on silver nanoparticles-induced ecotoxicity and the underlying toxicity mechanisms. *Regul. Toxicol. Pharmacol.* **2018**, *98*, 231–239. [CrossRef] [PubMed]
189. Contreras, E.Q.; Puppala, H.L.; Escalera, G.; Zhong, W.; Colvin, V.L. Size-dependent impacts of silver nanoparticles on the lifespan, fertility, growth, and locomotion of Caenorhabditis elegans. *Environ. Toxicol. Chem.* **2014**, *33*, 2716–2723. [CrossRef] [PubMed]
190. Contreras, M.; Posgai, R.; Gorey, T.J.; Nielsen, M.; Hussain, S.M.; Rowe, J.J. Silver nanoparticles induced heat shock protein 70, oxidative stress and apoptosis in Drosophila melanogaster. *Toxicol. Appl. Pharmacol.* **2010**, *242*, 263–269. [CrossRef]
191. Mao, B.; Chen, Z.Y.; Wang, Y.J.; Yan, S.J. Silver nanoparticles have lethal and sublethal adverse effects on development and longevity by inducing ROS-mediated stress responses. *Sci. Rep.* **2018**, *8*, 2445. [CrossRef] [PubMed]

192. Raj, A.; Shah, P.; Agrawal, N. Dose-dependent effect of silver nanoparticles (AgNPs) on fertility and survival of Drosophila: An in-vivo study. *PLoS ONE* **2017**, *12*, e0178051. [CrossRef] [PubMed]
193. Maurer, L.L.; Yang, X.; Schindler, A.J.; Taggart, R.K.; Jiang, C.; Hsu-Kim, H.; Sherwood, D.R.; Meyer, J.N. Intracellular trafficking pathways in silver nanoparticle uptake and toxicity in Caenorhabditis elegans. *Nanotoxicology* **2016**, *10*, 831–835. [CrossRef] [PubMed]
194. Alaraby, M.; Romero, S.; Hernández, A.; Marcos, R. Toxic and genotoxic effects of silver nanoparticles in Drosophila. *Environ. Mol. Mutagen.* **2019**, *60*, 277–285. [CrossRef] [PubMed]
195. Polishchuk, E.V.; Merolla, A.; Lichtmannegger, J.; Romano, A.; Indrieri, A.; Ilyechova, E.Y.; Concilli, M.; De Cegli, R.; Crispino, R.; Mariniello, M.; et al. Activation of autophagy, observed in liver tissues from patients with Wilson disease and from ATP7B-deficient animals, Protects hepatocytes from copper-induced apoptosis. *Gastroenterology* **2019**, *156*, 1173–1189. [CrossRef] [PubMed]
196. Chatterjee, N.; Eom, H.J.; Choi, J. Effects of silver nanoparticles on oxidative DNA damage-repair as a function of p38 MAPK status: A comparative approach using human Jurkat T cells and the nematode Caenorhabditis elegans. *Environ. Mol. Mutagen.* **2014**, *55*, 122–133. [CrossRef] [PubMed]
197. Lim, D.; Roh, J.Y.; Eom, H.J.; Choi, J.Y.; Hyun, J.; Choi, J. Oxidative stress-related PMK-1 P38 MAPK activation as a mechanism for toxicity of silver nanoparticles to reproduction in the nematode Caenorhabditis elegans. *Environ. Toxicol. Chem.* **2012**, *31*, 585–592. [CrossRef] [PubMed]
198. Chesi, G.; Hegde, R.N.; Iacobacci, S.; Concilli, M.; Parashuraman, S.; Festa, B.P.; Polishchuk, E.V.; Di Tullio, G.; Carissimo, A.; Montefusco, S.; et al. Identification of p38 MAPK and JNK as new targets for correction of Wilson disease-causing ATP7B mutants. *Hepatology* **2016**, *63*, 1842–1859. [CrossRef]
199. Armstrong, N.; Ramamoorthy, M.; Lyon, D.; Jones, K.; Duttaroy, A. Mechanism of silver nanoparticles action on insect pigmentation reveals intervention of copper homeostasis. *PLoS ONE* **2013**, *8*, e53186. [CrossRef]
200. Orlov, I.A.; Sankova, T.P.; Babich, P.S.; Sosnin, I.M.; Ilyechova, E.Y.; Kirilenko, D.A.; Brunkov, P.N.; Ataev, G.L.; Romanov, A.E.; Puchkova, L.V. New silver nanoparticles induce apoptosis-like process in *E. coli* and interfere with mammalian copper metabolism. *Int. J. Nanomed.* **2016**, *11*, 6561–6574. [CrossRef]
201. Kim, Y.; Suh, H.S.; Cha, H.J.; Kim, S.H.; Jeong, K.S.; Kim, D.H. A case of generalized argyria after ingestion of colloidal silver solution. *Am. J. Ind. Med.* **2009**, *52*, 246–250. [CrossRef]

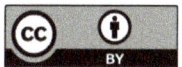

© 2019 by the authors. Licensee MDPI, Basel, Switzerland. This article is an open access article distributed under the terms and conditions of the Creative Commons Attribution (CC BY) license (http://creativecommons.org/licenses/by/4.0/).

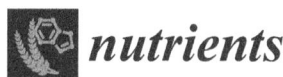

Review

Dietary and Sentinel Factors Leading to Hemochromatosis

Chang-Kyu Oh [1] and Yuseok Moon [1,2,3,*]

1. Laboratory of Mucosal Exposome and Biomodulation, Department of Biomedical Sciences, Pusan National University, Yangsan 50612, Korea; a_x_is@hanmail.net
2. BioMedical Research Institute, Pusan National University, Yangsan 50612, Korea
3. Program of Food Health Sciences, Busan 46241, Korea
* Correspondence: moon@pnu.edu; Tel.: +82-51-510-8094

Received: 15 February 2019; Accepted: 7 May 2019; Published: 10 May 2019

Abstract: Although hereditary hemochromatosis is associated with the mutation of genes involved in iron transport and metabolism, secondary hemochromatosis is due to external factors, such as intended or unintended iron overload, hemolysis-linked iron exposure or other stress-impaired iron metabolism. The present review addresses diet-linked etiologies of hemochromatosis and their pathogenesis in the network of genes and nutrients. Although the mechanistic association to diet-linked etiologies can be complicated, the stress sentinels are pivotally involved in the pathological processes of secondary hemochromatosis in response to iron excess and other external stresses. Moreover, the mutations in these sentineling pathway-linked genes increase susceptibility to secondary hemochromatosis. Thus, the crosstalk between nutrients and genes would verify the complex procedures in the clinical outcomes of secondary hemochromatosis and chronic complications, such as malignancy. All of this evidence provides crucial insights into comprehensive clinical or nutritional interventions for hemochromatosis.

Keywords: hemochromatosis; iron transport and metabolism; stress sentinel

---

1. Introduction: Regulation of Dietary Iron Metabolism

Iron is an essential metal nutrient required for all living organisms [1,2]. In response to various cues, including iron deficiency in the body, dietary iron ions can be absorbed in the apical site of duodenal enterocyte by two types of membrane proteins. One is duodenal cytochrome B (DcytB), which can reduce ferric Fe (III) ion to ferrous Fe (II) ion for transporting into the enterocytes. Another is divalent metal transporter-1 (DMT-1), which transports divalent metal ions into cells as the name implicates. Imported ferrous Fe (II) ions need to be intracellularly stored by binding to ferritin, due to the toxicity of the free form [3]. However, the stored irons can be released from enterocytes, which is facilitated by ferroportin (FPN, an iron transporter) and a ferroxidase such as hephaestin (HEPH) or ceruloplasmin on the basolateral membrane of duodenal enterocyte in response to signals from the deficient organs, including bone marrow. Exported ferrous Fe (II) ions are oxidized to ferric Fe (III) ion by HEPH and the oxidized ferric Fe (III) ion in a complex with transferrin is delivered via blood circulation to the target organs, such as the bone marrow for erythrocytosis, or liver for storage [4]. However, when stored, ferrous Fe (II) iron cannot be exported to blood vessels for various reasons and it accumulates in cells and organs, leading to iron overload (also known as hemochromatosis) in susceptible tissues, including the gut and liver (Figure 1).

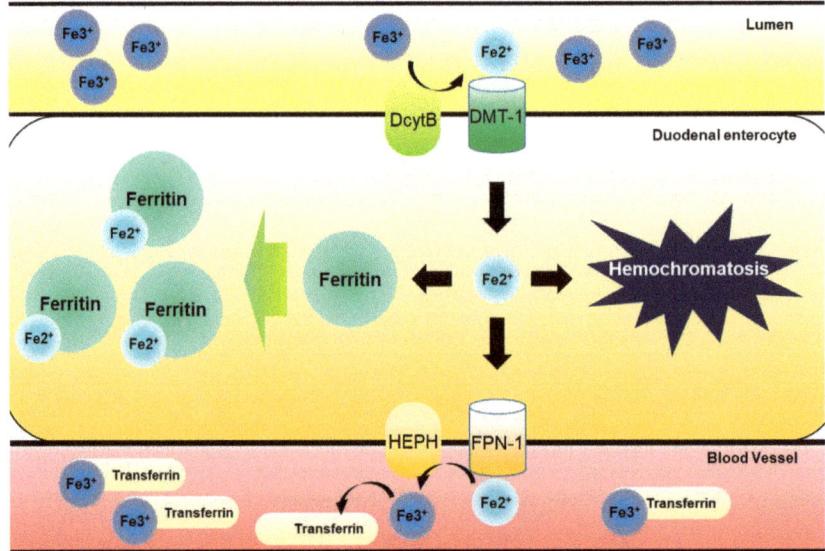

Figure 1. Dietary iron metabolism in gut. Luminal ferric Fe (III) ion from food intake is reduced to ferrous Fe (II) ion by DcytB in apical site of duodenal epithelia. After this, reduced ferrous Fe (II) ion is transported into gastrointestinal enterocytes by DMT-1. Imported ferrous Fe (II) ion have two pathways of modulation. One involves its binding to ferritin, which can store iron ions safely, preventing radial iron ion production, and another pathway involves FPN-1-mediated transport to bloodstream. Exported ferrous Fe (II) ion is then oxidized to ferric Fe (III) ion by HEPH in basolateral site of duodenal epithelial cells. Oxidized ferric Fe (III) ion binds to transferrin circulating bloodstream and is transported to bone marrow for erythrocytosis or liver for storage. However, free ferrous Fe (II) ions can accumulate in cells due to inhibition of the export to bloodstream or increase in import, leading to hemochromatosis.

Hemochromatosis in the liver, heart and endocrine glands has been associated with the triggering of liver cirrhosis, diabetes, cardiomyopathy or testicular failure [5–8]. In particular, genetic abnormalities in the iron transporting- or storage-linked genes may cause severe disorders of iron homeostasis and subsequent iron overload in most patients with primary hemochromatosis (also known as hereditary hemochromatosis) [5–8]. Most hereditary hemochromatosis is due to a mutation of the *HFE* gene, which can regulate iron uptake by interfering with the interactions between transferrin and transferrin receptor [9]. However, the primary action of HFE protein is the regulation of the iron storage hormone hepcidin [10], suggesting that it is involved in regulating systemic iron absorption rather than local iron uptake mediated by transferrin receptor. Moreover, hereditary hemochromatosis can be produced by other mutations in iron-modulating genes, such as hemojuvelin, hepcidin antimicrobial peptide (HAMP), transferrin receptor-2, ferroportin, ceruloplasmin and transferrin [11–13]. All of the genetic evidences in hereditary hemochromatosis provide insights into functions of iron metabolism-involved components in hemochromatosis. Conversely, there has been considerable clinical debate about whether hemochromatosis should be defined by genotype or presence of symptomatic iron excess independent of genotype [14,15]. There is non-mutagenic hemochromatosis, which is also called secondary hemochromatosis. Secondary hemochromatosis is mostly due to intended or unintended iron exposure to the body or the iron overload due to stress-impaired iron metabolism, which has not been well-addressed [16,17]. The potential causes of the systemic iron overload are transfusion, dietary iron excess, iron poisoning, massive hemolysis, ineffective erythropoiesis and underlying diseases, such as liver cirrhosis, steatohepatitis and porphyria cutanea tarda [17–20]. Transfusion has been well-addressed as a main cause of systemic iron overload. Repetitive transfusions within a short period of time lead to an accumulation of red blood cells (RBC), subsequent extraordinary burden of disrupted RBCs and subsequent release of heme with ferrous Fe (II). This acute overload from heme-bound iron can predispose a person to hemochromatosis and subsequent iron poisoning in severe cases [21,22]. Moreover, secondary hemochromatosis can be also caused by genetic disorders such as beta thalassemia especially if patients have received a large number of blood transfusions [23]. Many types of iron overload, other than the transfusion-linked hemochromatosis, are likely to be associated with diet- or other external factor-linked causes, such as dietary iron overload via consumption of high iron-containing food, hemolysis-linked iron overload via foodborne factors (infection and intoxication), and stress-impaired iron metabolism, all of which contribute to the disruption of iron homeostasis (Figure 2). The present review will address the diet- and stress-linked etiologies of secondary hemochromatosis and their mechanistic evidence in terms of human nutrition and metabolism. In particular, the crosstalk among the genes, nutrients and environment will give novel insights into the understanding of the pathogenesis of secondary hemochromatosis and provide a potential link to chronic complications in patients with hemochromatosis.

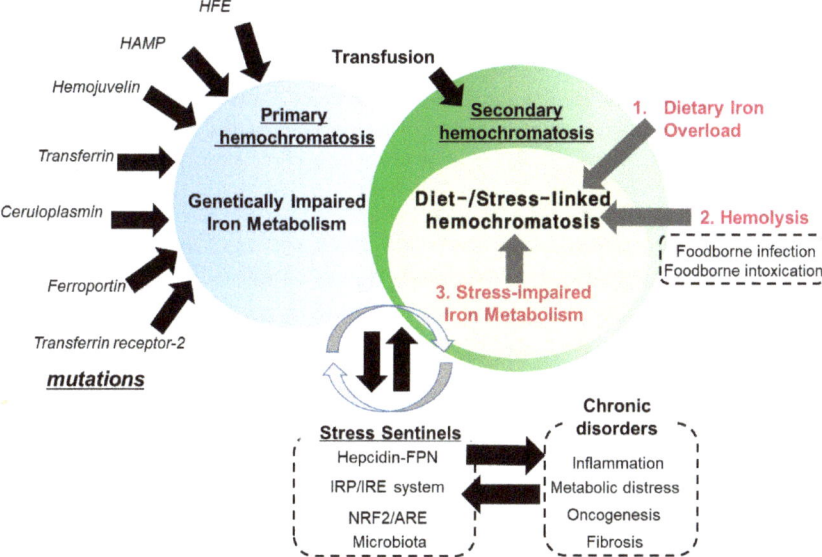

Figure 2. Etiological network in secondary hemochromatosis. Primary hemochromatosis is associated with mutation in genes involved in iron transport and metabolism, including HFE, hepcidin antimicrobial peptide (HAMP), hemojuvelin, transferrin, ceruloplasmin, ferroportin and transferrin receptor-2. Conversely, secondary hemochromatosis is linked to exposure to excess amounts of iron by transfusion or diet-associated etiologies including dietary iron overload via consumption of high iron-containing food, hemolysis-linked iron overload via foodborne factors (infection and intoxication), and stress-impaired iron metabolism. In particular, stress-impaired iron metabolism is closely associated with the stress responsive sentinels which are involved in the susceptibility to the hemochromatosis and other chronic distress. Some mutations in the sentinel-linked genes contribute to primary hemochromatosis.

2. Dietary Iron Overload

2.1. Iron Overload Via Consumption of High Iron-Containing Food

As mentioned, secondary hemochromatosis is due to either iron overload or iron metabolic impairment. In contrast with the blood transfusion-linked hemochromatosis, dietary iron excess tends to increase the systemic levels of both heme and nonheme irons, including circulating ferrous ion in some populations. In particular, it is common in sub-Saharan African populations who have the custom of drinking a fermented beverage with high nonheme iron content [24–26]. Dietary iron overload is more common in men than women, while the prevalence and severity increases with age [27]. As with hereditary hemochromatosis, different liver pathogenic processes, including hepatic portal fibrosis, micronodular cirrhosis and hepatocellular carcinoma (HCC), are notable sequelae of the dietary iron overload since the liver is the organ that is most likely to be inflicted by circulating iron [28–30]. In terms of histological patterns, the nonheme iron deposition shown in the African population is prominent in both cells of the mononuclear–phagocyte system and hepatic parenchymal cells, whereas hereditary hemochromatosis generally does not display elevated iron accumulation in the macrophages [27]. An exception concerns patients with ferroportin disease caused by mutations of the solute carrier family 40 member 1 gene (SLC40A1), who also display iron overload, primarily in Kupffer cells and other macrophages [31]. In addition to the hepatic lesions, dietary hemochromatosis has been linked to the development of metabolic disorders, including type 2 diabetes, chronic kidney disease and cardiomyopathy, using the experimental models [32–34]. In addition to the direct toxic actions of iron excess, the metabolic and inflammatory factors can mediate the age-linked pathological aggravation, which may contribute to the sequelae of the hemochromatosis. Although the mechanistic evidence still needs to be addressed, iron-induced oxidative/nitrative stress and reduced antioxidant capacity play important roles in mediating the pathologic events in the complications of dietary hemochromatosis. Moreover, nutritional iron overload-linked pathological patterns and complications in humans are similarly verified in the animal exposure model of dietary iron overload, supporting oxidative stress-associated disease severity [34].

2.2. Gene–Nutrient–Environment Interactions in Hemochromatosis

All clinical outcomes in African iron overload cannot be explained only by dietary factors. Since not all black Africans that consume large volumes of iron-rich fermented beverage have accumulated iron in the liver [24–26], it is expected that a genetic predisposition plays a role in the pathogenesis of African dietary hemochromatosis. The interaction between iron and genes can be implicated in a polymorphic variant (Gln248His) of the FPN-1-endocing SLC4A0A1 gene in African-Americans with their propensity to develop iron overload [35]. Although this variant was not yet identified in sub-Saharan African populations, it can suggest a potential crosstalk between genetic factors and dietary iron overload. Although typical patients with symptomatic iron overload have normal liver condition without alcoholism or viral hepatitis [15], intrahepatic iron overload by the genetic defects can promote the progression of the infective liver injuries. In particular, chronic hepatitis C tends to be aggravated by the presence of heterozygous HFE mutations, which leads to a high deposition of hepatic iron and advanced stages of fibrosis [36,37]. In addition to the viral infection, patients with hereditary hemochromatosis tend to display altered responses to other environmental factors, such as alcohol and smoking [38,39]. Among the non-genetic modifiers of hereditary hemochromatosis, reduced consumption of alcoholic beverages and body weight increase can explain decreased long-term iron load in hereditary hemochromatosis, while tobacco smoking may aggravate iron loading [39]. Mechanistically, these beneficial environmental modifiers can protect the progression of hereditary hemochromatosis-associated injuries in various organs via improved hepcidin production [39]. Animal studies also demonstrated that increased alcohol consumption down-regulates hepcidin mRNA expression, which was counteracted by blocking of alcohol metabolic enzymes [40,41]. Moreover, dietary antioxidants including vitamin E abolished down-regulation of hepcidin transcription [41], suggesting that alcohol metabolism-mediated oxidative stress aggravates hemochromatosis. Another nutritional supplementation with tannins via regular tea drinking is clinically associated with reduced iron absorption and the low frequency of phlebotomies in patients with hereditary hemochromatosis [42]. Whereas environmental factors may aggravate or ameliorate the progression of hereditary hemochromatosis, the only environmental or non-pharmacological interventions that are successfully proven are dietary restriction of iron availability and venesection.

3. Hemolysis-Associated Hemochromatosis during Foodborne Microbial Infection and Intoxication

Many biological (infection), chemical (toxins, metals) and physical factors (irradiation) from food may affect iron metabolism and iron-associated pathogenesis, such as hemolysis [43–47]. Heavy metals, including cadmium, mercury, lead, arsenic, manganese, chromium, cobalt, nickel, copper, zinc, selenium, silver, antimony and thallium, can be potential inducers of hemolysis when mammals are exposed to these toxic metals via circulation [48–50]. In particular, insufficient erythropoietin production and tissue iron accumulation are the central events in cadmium-induced hemolysis [49]. Although the mechanism of heavy metal-induced hemolysis is controversial, the increase of peroxide radicals play crucial roles in disruption of the RBC membrane [51]. Moreover, heavy metals lead to glutathione depletion [52] or disturbance in radical-metabolizing enzymes, such as superoxide dismutase, catalase or glutathione peroxidase [52,53], causing severe oxidative stress-associated massive hemolysis and subsequent hemochromatosis.

Foodborne infections and bacterial toxins also trigger massive hemolysis. Hemolytic uremic syndrome is a representative toxicoinfection by Shiga toxin-producing bacteria, such as enterohemorrhagic *Escherichia coli* and several *Shigella* species [54,55]. Shiga toxins can induce microangiopathic hemolysis by the activation of vascular endothelial cells, platelet and complement system [56,57]. Among them, the pathogenic events in the vascular tissues play key roles in determining the disease severity. There are two groups of Shiga toxins, which are namely, Shiga toxin type 1 and type 2 (Stx1 and 2) [58], which translocate to the ribosome via the retrograde translocation and specifically bind to and stall the ribosome during translation. The translational inhibition of global proteins in the ribosome activates the integrated stress responses, leading to various pathologic events, such as inflammation and sepsis [59–61]. In addition, some other microbial ribotoxins that include trichothecenes from grain-based foodstuff contaminated with the toxigenic molds, such as *Fusariun* species, are known to induce hemolysis [46,62,63]. Depending on the histological and toxicokinetic susceptibility, the fungal trichothecene mycotoxins, including T-2 toxin and deoxynivalenol, can induce differential levels of hemolysis in mammalians [46,63,64]. As implicated in the bacterial ribotoxins, an acute high level of exposure to the fungal trichothecenes produces the radiomimetic syndrome in patients acutely exposed to toxin-contaminated food [65,66]. In response to these foodborne infection or intoxication, the pathologic events such as leukopenia and hemolysis may discharge heme into the blood circulation, resulting in the accumulation of an excessive amount of iron ions in many organs. Foodborne infection- or intoxication-linked hemolysis as a cause of hemochromatosis can increase the systemic levels of irons in the circulation, which increases the risk of iron deposition and toxicities in a broad range of tissues. In addition to hemochromatosis via hemolysis, ribotoxins can cause hemolysis-independent disruption of iron metabolism, which will be discussed in Section 4.

4. Stress-Impaired Iron Metabolism

4.1. Hepcidin-FPN Axis as the Environmental Sentinel

As mentioned earlier parts, hepcidin is a key regulator of dietary iron uptake in response to systemic iron status, In particular, the hepatic hepcidin is the main negative modulator of the posttranslational control of FPN-1 in the liver–target organ axis [67–69]. Hepcidin is a peptide hormone that is encoded by HAMP gene and is a key regulator in iron homeostasis [70]. The hepcidin level is increased by increased iron loading, which is a homeostatic response of the body to restrict iron absorption. However, abnormally high levels of hepcidin under the pathologic conditions lead to anemia due to iron deficiency. In contrast, dietary iron deficiency decreases hepcidin production, leading to intestinal iron absorption and iron release from macrophages so that more iron is available for the body's needs [10,71,72]. In response to external insults, such as infections, the hepcidin–FPN axis provides an antimicrobial machinery by blocking the iron supply to the blood vessel, which is available for microbial growth [73]. Likewise, other environmental factors, including metals, can disrupt the hepcidin–FPN axis and induce hemochromatosis [74–76]. Moreover, FPN1 expression can be transcriptionally regulated by iron and other transition metals. For instance, metals, such as zinc and cadmium, can activate the metal response element-binding transcription factor-1 (MTF-1), which can promote the expression of FPN-1 and metal efflux from the cells for protection [76]. As a counteracting response to metal influx in the circulation, treatment with heavy metals, such as lead, can enhance the production of hepcidin and consequent sequestering of splenic irons, resulting in reduced iron availability for erythropoiesis and metal-induced hemolytic anemia in severe cases [50]. Mechanistically, FPN-1 is internalized without phosphorylation in response to hepcidin binding [77]. Hepcidin-induced endocytosis of FPN-1 is highly dependent on ubiquitination in lysine residues of FPN-1 [78] Internalized FPN-1 cannot be available for iron export from intracellular space to the circulation. Various environmental factors, such as infections, may influence hepcidin expression and subsequent hemochromatosis in the extrahepatic regions, including the brain. For example, bacterial lipopolysaccharide induces the hepatic hepcidin production, which downregulates the bioavailable FPN-1, leading to intracellular iron accumulation in the brain [79,80]. Perturbations in iron homeostasis and iron accumulation are observed in the neurodegenerative disorders, including Alzheimer's disease and Parkinson's disease [79]. When taken together, the hepcidin–FPN axis is a crucial sentinel in response to internal and external stressors, including infection, inflammatory or inorganic toxic insults. Disruption in this axis of sentinel leads to hemochromatosis.

4.2. IRP/IRE System as the Environmental Sentinel

The iron responsive element binding protein (IRP) binds to the iron responsive element (IRE), a short conserved stem-loop cis-element. This protein is crucial in iron metabolism because of the translational regulation of ferritin and transferrin receptor (TfR), which is needed for the import of iron into the cell [81,82]. IRP is the functional complex that consists of IRP1 and IRP2 as the Fe-S cluster assembly, which binds to the 5'- and 3'-untranslated regions (UTRs) of the mRNA of target genes. Iron deficiency allows the regulatory action of IRP. Binding of IRP to the 3'-UTR stabilizes TfR1 mRNA whereas binding to the 5'-UTR halts translation of the mRNAs of FPN-1 and ferritin. In contrast, excess iron ions bind to F-box/LRR-receptor protein 5 (FBLX5) and induce protein degradation of IRP via proteasomal activation, leading to induction of ferritin and reduction of TfR [83,84]. Depending on the relative location of IRE and the open reading frame, the translation will be differentially regulated [85]. When cellular iron is scarce, IRP molecules are available for binding to the 5'-IRE and the initiation of translation of ferritin or ferroportin 1 is blocked. In contrast, when 3'-IRE is occupied by available IRPs, this enhances the stability of the TfR transcript. When iron is abundant, very few IREs are occupied by IRPs and TfR mRNA is rapidly degraded, but more ferritin translation occurs [81]. Ultimately, iron excess downregulates TfR-mediated iron acquisition, while promoting ferritin-mediated storage and FPN-mediated export. Therefore, ferritin is a representative marker of iron overload diseases, such as hemochromatosis. Furthermore, the IRP/IRE system also regulates the level of ferritin mRNA, which is responsible for iron storage in cells and works as a buffer for iron deficiency. Because ferritin stores iron ions in a non-toxic form, the degradation of ferritin mRNA can aggravate hemochromatosis-related pathologies. Although ferritin can be used as a potential marker of hemochromatosis, some of inflammatory or metabolic stressors can elevate ferritin levels irrespective of iron overload. For example, ferritin levels are high in patients with infections, such as pulmonary tuberculosis [86,87]. Moreover, ferritin can be a potential biomarker of metabolic stress. Ferritin levels throughout childhood are positively associated with cardiometabolic risk in adolescence [88]. In addition to the metabolic diseases, some degenerative disorders display abnormal iron metabolism of IRP-ferritin, which can be associated with oxidative stress during prion infection [89,90]. However, activation of IRP by *Salmonella* infection can promote host innate immunity by inducing expression of antimicrobial proteins such as lipocalin 2 [91]. Moreover, dietary supplements such as phytochemicals can modulate hemochromatosis. Exposure to dietary curcumin known as a biologically active iron chelator perturbs all parameters of iron metabolism, particularly in mice that are fed a low-iron diet and when the animals display a phenotype of iron deficiency anemia, including a decline in serum iron and decreased transferrin saturation [92]. Iron chelation is important for managing patients with iron overload since returning tissue iron levels to normal levels attenuates iron excess-related toxicity. In particular, curcumin treatment activates IRP and TfR1 while downregulating ferritin and hepcidin levels in liver or hepatocytes without a consequence of gastrointestinal toxicity [92,93]. Therefore, although the phytochemical curcumin can facilitate the development of anemia in patients with marginal iron status, it can potently contribute to intervention with hemochromatosis. Taken together, the environmental cue-induced alteration of IRP/IRE system is a hallmark of some inflammatory and metabolic diseases as well as hemochromatosis. However, the disruption of IRE/IRP-linked iron metabolism may aggravate the disease progression.

4.3. NRF/ARE System as the Environmental Sentinel

Although the posttranslational regulation of FPN-1 has been extensively studied, the transcriptional regulation by nuclear respiratory factor (NRF) also plays a crucial role in iron regulation [94]. As transcription factors, NFR1 and NFR2 bind to ARE and regulate the expression of target genes, including cytoprotective factors, such as NAD(P)H quinone dehydrogenase 1, heme oxygenase 1 or Glutamate—cysteine ligase catalytic subunit and FPN-1 [94–96]. Usually, NRF2 that is bound to Kelch ECH associating protein1 (KEAP1) cannot bind to the antioxidant responsive element (ARE) and the hijacked NRF2 is degraded through the proteasomal pathway. Oxidative or electrophilic stress stimulates KEAP1, which releases NRF2 that becomes available for a heterodimer formation with small musculoaponeurotic fibrosarcoma (sMAF). Following this, the NRF2/sMAF heterodimer is transported into nucleus and binds to ARE for gene induction [97,98]. Various environmental factors produce oxidative stress, which would modulate NRF2/ARE-linked biological events. For example, ochratoxin A, a type of toxin produced by *Aspergillus ochraceus*, can block the NRF2 pathway in various ways. Foodborne oncogenic ochratoxin A (OTA) can block the translation of NRF2 through miR-132 in LLC-PK1 cells [99–101]. As a result, chronic exposure to OTA depletes the protein pools of NRF2 in cells. Besides, OTA also interferes with the translocation of NRF2 into nucleus, the nuclear accumulation of NRF2 under the oxidative stress and the binding of NRF2 to ARE [100,102,103]. Moreover, ribotoxic stress downregulates NRF2 through p38 MAPK, leading to the suppression of FPN 1 in human enterocytes *in vitro* and nematode gut [47]. Murine genetic ablation models demonstrate that regulation of NRF-linked sentinel have potential to contribute to iron metabolism and hemochromatosis. [104,105].

In addition to involvement in FPN1 induction and iron efflux, NRF2-ARE pathways can be crucial in ameliorating tissue injuries such as oxidative stress during hemochromatosis. Extended exposure to ribotoxic stress enhances NRF2-linked protection against the oxidative stress in the murine liver and placenta during the gestational period in mice [106,107]. Moreover, the perylene quinone-type mycotoxins trigger a concentration-dependent increase in NRF2-ARE-dependent promoter activity for genes of antioxidant enzymes [108]. In addition, several dietary phytochemicals that are widely distributed in fruits and vegetables can induce NRF-mediated antioxidant and detoxification enzymes in a variety of mode of actions, including Keap1-dependent and Keap1-independent cascades and epigenetic pathways [109]. Therefore, diet-linked hemochromatosis and related disorders can be potentially counteracted by antioxidant responses of natural NRF modulators. Therefore, the ultimate risk of diet-linked hemochromatosis needs to be carefully assessed based on food composition and the complex interaction between components with opposite regulatory action in the NRF/ARE-linked sentinels.

4.4. Gut Microbiota, a Crucial Mucosal Sentinel of Hemochromatosis

Iron homeostasis is the important regulatory factor of bacterial infections, colonization and community in the mucosal ecology. Therefore, patients with hemochromatosis would have altered responses to infection and immunity. In particular, luminal iron levels affect the composition of gut microbiota. The epidemic investigation in the gut iron-overloaded population shows a significant reduction in the beneficial *lactobacilli* and increased levels of enteropathogens, such as *Escherichia coli* and *Salmonella* species [110]. As described in the environmental sentinel of the hemochromatosis, the IRP2 and Hfe are important regulators of iron homeostasis and their mutations are closely associated with hereditary hemochromatosis. In the murine model, a deficiency in IRP2 elevates fecal iron concentrations, which may determine the abundance of some gut bacteria [111]. Although *Lactobacillus (L.) murinus* and *L. intestinalis* are highly abundant in Irp2−/− mice, *Enterococcus faecium* and a species similar to *Olsenella* are highly abundant in Hfe-/- mice. Moreover, *in vitro* evaluation suggested that that the iron supplementation increases the growth rate and health benefits of some lactobacillus strains [112]. However, these experimental results are in contrast to the epidemiological evidence on the suppressive effects of hemochromatosis on the beneficial lactobacillus. Thus, there remains the need to address the complicated mechanisms of iron overload-induced dysbiosis between the genetic and environmental etiologies. In terms of intervention, dietary factors are very important in improving the abnormal composition of microbiota and detrimental metabolism by dysbiosis in patients with hemochromatosis. In addition to controlling a high iron content diet, microbiota-targeted nutritional interventions could be another innovative opportunity to improve hemochromatosis.

5. Chronic Predisposing Factors

From the analyzed evidence, direct nutritional iron overload and hemolysis-inducing foodborne factors appear to substantially contribute to most cases of clinical outcomes of hemochromatosis. However, the stress-impaired iron metabolism is another considerable risk factor of secondary hemochromatosis. Moreover, the stress-responsive sentinels leading to hemochromatosis are also involved in various types of chronic diseases inflammatory, fibrogenic and oncogenic disorders [113–116]. Conversely, environmental sentinel-linked aggravation of iron metabolism may predispose patients with chronic diseases to hemochromatosis although they have not experienced excessive exposure to external iron and hemolysis.

Various reports have suggested that patients with hemochromatosis are also susceptible to the development and progression of these chronic diseases, including metabolic diseases, cancer and inflammation [117–119]. Untreated hereditary hemochromatosis can be associated with considerable morbidity due to liver cirrhosis, arthritis and diabetes mellitus and increased mortality [120]. The association of hemochromatosis with type 2 diabetes is mechanistically linked to β-cell dysfunction and apoptosis, based on the experimental model using Hfe knockout mice, which is mediated by elevated oxidative stress [121]. Limited studies have linked hemochromatosis to hepatic and extrahepatic malignancies, including esophageal cancer, colorectal cancer, malignant melanoma and lung cancer, despite the conflicting evidence [122–126]. Iron reduction by phlebotomy not only decreased visceral cancer risk by 35% but also decreased mortality in cancer patients by 60% in a supposedly normal population with peripheral arterial disease [127]. As mentioned in Section 2, dietary iron overload in black Africans has been positively associated with progression of the hepatocellular carcinoma (HCC). The risk of HCC development is 4.1 in black patients in southern Africa with dietary iron overload relative to individuals with normal iron status after adjusting for the confounding factors, such as alcohol consumption, hepatic viral infections, cirrhosis and dietary exposure to hepatocarcinogenic aflatoxin B1 [128]. It was also consistent with other observations in Africans that consider the confounding effects of viral infections [129,130]. Among cancers, HCC is one of the most susceptible tumors to iron disorders, which demonstrates the roles of the iron-linked sentineling pathways in the cancer prognosis based on the clinical gene profiling in HCC patients using a public dataset (Figure 3). Regardless of their mode of action in iron metabolism, a lower level of expression of sentineling pathway-linked genes (hepcidin, ferroportin, IRP1/2 and NRF1) was associated with worse prognosis in HCC, which indicates the regulatory actions of the sentineling pathways against the tumorigenesis. Consistent with the analysis in HCC, high ferroportin is a strong and independent predictor of good prognosis of patients with the breast cancer [131]. Thus, all of this evidence suggests that disruption of these iron-linked sentineling pathways is supposed to be detrimental to cancer patients. However, experimental evidence indicates the positive association between iron overload and oncogenic processes, including tumor initiation and promotion. Mechanistically, the local deposition of an excess amount of iron induces toxicity via oxidative radical production and peroxidation of lipids and DNA in cells [132,133]. Furthermore, lipid peroxidation can induce the activation of growth factors, such as TGF-β1, which is a driver of fibrosis through enhanced collagen accumulation and organelle damage [134]. Although the most well-known mediator between iron overload and chronic diseases, including tumors, is oxidative stress, additional mechanistic evidence needs to be identified in the biological network that leads to the redox disturbance. Taken together, while the iron overload can promote tumor initiation and progression, the iron-linked sentinels can exert regulatory actions against the malignancy-associated outcomes in patients. However, systematic investigations and tracking of diverse phases in secondary hemochromatosis are further warranted for better understanding of the interplay between gene and nutrients via stress sentineling pathways in the malignant complications.

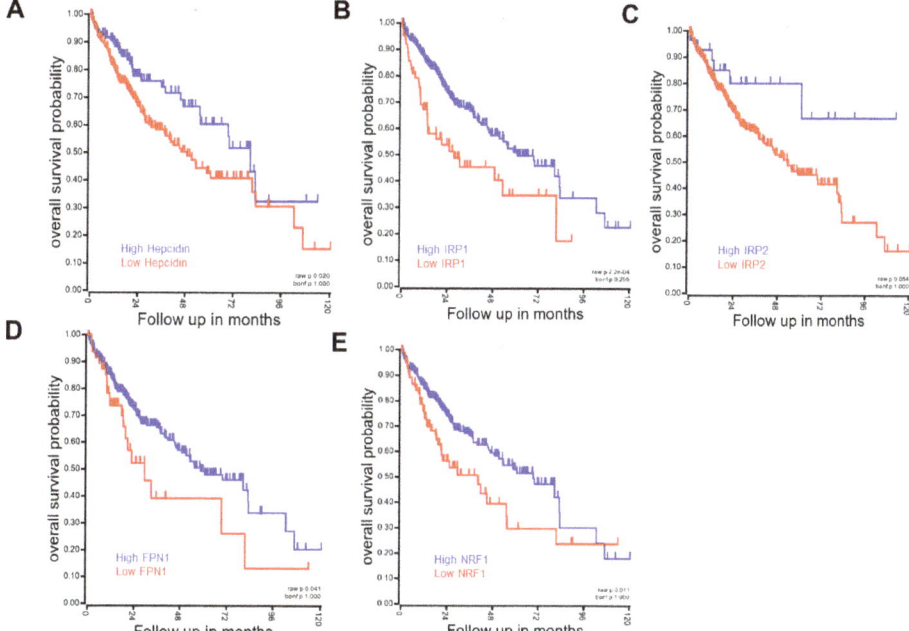

Figure 3. Examples for roles of iron stress sentinels in hepatocellular carcinoma (HCC) survival. The Kaplan–Meier survival plots based on the expression of genes (Hepcidin (cutoff=395.45, (A)), IRP1 (cutoff = 2167.24, (B)), IRP2 (cutoff = 1563.70, (C)), FPN (cutoff = 2757.82, (D)) and NRF1 (cutoff = 6179.32, (E)), which were obtained from tissues in the patients with HCC (TCGA-LIHC, n = 371). This was generated by the Cancer Genome Atlas (TCGA) Research Network: http://cancergenome.nih.gov/. NRF2 did not display significant patterns of gene-associated survival in the present dataset.

6. Conclusions

In addition to the direct dietary iron exposure, various disease states, including infection, hemolysis and chronic distress, disturb iron homeostasis, which is comprehensively associated with sporadic cases of hemochromatosis. Although the mechanistic links could be complicated, the stress-responsive sentinels support the prediction or monitoring of the outcomes of nutritional hemochromatosis in association with genetic mutations. Many metabolic, inflammatory and other pathologic insults can alter the stress sentineling pathways, leading to hemochromatosis, irrespective of external iron overload. While the stress sentinel-linked molecular events mediate the initiation and progression of secondary hemochromatosis, mutations in these sentineling pathway-linked genes are also involved in hereditary hemochromatosis. Therefore, the crosstalk between the hereditary and environmental etiologies via stress sentineling need to be assessed in order to understand the complex procedure, which leads to the clinical outcomes of hemochromatosis. Environmental stress sentinels and other external factors provide potential clues for secondary hemochromatosis and associated complications. Based on mechanistic evidence, more comprehensive and integrated clinical or nutritional interventions need to be developed.

Author Contributions: Project design and hypotheses were made by Y.M. and C.-K.O. Y.M. and C.-K.O. conducted systemic reviewing. Y.M. and C.-K.O. prepared the manuscript. Y.M. supervised the overall project.

Acknowledgments: This research was supported by the Basic Science Research Program through the National Research Foundation of Korea (NRF) funded by the Ministry of Education (2018R1D1A3B05041889).

Conflicts of Interest: The authors declare that they have no conflict of interest associated with the contents of this article.

References

1. Siah, C.W.; Ombiga, J.; Adams, L.A.; Trinder, D.; Olynyk, J.K. Normal iron metabolism and the pathophysiology of iron overload disorders. *Clin. Biochem. Rev.* **2006**, *27*, 5–16. [PubMed]
2. Wang, J.; Pantopoulos, K. Regulation of cellular iron metabolism. *Biochem. J.* **2011**, *434*, 365–381. [CrossRef] [PubMed]
3. Orino, K.; Lehman, L.; Tsuji, Y.; Ayaki, H.; Torti, S.V.; Torti, F.M. Ferritin and the response to oxidative stress. *Biochem. J.* **2001**, *357*, 241–247. [CrossRef]
4. von Drygalski, A.; Adamson, J.W. Iron metabolism in man. *JPEN J. Parenter Enteral Nutr.* **2013**, *37*, 599–606. [CrossRef]
5. Lu, J.P.; Hayashi, K. Selective iron deposition in pancreatic islet B cells of transfusional iron-overloaded autopsy cases. *Pathol. Int.* **1994**, *44*, 194–199. [CrossRef] [PubMed]
6. Pietrangelo, A. Hereditary hemochromatosis–a new look at an old disease. *N. Engl. J. Med.* **2004**, *350*, 2383–2397. [CrossRef]
7. Mendes, A.I.; Ferro, A.; Martins, R.; Picanco, I.; Gomes, S.; Cerqueira, R.; Correia, M.; Nunes, A.R.; Esteves, J.; Fleming, R.; et al. Non-classical hereditary hemochromatosis in Portugal: Novel mutations identified in iron metabolism-related genes. *Ann. Hematol.* **2009**, *88*, 229–234. [CrossRef]
8. Finch, S.C.; Finch, C.A. Idiopathic hemochromatosis, an iron storage disease. A. Iron metabolism in hemochromatosis. *Medicine* **1955**, *34*, 381–430. [CrossRef]
9. European Association For The Study Of The Liver. EASL clinical practice guidelines for HFE hemochromatosis. *J. Hepatol.* **2010**, *53*, 3–22. [CrossRef]
10. Nemeth, E.; Ganz, T. Regulation of iron metabolism by hepcidin. *Annu. Rev. Nutr.* **2006**, *26*, 323–342. [CrossRef] [PubMed]
11. Njajou, O.T.; Vaessen, N.; Joosse, M.; Berghuis, B.; van Dongen, J.W.; Breuning, M.H.; Snijders, P.J.; Rutten, W.P.; Sandkuijl, L.A.; Oostra, B.A.; et al. A mutation in SLC11A3 is associated with autosomal dominant hemochromatosis. *Nat. Genet.* **2001**, *28*, 213–214. [CrossRef]
12. Pietrangelo, A. Non-HFE hemochromatosis. *Hepatology* **2004**, *39*, 21–29. [CrossRef]
13. Camaschella, C.; Fargion, S.; Sampietro, M.; Roetto, A.; Bosio, S.; Garozzo, G.; Arosio, C.; Piperno, A. Inherited HFE-unrelated hemochromatosis in Italian families. *Hepatology* **1999**, *29*, 1563–1564. [CrossRef]

14. Adams, P.C. Hemochromatosis case definition: Out of focus? *Nat. Clin. Pract. Gastroenterol. Hepatol.* **2006**, *3*, 178–179. [CrossRef]
15. Beaton, M.D.; Adams, P.C. The myths and realities of hemochromatosis. *Can. J. Gastroenterol.* **2007**, *21*, 101–104. [CrossRef]
16. Jaeger, M.; Aul, C.; Sohngen, D.; Germing, U.; Schneider, W. Secondary hemochromatosis in polytransfused patients with myelodysplastic syndromes. *Beitr. Infusionsther.* **1992**, *30*, 464–468.
17. Lichtman, S.M.; Attivissimo, L.; Goldman, I.S.; Schuster, M.W.; Buchbinder, A. Secondary hemochromatosis as a long-term complication of the treatment of hematologic malignancies. *Am. J. Hematol* **1999**, *61*, 262–264. [CrossRef]
18. Wallerstein, R.O.; Robbins, S.L. Hemochromatosis after prolonged oral iron therapy in a patient with chronic hemolytic anemia. *Am. J. Med.* **1953**, *14*, 256–260. [CrossRef]
19. Piperno, A. Classification and diagnosis of iron overload. *Haematologica* **1998**, *83*, 447–455.
20. Banner, W., Jr.; Tong, T.G. Iron poisoning. *Pediatr. Clin. N. Am.* **1986**, *33*, 393–409. [CrossRef]
21. Ponka, P. Tissue-specific regulation of iron metabolism and heme synthesis: Distinct control mechanisms in erythroid cells. *Blood* **1997**, *89*, 1–25. [PubMed]
22. Bottomley, S.S. Porphyrin and iron metabolism in sideroblastic anemia. *Semin. Hematol.* **1977**, *14*, 169–185. [PubMed]
23. Rotaru, I.; Gaman, A.; Gaman, G. Secondary haemochromatosis in a patient with thalassemia intermedia. *Curr. Health Sci. J.* **2014**, *40*, 67–70. [CrossRef] [PubMed]
24. Gangaidzo, I.T.; Gordeuk, V.R. Hepatocellular carcinoma and African iron overload. *Gut* **1995**, *37*, 727–730. [CrossRef] [PubMed]
25. Gordeuk, V.R. African iron overload. *Semin. Hematol.* **2002**, *39*, 263–269. [CrossRef] [PubMed]
26. MacPhail, A.P.; Mandishona, E.M.; Bloom, P.D.; Paterson, A.C.; Rouault, T.A.; Gordeuk, V.R. Measurements of iron status and survival in African iron overload. *S. Afr. Med. J.* **1999**, *89*, 966–972.
27. Brink, B.; Disler, P.; Lynch, S.; Jacobs, P.; Charlton, R.; Bothwell, T. Patterns of iron storage in dietary iron overload and idiopathic hemochromatosis. *J. Lab. Clin. Med.* **1976**, *88*, 725–731.
28. Kowdley, K.V. Iron, hemochromatosis, and hepatocellular carcinoma. *Gastroenterology* **2004**, *127*, S79–S86. [CrossRef] [PubMed]
29. Park, C.H.; Bacon, B.R.; Brittenham, G.M.; Tavill, A.S. Pathology of dietary carbonyl iron overload in rats. *Lab. Investig.* **1987**, *57*, 555–563.
30. Pearson, E.G.; Hedstrom, O.R.; Poppenga, R.H. Hepatic cirrhosis and hemochromatosis in three horses. *J. Am. Vet. Med. Assoc.* **1994**, *204*, 1053–1056.
31. Sabelli, M.; Montosi, G.; Garuti, C.; Caleffi, A.; Oliveto, S.; Biffo, S.; Pietrangelo, A. Human macrophage ferroportin biology and the basis for the ferroportin disease. *Hepatology* **2017**, *65*, 1512–1525. [CrossRef]
32. Fu, S.; Li, F.; Zhou, J.; Liu, Z. The Relationship Between Body Iron Status, Iron Intake And Gestational Diabetes: A Systematic Review and Meta-Analysis. *Medicine* **2016**, *95*, e2383. [CrossRef] [PubMed]
33. Gao, W.; Li, X.; Gao, Z.; Li, H. Iron increases diabetes-induced kidney injury and oxidative stress in rats. *Biol. Trace Elem. Res.* **2014**, *160*, 368–375. [CrossRef] [PubMed]
34. Sukumaran, A.; Chang, J.; Han, M.; Mintri, S.; Khaw, B.A.; Kim, J. Iron overload exacerbates age-associated cardiac hypertrophy in a mouse model of hemochromatosis. *Sci. Rep.* **2017**, *7*, 5756. [CrossRef]
35. Beutler, E.; Barton, J.C.; Felitti, V.J.; Gelbart, T.; West, C.; Lee, P.L.; Waalen, J.; Vulpe, C. Ferroportin 1 (SCL40A1) variant associated with iron overload in African-Americans. *Blood Cells Mol. Dis.* **2003**, *31*, 305–309. [CrossRef]
36. Smith, B.C.; Gorve, J.; Guzail, M.A.; Day, C.P.; Daly, A.K.; Burt, A.D.; Bassendine, M.F. Heterozygosity for hereditary hemochromatosis is associated with more fibrosis in chronic hepatitis C. *Hepatology* **1998**, *27*, 1695–1699. [CrossRef]
37. Kazemi-Shirazi, L.; Datz, C.; Maier-Dobersberger, T.; Kaserer, K.; Hackl, F.; Polli, C.; Steindl, P.E.; Penner, E.; Ferenci, P. The relation of iron status and hemochromatosis gene mutations in patients with chronic hepatitis C. *Gastroenterology* **1999**, *116*, 127–134. [CrossRef]
38. Barton, J.C.; McLaren, C.E.; Chen, W.P.; Ramm, G.A.; Anderson, G.J.; Powell, L.W.; Subramaniam, V.N.; Adams, P.C.; Phatak, P.D.; Gurrin, L.C.; et al. Cirrhosis in Hemochromatosis: Independent Risk Factors in 368 HFE p.C282Y Homozygotes. *Ann. Hepatol* **2018**, *17*, 871–879. [CrossRef]

39. Deugnier, Y.; Morcet, J.; Laine, F.; Hamdi-Roze, H.; Bollard, A.S.; Guyader, D.; Moirand, R.; Bardou-Jacquet, E. Reduced phenotypic expression in genetic hemochromatosis with time: Role of exposure to nongenetic modifiers. *J. Hepatol.* **2018**. [CrossRef]
40. Bridle, K.; Cheung, T.K.; Murphy, T.; Walters, M.; Anderson, G.; Crawford, D.G.; Fletcher, L.M. Hepcidin is down-regulated in alcoholic liver injury: Implications for the pathogenesis of alcoholic liver disease. *Alcohol. Clin. Exp. Res.* **2006**, *30*, 106–112. [CrossRef]
41. Harrison-Findik, D.D.; Schafer, D.; Klein, E.; Timchenko, N.A.; Kulaksiz, H.; Clemens, D.; Fein, E.; Andriopoulos, B.; Pantopoulos, K.; Gollan, J. Alcohol metabolism-mediated oxidative stress down-regulates hepcidin transcription and leads to increased duodenal iron transporter expression. *J. Biol. Chem.* **2006**, *281*, 22974–22982. [CrossRef]
42. Kaltwasser, J.P.; Werner, E.; Schalk, K.; Hansen, C.; Gottschalk, R.; Seidl, C. Clinical trial on the effect of regular tea drinking on iron accumulation in genetic haemochromatosis. *Gut* **1998**, *43*, 699–704. [CrossRef]
43. Saleem, K.; Wani, W.A.; Haque, A.; Lone, M.N.; Hsieh, M.F.; Jairajpuri, M.A.; Ali, I. Synthesis, DNA binding, hemolysis assays and anticancer studies of copper(II), nickel(II) and iron(III) complexes of a pyrazoline-based ligand. *Future Med. Chem.* **2013**, *5*, 135–146. [CrossRef]
44. Ko, H.; Maymani, H.; Rojas-Hernandez, C. Hemolytic uremic syndrome associated with *Escherichia coli* O157:H7 infection in older adults: A case report and review of the literature. *J. Med. Case Rep.* **2016**, *10*, 175. [CrossRef]
45. Puchala, M.; Szweda-Lewandowska, Z.; Kiefer, J. The influence of radiation quality on radiation-induced hemolysis and hemoglobin oxidation of human erythrocytes. *J. Radiat. Res.* **2004**, *45*, 275–279. [CrossRef]
46. DeLoach, J.R.; Gyongyossy-Issa, M.I.; Khachatourians, G.G. Species-specific hemolysis of erythrocytes by T-2 toxin. *Toxicol. Appl. Pharmacol.* **1989**, *97*, 107–112. [CrossRef]
47. Oh, C.K.; Park, S.H.; Kim, J.; Moon, Y. Non-mutagenic Suppression of Enterocyte Ferroportin 1 by Chemical Ribosomal Inactivation via p38 Mitogen-activated Protein Kinase (MAPK)-mediated Regulation: Evidence for environmental hemochromatosis. *J. Biol. Chem.* **2016**, *291*, 19858–19872. [CrossRef]
48. Brandao, R.; Lara, F.S.; Pagliosa, L.B.; Soares, F.A.; Rocha, J.B.; Nogueira, C.W.; Farina, M. Hemolytic effects of sodium selenite and mercuric chloride in human blood. *Drug Chem. Toxicol.* **2005**, *28*, 397–407. [CrossRef]
49. Horiguchi, H.; Oguma, E.; Kayama, F. Cadmium induces anemia through interdependent progress of hemolysis, body iron accumulation, and insufficient erythropoietin production in rats. *Toxicol. Sci.* **2011**, *122*, 198–210. [CrossRef]
50. Wang, X.; Wang, L.; Liu, S. Heme-regulated eIF2alpha kinase plays a crucial role in protecting erythroid cells against Pb-induced hemolytic stress. *Chem. Res. Toxicol.* **2015**, *28*, 460–469. [CrossRef]
51. Ribarov, S.R.; Benov, L.C. Relationship between the hemolytic action of heavy metals and lipid peroxidation. *Biochim. Biophys. Acta* **1981**, *640*, 721–726. [CrossRef]
52. Jozefczak, M.; Remans, T.; Vangronsveld, J.; Cuypers, A. Glutathione is a key player in metal-induced oxidative stress defenses. *Int. J. Mol. Sci.* **2012**, *13*, 3145–3175. [CrossRef] [PubMed]
53. Valko, M.; Jomova, K.; Rhodes, C.J.; Kuca, K.; Musilek, K. Redox- and non-redox-metal-induced formation of free radicals and their role in human disease. *Arch. Toxicol.* **2016**, *90*, 1–37. [CrossRef] [PubMed]
54. Beutin, L. Emerging enterohaemorrhagic Escherichia coli, causes and effects of the rise of a human pathogen. *J. Vet. Med. B Infect. Dis. Vet. Public Health* **2006**, *53*, 299–305. [CrossRef]
55. Spears, K.J.; Roe, A.J.; Gally, D.L. A comparison of enteropathogenic and enterohaemorrhagic *Escherichia coli* pathogenesis. *FEMS Microbiol. Lett.* **2006**, *255*, 187–202. [CrossRef] [PubMed]
56. Orth, D.; Wurzner, R. Complement in typical hemolytic uremic syndrome. *Semin. Thromb. Hemost.* **2010**, *36*, 620–624. [CrossRef] [PubMed]
57. Stahl, A.L.; Sartz, L.; Karpman, D. Complement activation on platelet-leukocyte complexes and microparticles in enterohemorrhagic Escherichia coli-induced hemolytic uremic syndrome. *Blood* **2011**, *117*, 5503–5513. [CrossRef]
58. Friedman, D.I.; Court, D.L. Bacteriophage lambda: Alive and well and still doing its thing. *Curr. Opin. Microbiol.* **2001**, *4*, 201–207. [CrossRef]
59. Mayer, C.L.; Leibowitz, C.S.; Kurosawa, S.; Stearns-Kurosawa, D.J. Shiga toxins and the pathophysiology of hemolytic uremic syndrome in humans and animals. *Toxins* **2012**, *4*, 1261–1287. [CrossRef]
60. Moon, Y. Cellular alterations of mucosal integrity by ribotoxins: Mechanistic implications of environmentally-linked epithelial inflammatory diseases. *Toxicon* **2012**, *59*, 192–204. [CrossRef]

61. Park, S.H.; Moon, Y. Integrated stress response-altered pro-inflammatory signals in mucosal immune-related cells. *Immunopharmacol. Immunotoxicol.* **2013**, *35*, 205–214. [CrossRef] [PubMed]
62. Gyongyossy-Issa, M.I.; Khanna, V.; Khachatourians, G.G. Characterisation of hemolysis induced by T-2 toxin. *Biochim. Biophys. Acta* **1985**, *838*, 252–256. [CrossRef]
63. Segal, R.; Milo-Goldzweig, I.; Joffe, A.Z.; Yagen, B. Trichothecene-induced hemolysis. I. The hemolytic activity of T-2 toxin. *Toxicol. Appl. Pharmacol.* **1983**, *70*, 343–349. [CrossRef]
64. Rizzo, A.F.; Atroshi, F.; Hirvi, T.; Saloniemi, H. The hemolytic activity of deoxynivalenol and T-2 toxin. *Nat. Toxins* **1992**, *1*, 106–110. [CrossRef]
65. Gyongyossy-Issa, M.I.; Khachatourians, G.G. Interaction of T-2 toxin and murine lymphocytes and the demonstration of a threshold effect on macromolecular synthesis. *Biochim. Biophys. Acta* **1985**, *844*, 167–173. [CrossRef]
66. Schiefer, H.B.; Hancock, D.S. Systemic effects of topical application of T-2 toxin in mice. *Toxicol. Appl. Pharmacol.* **1984**, *76*, 464–472. [CrossRef]
67. Ward, D.M.; Kaplan, J. Ferroportin-mediated iron transport: Expression and regulation. *Biochim. Biophys. Acta* **2012**, *1823*, 1426–1433. [CrossRef]
68. Nemeth, E.; Tuttle, M.S.; Powelson, J.; Vaughn, M.B.; Donovan, A.; Ward, D.M.; Ganz, T.; Kaplan, J. Hepcidin regulates cellular iron efflux by binding to ferroportin and inducing its internalization. *Science* **2004**, *306*, 2090–2093. [CrossRef]
69. De Domenico, I.; Ward, D.M.; Langelier, C.; Vaughn, M.B.; Nemeth, E.; Sundquist, W.I.; Ganz, T.; Musci, G.; Kaplan, J. The molecular mechanism of hepcidin-mediated ferroportin down-regulation. *Mol. Biol. Cell* **2007**, *18*, 2569–2578. [CrossRef]
70. Bridle, K.R.; Frazer, D.M.; Wilkins, S.J.; Dixon, J.L.; Purdie, D.M.; Crawford, D.H.; Subramaniam, V.N.; Powell, L.W.; Anderson, G.J.; Ramm, G.A. Disrupted hepcidin regulation in HFE-associated haemochromatosis and the liver as a regulator of body iron homoeostasis. *Lancet* **2003**, *361*, 669–673. [CrossRef]
71. Nemeth, E.; Rivera, S.; Gabayan, V.; Keller, C.; Taudorf, S.; Pedersen, B.K.; Ganz, T. IL-6 mediates hypoferremia of inflammation by inducing the synthesis of the iron regulatory hormone hepcidin. *J. Clin. Investig.* **2004**, *113*, 1271–1276. [CrossRef]
72. Ganz, T. Hepcidin, a key regulator of iron metabolism and mediator of anemia of inflammation. *Blood* **2003**, *102*, 783–788. [CrossRef]
73. Rodrigues, P.N.; Vazquez-Dorado, S.; Neves, J.V.; Wilson, J.M. Dual function of fish hepcidin: Response to experimental iron overload and bacterial infection in sea bass (Dicentrarchus labrax). *Dev. Comp. Immunol.* **2006**, *30*, 1156–1167. [CrossRef]
74. Chen, J.; Shi, Y.H.; Li, M.Y. Changes in transferrin and hepcidin genes expression in the liver of the fish Pseudosciaena crocea following exposure to cadmium. *Arch. Toxicol.* **2008**, *82*, 525–530. [CrossRef]
75. Ilback, N.G.; Frisk, P.; Tallkvist, J.; Gadhasson, I.L.; Blomberg, J.; Friman, G. Gastrointestinal uptake of trace elements are changed during the course of a common human viral (Coxsackievirus B3) infection in mice. *J. Trace Elem. Med. Biol.* **2008**, *22*, 120–130. [CrossRef]
76. Troadec, M.B.; Ward, D.M.; Lo, E.; Kaplan, J.; De Domenico, I. Induction of FPN1 transcription by MTF-1 reveals a role for ferroportin in transition metal efflux. *Blood* **2010**, *116*, 4657–4664. [CrossRef]
77. Ross, S.L.; Tran, L.; Winters, A.; Lee, K.J.; Plewa, C.; Foltz, I.; King, C.; Miranda, L.P.; Allen, J.; Beckman, H.; et al. Molecular mechanism of hepcidin-mediated ferroportin internalization requires ferroportin lysines, not tyrosines or JAK-STAT. *Cell Metab.* **2012**, *15*, 905–917. [CrossRef]
78. Qiao, B.; Sugianto, P.; Fung, E.; Del-Castillo-Rueda, A.; Moran-Jimenez, M.J.; Ganz, T.; Nemeth, E. Hepcidin-induced endocytosis of ferroportin is dependent on ferroportin ubiquitination. *Cell Metab.* **2012**, *15*, 918–924. [CrossRef]
79. Masaldan, S.; Bush, A.I.; Devos, D.; Rolland, A.S.; Moreau, C. Striking while the iron is hot: Iron metabolism and Ferroptosis in neurodegeneration. *Free Radic. Biol. Med.* **2018**. [CrossRef]
80. Wang, Q.; Du, F.; Qian, Z.M.; Ge, X.H.; Zhu, L.; Yung, W.H.; Yang, L.; Ke, Y. Lipopolysaccharide induces a significant increase in expression of iron regulatory hormone hepcidin in the cortex and substantia nigra in rat brain. *Endocrinology* **2008**, *149*, 3920–3925. [CrossRef]
81. Bayeva, M.; Chang, H.C.; Wu, R.; Ardehali, H. When less is more: Novel mechanisms of iron conservation. *Trends Endocrinol. Metab.* **2013**, *24*, 569–577. [CrossRef]

82. Zhou, Z.D.; Tan, E.K. Iron regulatory protein (IRP)-iron responsive element (IRE) signaling pathway in human neurodegenerative diseases. *Mol. Neurodegener.* **2017**, *12*, 75. [CrossRef]
83. Kim, S.; Wing, S.S.; Ponka, P. S-nitrosylation of IRP2 regulates its stability via the ubiquitin-proteasome pathway. *Mol. Cell Biol.* **2004**, *24*, 330–337. [CrossRef]
84. Wang, J.; Chen, G.; Muckenthaler, M.; Galy, B.; Hentze, M.W.; Pantopoulos, K. Iron-mediated degradation of IRP2, an unexpected pathway involving a 2-oxoglutarate-dependent oxygenase activity. *Mol. Cell Biol.* **2004**, *24*, 954–965. [CrossRef]
85. Cazzola, M.; Skoda, R.C. Translational pathophysiology: A novel molecular mechanism of human disease. *Blood* **2000**, *95*, 3280–3288.
86. Birgegard, G.; Hallgren, R.; Killander, A.; Stromberg, A.; Venge, P.; Wide, L. Serum ferritin during infection. A longitudinal study. *Scand. J. Haematol.* **1978**, *21*, 333–340. [CrossRef]
87. Friis, H.; Range, N.; Braendgaard Kristensen, C.; Kaestel, P.; Changalucha, J.; Malenganisho, W.; Krarup, H.; Magnussen, P.; Bengaard Andersen, A. Acute- phase response and iron status markers among pulmonary tuberculosis patients: A cross-sectional study in Mwanza, Tanzania. *Br. J. Nutr.* **2009**, *102*, 310–317. [CrossRef]
88. Suarez-Ortegon, M.F.; Blanco, E.; McLachlan, S.; Fernandez-Real, J.M.; Burrows, R.; Wild, S.H.; Lozoff, B.; Gahagan, S. Ferritin levels throughout childhood and metabolic syndrome in adolescent stage. *Nutr. Metab. Cardiovasc. Dis.* **2018**. [CrossRef]
89. Fernaeus, S.; Halldin, J.; Bedecs, K.; Land, T. Changed iron regulation in scrapie-infected neuroblastoma cells. *Brain Res. Mol. Brain Res.* **2005**, *133*, 266–273. [CrossRef]
90. Kim, B.H.; Jun, Y.C.; Jin, J.K.; Kim, J.I.; Kim, N.H.; Leibold, E.A.; Connor, J.R.; Choi, E.K.; Carp, R.I.; Kim, Y.S. Alteration of iron regulatory proteins (IRP1 and IRP2) and ferritin in the brains of scrapie-infected mice. *Neurosci. Lett.* **2007**, *422*, 158–163. [CrossRef]
91. Nairz, M.; Ferring-Appel, D.; Casarrubea, D.; Sonnweber, T.; Viatte, L.; Schroll, A.; Haschka, D.; Fang, F.C.; Hentze, M.W.; Weiss, G.; et al. Iron Regulatory Proteins Mediate Host Resistance to Salmonella Infection. *Cell Host. Microbe* **2015**, *18*, 254–261. [CrossRef]
92. Jiao, Y.; Wilkinson, J.T.; Di, X.; Wang, W.; Hatcher, H.; Kock, N.D.; D'Agostino, R., Jr.; Knovich, M.A.; Torti, F.M.; Torti, S.V. Curcumin, a cancer chemopreventive and chemotherapeutic agent, is a biologically active iron chelator. *Blood* **2009**, *113*, 462–469. [CrossRef]
93. Jiao, Y.; Wilkinson, J.t.; Christine Pietsch, E.; Buss, J.L.; Wang, W.; Planalp, R.; Torti, F.M.; Torti, S.V. Iron chelation in the biological activity of curcumin. *Free Radic. Biol. Med.* **2006**, *40*, 1152–1160. [CrossRef]
94. Pietsch, E.C.; Chan, J.Y.; Torti, F.M.; Torti, S.V. Nrf2 mediates the induction of ferritin H in response to xenobiotics and cancer chemopreventive dithiolethiones. *J. Biol Chem.* **2003**, *278*, 2361–2369. [CrossRef]
95. Yang, C.; Zhang, X.; Fan, H.; Liu, Y. Curcumin upregulates transcription factor Nrf2, HO-1 expression and protects rat brains against focal ischemia. *Brain Res.* **2009**, *1282*, 133–141. [CrossRef]
96. Tanigawa, S.; Fujii, M.; Hou, D.X. Action of Nrf2 and Keap1 in ARE-mediated NQO1 expression by quercetin. *Free Radic. Biol. Med.* **2007**, *42*, 1690–1703. [CrossRef]
97. Afonyushkin, T.; Oskolkova, O.V.; Philippova, M.; Resink, T.J.; Erne, P.; Binder, B.R.; Bochkov, V.N. Oxidized phospholipids regulate expression of ATF4 and VEGF in endothelial cells via NRF2-dependent mechanism: Novel point of convergence between electrophilic and unfolded protein stress pathways. *Arterioscler. Thromb. Vasc. Biol.* **2010**, *30*, 1007–1013. [CrossRef]
98. Motohashi, H.; Yamamoto, M. Nrf2-Keap1 defines a physiologically important stress response mechanism. *Trends Mol. Med.* **2004**, *10*, 549–557. [CrossRef]
99. Boesch-Saadatmandi, C.; Wagner, A.E.; Graeser, A.C.; Hundhausen, C.; Wolffram, S.; Rimbach, G. Ochratoxin A impairs Nrf2-dependent gene expression in porcine kidney tubulus cells. *J. Anim. Physiol. Anim. Nutr.* **2009**, *93*, 547–554. [CrossRef]
100. Limonciel, A.; Jennings, P. A review of the evidence that ochratoxin A is an Nrf2 inhibitor: Implications for nephrotoxicity and renal carcinogenicity. *Toxins* **2014**, *6*, 371–379. [CrossRef]
101. Stachurska, A.; Ciesla, M.; Kozakowska, M.; Wolffram, S.; Boesch-Saadatmandi, C.; Rimbach, G.; Jozkowicz, A.; Dulak, J.; Loboda, A. Cross-talk between microRNAs, nuclear factor E2-related factor 2, and heme oxygenase-1 in ochratoxin A-induced toxic effects in renal proximal tubular epithelial cells. *Mol. Nutr. Food Res.* **2013**, *57*, 504–515. [CrossRef] [PubMed]

102. Ramyaa, P.; Krishnaswamy, R.; Padma, V.V. Quercetin modulates OTA-induced oxidative stress and redox signalling in HepG2 cells—Up regulation of Nrf2 expression and down regulation of NF-kappaB and COX-2. *Biochim. Biophys. Acta* **2014**, *1840*, 681–692. [CrossRef] [PubMed]
103. Cavin, C.; Delatour, T.; Marin-Kuan, M.; Holzhauser, D.; Higgins, L.; Bezencon, C.; Guignard, G.; Junod, S.; Richoz-Payot, J.; Gremaud, E.; et al. Reduction in antioxidant defenses may contribute to ochratoxin A toxicity and carcinogenicity. *Toxicol. Sci.* **2007**, *96*, 30–39. [CrossRef] [PubMed]
104. Harada, N.; Kanayama, M.; Maruyama, A.; Yoshida, A.; Tazumi, K.; Hosoya, T.; Mimura, J.; Toki, T.; Maher, J.M.; Yamamoto, M.; et al. Nrf2 regulates ferroportin 1-mediated iron efflux and counteracts lipopolysaccharide-induced ferroportin 1 mRNA suppression in macrophages. *Arch. Biochem. Biophys.* **2011**, *508*, 101–109. [CrossRef] [PubMed]
105. Tanaka, Y.; Ikeda, T.; Yamamoto, K.; Ogawa, H.; Kamisako, T. Dysregulated expression of fatty acid oxidation enzymes and iron-regulatory genes in livers of Nrf2-null mice. *J. Gastroenterol. Hepatol.* **2012**, *27*, 1711–1717. [CrossRef] [PubMed]
106. Yu, M.; Chen, L.; Peng, Z.; Wang, D.; Song, Y.; Wang, H.; Yao, P.; Yan, H.; Nussler, A.K.; Liu, L.; et al. Embryotoxicity Caused by DON-Induced Oxidative Stress Mediated by Nrf2/HO-1 Pathway. *Toxins* **2017**, *9*, 188. [CrossRef] [PubMed]
107. Yu, M.; Peng, Z.; Liao, Y.; Wang, L.; Li, D.; Qin, C.; Hu, J.; Wang, Z.; Cai, M.; Cai, Q.; et al. Deoxynivalenol-induced oxidative stress and Nrf2 translocation in maternal liver on gestation day 12.5d and 18.5d. *Toxicon* **2019**, *161*, 17–22. [CrossRef]
108. Jarolim, K.; Del Favero, G.; Pahlke, G.; Dostal, V.; Zimmermann, K.; Heiss, E.; Ellmer, D.; Stark, T.D.; Hofmann, T.; Marko, D. Activation of the Nrf2-ARE pathway by the Alternaria alternata mycotoxins altertoxin I and II. *Arch. Toxicol.* **2017**, *91*, 203–216. [CrossRef]
109. Qin, S.; Hou, D.X. Multiple regulations of Keap1/Nrf2 system by dietary phytochemicals. *Mol. Nutr. Food Res.* **2016**, *60*, 1731–1755. [CrossRef]
110. Zimmermann, M.B.; Chassard, C.; Rohner, F.; N'Goran, E.K.; Nindjin, C.; Dostal, A.; Utzinger, J.; Ghattas, H.; Lacroix, C.; Hurrell, R.F. The effects of iron fortification on the gut microbiota in African children: A randomized controlled trial in Cote d'Ivoire. *Am. J. Clin. Nutr* **2010**, *92*, 1406–1415. [CrossRef]
111. Buhnik-Rosenblau, K.; Moshe-Belizowski, S.; Danin-Poleg, Y.; Meyron-Holtz, E.G. Genetic modification of iron metabolism in mice affects the gut microbiota. *Biometals* **2012**, *25*, 883–892. [CrossRef]
112. Bailey, J.R.; Probert, C.S.; Cogan, T.A. Identification and characterisation of an iron-responsive candidate probiotic. *PLoS ONE* **2011**, *6*, e26507. [CrossRef]
113. Funakoshi, N.; Chaze, I.; Alary, A.S.; Tachon, G.; Cunat, S.; Giansily-Blaizot, M.; Bismuth, M.; Larrey, D.; Pageaux, G.P.; Schved, J.F.; et al. The role of genetic factors in patients with hepatocellular carcinoma and iron overload—A prospective series of 234 patients. *Liver Int.* **2016**, *36*, 746–754. [CrossRef]
114. Hino, K.; Nishina, S.; Sasaki, K.; Hara, Y. Mitochondrial damage and iron metabolic dysregulation in hepatitis C virus infection. *Free Radic. Biol. Med.* **2018**. [CrossRef]
115. Jiang, J.W.; Chen, X.H.; Ren, Z.G.; Zheng, S.S. Gut microbial dysbiosis associates hepatocellular carcinoma via the gut-liver axis. *Hepatobiliary Pancreat. Dis. Int.* **2018**. [CrossRef]
116. Nanba, S.; Ikeda, F.; Baba, N.; Takaguchi, K.; Senoh, T.; Nagano, T.; Seki, H.; Takeuchi, Y.; Moritou, Y.; Yasunaka, T.; et al. Association of hepatic oxidative stress and iron dysregulation with HCC development after interferon therapy in chronic hepatitis C. *J. Clin. Pathol.* **2016**, *69*, 226–233. [CrossRef]
117. Harrison, S.A.; Bacon, B.R. Relation of hemochromatosis with hepatocellular carcinoma: Epidemiology, natural history, pathophysiology, screening, treatment, and prevention. *Med. Clin. N. Am.* **2005**, *89*, 391–409. [CrossRef]
118. Mallory, M.A.; Kowdley, K.V. Hereditary hemochromatosis and cancer risk: More fuel to the fire? *Gastroenterology* **2001**, *121*, 1253–1254. [CrossRef]
119. Toyokuni, S. Mysterious link between iron overload and CDKN2A/2B. *J. Clin. Biochem. Nutr.* **2011**, *48*, 46–49. [CrossRef]
120. Utzschneider, K.M.; Kowdley, K.V. Hereditary hemochromatosis and diabetes mellitus: Implications for clinical practice. *Nat. Rev. Endocrinol.* **2010**, *6*, 26–33. [CrossRef]
121. Cooksey, R.C.; Jouihan, H.A.; Ajioka, R.S.; Hazel, M.W.; Jones, D.L.; Kushner, J.P.; McClain, D.A. Oxidative stress, beta-cell apoptosis, and decreased insulin secretory capacity in mouse models of hemochromatosis. *Endocrinology* **2004**, *145*, 5305–5312. [CrossRef]

122. Ammann, R.W.; Muller, E.; Bansky, J.; Schuler, G.; Hacki, W.H. High incidence of extrahepatic carcinomas in idiopathic hemochromatosis. *Scand. J. Gastroenterol.* **1980**, *15*, 733–736. [CrossRef]
123. Elmberg, M.; Hultcrantz, R.; Ekbom, A.; Brandt, L.; Olsson, S.; Olsson, R.; Lindgren, S.; Loof, L.; Stal, P.; Wallerstedt, S.; et al. Cancer risk in patients with hereditary hemochromatosis and in their first-degree relatives. *Gastroenterology* **2003**, *125*, 1733–1741. [CrossRef]
124. Hsing, A.W.; McLaughlin, J.K.; Olsen, J.H.; Mellemkjar, L.; Wacholder, S.; Fraumeni, J.F., Jr. Cancer risk following primary hemochromatosis: A population-based cohort study in Denmark. *Int. J. Cancer* **1995**, *60*, 160–162. [CrossRef]
125. Shaheen, N.J.; Silverman, L.M.; Keku, T.; Lawrence, L.B.; Rohlfs, E.M.; Martin, C.F.; Galanko, J.; Sandler, R.S. Association between hemochromatosis (HFE) gene mutation carrier status and the risk of colon cancer. *J. Natl. Cancer Inst.* **2003**, *95*, 154–159. [CrossRef]
126. Tiniakos, G.; Williams, R. Cirrhotic process, liver cell carcinoma and extrahepatic malignant tumors in idiopathic haemochromatosis. Study of 71 patients treated with venesection therapy. *Appl. Pathol.* **1988**, *6*, 128–138.
127. Zacharski, L.R.; Chow, B.K.; Howes, P.S.; Shamayeva, G.; Baron, J.A.; Dalman, R.L.; Malenka, D.J.; Ozaki, C.K.; Lavori, P.W. Decreased cancer risk after iron reduction in patients with peripheral arterial disease: Results from a randomized trial. *J. Natl. Cancer Inst.* **2008**, *100*, 996–1002. [CrossRef]
128. Mandishona, E.; MacPhail, A.P.; Gordeuk, V.R.; Kedda, M.A.; Paterson, A.C.; Rouault, T.A.; Kew, M.C. Dietary iron overload as a risk factor for hepatocellular carcinoma in Black Africans. *Hepatology* **1998**, *27*, 1563–1566. [CrossRef]
129. Gordeuk, V.R.; McLaren, C.E.; MacPhail, A.P.; Deichsel, G.; Bothwell, T.H. Associations of iron overload in Africa with hepatocellular carcinoma and tuberculosis: Strachan's 1929 thesis revisited. *Blood* **1996**, *87*, 3470–3476.
130. Moyo, V.M.; Makunike, R.; Gangaidzo, I.T.; Gordeuk, V.R.; McLaren, C.E.; Khumalo, H.; Saungweme, T.; Rouault, T.; Kiire, C.F. African iron overload and hepatocellular carcinoma (HA-7-0-080). *Eur. J. Haematol.* **1998**, *60*, 28–34. [CrossRef]
131. Pinnix, Z.K.; Miller, L.D.; Wang, W.; D'Agostino, R., Jr.; Kute, T.; Willingham, M.C.; Hatcher, H.; Tesfay, L.; Sui, G.; Di, X.; et al. Ferroportin and iron regulation in breast cancer progression and prognosis. *Sci. Transl. Med.* **2010**, *2*, 43ra56. [CrossRef]
132. Gutteridge, J.M.; Fu, X.C. Enhancement of bleomycin-iron free radical damage to DNA by antioxidants and their inhibition of lipid peroxidation. *FEBS Lett.* **1981**, *123*, 71–74. [CrossRef]
133. Gutteridge, J.M. Iron promoters of the Fenton reaction and lipid peroxidation can be released from haemoglobin by peroxides. *FEBS Lett.* **1986**, *201*, 291–295. [CrossRef]
134. Kershenobich Stalnikowitz, D.; Weissbrod, A.B. Liver fibrosis and inflammation. A review. *Ann. Hepatol.* **2003**, *2*, 159–163.

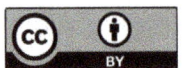

© 2019 by the authors. Licensee MDPI, Basel, Switzerland. This article is an open access article distributed under the terms and conditions of the Creative Commons Attribution (CC BY) license (http://creativecommons.org/licenses/by/4.0/).

MDPI
St. Alban-Anlage 66
4052 Basel
Switzerland
Tel. +41 61 683 77 34
Fax +41 61 302 89 18
www.mdpi.com

Nutrients Editorial Office
E-mail: nutrients@mdpi.com
www.mdpi.com/journal/nutrients